Advanced Practice in Healthcare

Advanced Practice in Healthcare

DYNAMIC DEVELOPMENTS IN NURSING
AND ALLIED HEALTH PROFESSIONS

Fourth Edition

Edited by

Paula McGee
Emeritus Professor
Birmingham City University
Birmingham, UK

Chris Inman
Birmingham City University
Birmingham, UK

WILEY Blackwell

This edition first published 2019
© 2019 John Wiley and Sons Ltd

Edition History
John Wiley and Sons (3e, 2009)

Registered Office(s)
John Wiley & Sons, Inc., 111 River Street, Hoboken, NJ 07030, USA
John Wiley & Sons Ltd, The Atrium, Southern Gate, Chichester, West Sussex, PO19 8SQ, UK

Editorial Office
9600 Garsington Road, Oxford, OX4 2DQ, UK

For details of our global editorial offices, customer services, and more information about Wiley products visit us at www.wiley.com.

Wiley also publishes its books in a variety of electronic formats and by print-on-demand. Some content that appears in standard print versions of this book may not be available in other formats.

Library of Congress Cataloging-in-Publication Data

Names: McGee, Paula, editor. Title: Advanced practice in healthcare : dynamic developments in nursing and allied health professions / edited by Paula McGee, Emeritus Professor, Birmingham City University, Birmingham, UK, Chris Inman, Birmingham City University, Birmingham UK, AAPE UK longstanding committee member.
Other titles: Advanced practice in nursing and the allied health professions.Description: 4th edition. | Hoboken, NJ : Wiley-Blackwell, 2019. | Revision of: Advanced practice in nursing and the allied health professions / edited by Paula McGee. 2009. 3rd ed. | Includes bibliographical references and index. |
Identifiers: LCCN 2019001698 (print) | LCCN 2019003059 (ebook) | ISBN 9781119439127 (Adobe PDF) | ISBN 9781119439110 (ePub) | ISBN 9781119439097 (pbk.)
Subjects: LCSH: Nurse practitioners–Great Britain. | Nursing–Great Britain.
Classification: LCC RT82.8 (ebook) | LCC RT82.8 .A365 2019 (print) | DDC 610.73/7–dc23
LC record available at https://lccn.loc.gov/2019001698

Cover Design: Wiley
Cover Image: © Pobytov / Getty Images

Set in 10/12pt New Baskerville by SPi Global, Pondicherry, India

10 9 8 7 6 5 4 3 2 1

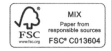

CONTENTS

Note on Contributors   xi

Introduction   xv

Part 1   Advanced Practice as a Global Phenomenon

1 The Conceptualization of Advanced Practice   3
Paula McGee and Chris Inman
  1.1 Introduction   3
  1.2 Competence   5
  1.3 Variations in Advanced Practice   12
  1.4 Conclusion   15
  References   16

2 An International Perspective of Advanced
Nursing Practice   19
Madrean Schober
  2.1 Introduction: Overview of Advanced Nursing Practice   20
  2.2 Advanced Nursing Practice Defined:
       An International Position   20
  2.3 Drivers and Motivation   23
  2.4 Influence of International Organizations   24
  2.5 Regional and Country Profiles of Advanced
       Nursing Practice   26
  2.6 Country-specific Initiatives   28
  2.7 International Collaboration for a New Initiative   30
  2.8 Controversial Issues   31
  2.9 Challenges   33
  2.10 Conclusion   36
  References   37

3 Development of Advanced Practice Nursing Roles
in the Netherlands   39
Christine de Vries de Winter
  3.1 Introduction   39
  3.2 The Dutch Healthcare System   40
  3.3 Development of Advanced Nursing Practice
       in the Netherlands   41
  3.4 Regulation of Advanced Practice   42

3.5 Preparation of Advanced Nurse Practitioners   42
3.6 Issues in Advanced Practice in the Netherlands   45
3.7 Education   46
3.8 The Future of Advanced Nursing Practice: Innovation
    in Healthcare and Education   46
3.9 Conclusion   48
References   49

4 Advanced Practice in Nursing and Midwifery:
The Contribution to Healthcare in Australia   51
Grainne Lowe and Virginia Plummer
4.1 Introduction   51
4.2 Advanced Practice in Australia   52
4.3 Current Issues in Advanced Practice in Australia   57
4.4 Advanced Practice in Midwifery   60
4.5 Conclusion   61
References   62

5 Influences on the Development of Advanced
Nursing Practice in the UK   65
Paula McGee
5.1 Introduction   65
5.2 The National Health Service in the UK   66
5.3 Health Policy   67
5.4 Influence of Health Policies and Reform
    of the National Health Service   67
5.5 Influence of Nursing Strategies   71
5.6 Influence of Nursing Organizations   73
5.7 Conclusion   79
References   80

Part 2   Advanced Practice in Allied Health Professions

6 The Development of Advanced Practice in the Allied
Health Professions in the UK   85
Paula McGee
6.1 Introduction   85
6.2 Background to the Development of Advanced
    Practice in Allied Health Professions   87
6.3 Advanced Practice in Allied Health Professions   90
6.4 Advanced Practice in Physiotherapy   90
6.5 Advanced Practice Paramedics   91
6.6 Current Issues in Advanced Practice in Allied
    Health Professions   92
6.7 Conclusion   98
References   99

7 Advanced Practice in the Radiography Professions   101
Nick White and Helen White

7.1 Introduction   101
7.2 Worldwide Variation in the Adoption of Advanced
      Practice in Radiography   102
7.3 Four-tier Service and Advanced
      Practice in Radiography   102
7.4 Educational Preparation for Advanced
      Practice Roles in Radiography   104
7.5 Defining Advanced Practice – Do Role Specialism
      and Role Extension in Radiography Truly Lead
      to "Advanced Practice"?   105
7.6 Taking Stock: The Deployment of Advanced
      Practitioners within the Diagnostic Imaging,
      Radiotherapy, and Ultrasound Communities
      of Practice   107
7.7 Future Developments and Opportunities   110
7.8 Conclusion   112
References   113

8 Advanced Practice in Speech and Language Therapy   115
Susan Beaumont

8.1 Introduction   115
8.2 The Role of the Advanced Practitioner Speech
      and Language Therapist   120
8.3 Current Challenges in Advanced Speech
      and Language Therapy   123
8.4 Conclusion   124
References   125

Part 3   The Advanced Practitioner in Direct Patient Care

9 Prescribing and Advanced Practice   131
Andrew Campbell

9.1 Introduction   131
9.2 The History of Non-medical Prescribing
      in the UK   132
9.3 Registered Non-medical Prescribers
      in England   133
9.4 Preparing for Prescribing   133
9.5 Who May Prescribe What?   135
9.6 The Principles of Effective Prescribing   138
9.7 Safety and Clinical Governance   141
9.8 The Future of Non-medical Prescribing   142
9.9 Conclusion   144
References   145

10 The Advanced Clinical Nurse Practitioner and Direct Care   147
Mary Hutchinson
    10.1 Introduction   147
    10.2 Holistic Health Assessment   154
    10.3 Conclusion   155
    References   156

11 The Advanced Critical Care Practitioner   159
Paula McGee and Jonathan Downham
    11.1 Introduction   159
    11.2 The Advanced Critical Care Practitioner Role   160
    11.3 Scope of Practice   161
    11.4 Competences for the Advanced Critical Care
         Practitioner Role   164
    11.5 Processes in the Development of the Advanced
         Critical Care Practitioner Role   165
    11.6 Current Issues in Advanced Critical Practice   169
    11.7 Conclusion   170
    References   171

12 The Interface between Advanced Nursing
    and Medical Practice   173
Lesley Kavi and Paula McGee
    12.1 Introduction   173
    12.2 General Practice in the UK   174
    12.3 Current Issues in General Practice   175
    12.4 Advanced Nursing Practice   176
    12.5 The Advantages and Disadvantages of
         Advanced Nursing Practice in General Practice   181
    12.6 Conclusion   184
    References   185

Part 4   Developing Advanced Practitioners' Skills

13 Legal and Ethical Issues Related to Professional Practice   189
Nicola J Stock
    13.1 Introduction   190
    13.2 Ethical Theories   190
    13.3 The Mental Capacity Act   194
    13.4 Deprivation of Liberty Safeguards   195
    13.5 Consent, Autonomy, and Advocacy   196
    13.6 Negligence   197
    13.7 Handling Complaints   199
    13.8 Whistleblowing   200
    13.9 Duty of Candor   201
    13.10 Improving Care Quality   202
    13.11 Conclusion   202
    References   204

14 Advanced Practice in a Diverse Society   205
Paula McGee
14.1 Introduction   205
14.2 Human Rights   206
14.3 Tackling Discrimination   209
14.4 Advanced Practice Competences   213
14.5 A Way Forward – Having That Difficult Conversation   217
14.6 Conclusion   218
References   220

15 Educational and Professional Influences on Advanced
and Consultant Practitioners   223
Chris Inman
15.1 Introduction   223
15.2 The Education of Advanced Practitioners in the UK   224
15.3 Collaboration with the Netherlands   225
15.4 Consultant Practitioners   227
15.5 Consultant Roles and Research   228
15.6 The Interface between Medicine and Advanced
and Consultant Practitioners   229
15.7 The Advanced Practitioner's Role – Enhancing
the Impact on Care   230
15.8 Conclusion   231
References   232

16 Assessment of Advanced Practice   235
Chris Inman
16.1 Introduction   235
16.2 Stages and Subject Areas of Advanced
Practice Master's Courses in the UK   237
16.3 Advanced Health Assessments and OSCEs
in Universities in the UK   239
16.4 OSCEs – Recent Published Research   241
16.5 Practice Assessments and Requirements
for a Portfolio of Evidence   244
16.6 The Second and Third Stages of Assessment
for a Master's Degree   246
16.7 End-point Assessment – Master's-degree
Apprenticeship   246
16.8 Conclusion   247
References   248

17 Leadership in Advanced Practice   251
Paula McGee
17.1 Introduction   251
17.2 The Nature of Leadership   252
17.3 Attributes of the Leader   253
17.4 Leadership and Management   255

17.5 Leadership in Advanced Practice   255
17.6 Conclusion   262
References   263

18 Research Competence in Advanced Practice   265
Paula McGee
18.1 Introduction   265
18.2 Research Competence in Advanced Practice   266
18.3 Direct Patient Care   270
18.4 Publication of Research Results   273
18.5 An Agenda for Research   277
18.6 Conclusion   278
References   279

19 Conclusion: The Future for Advanced Practice   281
Paula McGee and Chris Inman
19.1 Introduction   281
19.2 Full Practice Authority   283
19.3 The Relationship with Medicine   284
19.4 The Preparation of Advanced Practitioners   285
References   286

Index   287

Susan Beaumont, BSc Speech Pathology and Therapeutics, MSc Advanced Practice, MRCSLT, HCPC Reg

Principal Speech and Language Therapist, Worcestershire Health and Care NHS Trust, UK

Sue Beaumont has worked in the field of dysphagia (swallowing disorders) for 18 years and leads this specialism for the pediatric speech and language therapy service across Worcestershire Health and Care NHS Trust. During this time, she has significantly developed the service. She is well known for her clinical expertise and as a resource for advice within the Trust and regionally through her links with other Acute and Community NHS Trusts. She chaired the Speech and Language Therapy Clinical Excellence Network and continues to serve as a member. She is passionate about improving both care for children with dysphagia and support for their parents. She is fascinated by the challenges presented by increasingly complex cases and the ethical dilemmas they present in health and social care.

Andrew Campbell, BSc (Hons) Pharmacy, PG Dip. Clinical Pharmacy, PG Cert. Psychiatric Therapeutics, MSc Clinical Pharmacy, PG Cert. Independent Prescribing, Professional Doctorate in Pharmacy

Chief Pharmacist, Dudley & Walsall Mental Health Partnership NHS Trust, UK

Andrew Campbell is currently the Chief Pharmacist for Dudley and Walsall Mental Health Partnership Trust and is a qualified non-medical prescriber. He has several years' experience as a visiting lecturer on the non-medical prescribing program at Birmingham City University, and was formerly the West Midlands regional Non-Medical Prescribing Lead. Andrew is committed to education and training and has recently completed his professional doctorate, which explored attitudes to prescribing practice in a mental health context.

Jonathan Downham, RN, ACCNP, MSc

Advanced Critical Care Nurse Practitioner, Intensive Care, Warwick Foundation NHS Trust, UK

Jonathan Downham holds a Master's degree in anesthetic practice and provides a wide range of educative materials for critical care practitioners at Critical Care Practitioner, www.criticalcarepractitioner.co.uk.

Mary Hutchinson, RGN, BSc (Hons), MSc, FFEN

Senior Lecturer, Birmingham City University, and Advanced Nurse Practitioner, BADGER Medical Services, UK

Mary Hutchinson has a dual role as a Senior Lecturer in Advanced Clinical Practice and an Advanced Nurse Practitioner (ANP) with an out-of-hours service co-located with a local Emergency Department. Her clinical career encompasses many aspects of urgent and emergency care, from Staff Nurse in a community hospital Casualty Department to eight years as Sister in an Emergency Department, during which time she project-managed development of the Emergency Nurse Practitioner role. Mary has been Service Manager/Professional Lead of two long-established Minor Injury Units and a Community Rapid Response Team. She served for two years as an ANP in primary care, and latterly has worked as Clinical Lead in a nurse-led Urgent Care Centre. As a Founding Fellow and Board Member of the Faculty of Emergency Nursing (FEN), and a committee member of the Royal College of Nursing (RCN) Advanced Nurse Practitioner Forum, she continues to work to update the FEN career and competence framework, and is an active participant in the RCN ANP credentialing process.

Chris Inman, RN, DEd, MSc

Former long-standing Program Director, Master's in Advanced Practice, Birmingham City University, UK

Having consolidated her nursing qualification for 18 years with experience in a variety of clinical and educational settings and locations, Chris Inman completed an MSc in Sociological Research Methods at Warwick University and became a lecturer at Hull University. She then accepted a post as Head of Nursing developments at the Open University, and was subsequently appointed Program Director for the first MSC Advanced Practice course in the UK. This course developed dynamically over several years, expanded to recruit students from The Netherlands, and continues to produce high-flying graduates, many of whom have become non-medical consultants and leaders in healthcare. Christine's doctoral research at King's College London explored the learning needs of senior healthcare professionals undertaking PhD study. Later investigation involved exploration into the syllabi of advanced practice programs in the UK, which challenged the assumption that courses were consistent across the country. Her recent interest is in exploring the assessment of advanced practitioners and variations in examination. Chris is a long-standing committee member of the Association of Advanced Practice Educators UK.

Lesley Kavi, MB ChB, DRCOG, DFSRH

General Practitioner (primary care physician), Birmingham, UK.

Lesley Kavi obtained her medical degree at Glasgow University in 1983 and undertook GP training in the Lake District. Having previously worked as a GP partner in inner-city Dundee, she is currently practicing in Birmingham. Lesley holds postgraduate diplomas in syncope and related disorders, obstetrics and gynecology, and contraception. In addition, she has an interest in heritable connective tissue disorders. She currently teaches physical examination techniques and differential diagnosis on the MSc in Advanced Practice at Birmingham City University. Lesley is a volunteer managing trustee and chair of PoTS UK, a charity that supports patients with postural tachycardia syndrome. She has written a number of journal papers on PoTS and syncope in primary care.

Grainne Lowe, RN, PhD

Lecturer, Deakin University, Australia

Grainne Lowe is a Nurse Practitioner in the specialty area of emergency nursing. She has over 30 years' experience in a variety of nursing positions, including clinical practice, research, and education, with her current role as a Lecturer at Deakin University. Grainne has researched the Nurse Practitioner role over a number of years, including completion of her doctoral thesis specifically focusing on the integration of Nurse Practitioners into the Australian health-care system.

Paula McGee, RN, RNT, PhD, MA, BA, Cert. Ed.

Emeritus Professor of Nursing, Birmingham City University, UK

Paula McGee has researched and published about advanced practice for many years and is committed to advancing expertise in this developing field of nursing. She has launched and edited several professional journals, including the *British Journal of Nursing*, *Research Ethics*, and *Diversity in Health and Care*. She has also been an associate editor of the *Journal of Transcultural Nursing* and has guest edited other journal publications.

Virginia Plummer, RN, RM, PhD

Associate Professor, Director of International Engagement, Monash University and Peninsula Health, Australia

Virginia Plummer's research interests include local and international approaches to health service management, the nursing workforce, and costing studies. During her PhD she undertook an analysis of nearly two million nursing hours in three countries in a study of patient dependency and nurse–patient ratios. Virginia received an Australian Research Council Linkage grant toward enhancing patient management at point of care using electronic-based clinical pathways. She has supervised more than 50 Honors, Master's, and PhD students to completion in research related to midwifery, emergency care, critical care, disaster management, advanced practice roles, and health service evaluation. Virginia is Chair of the Human Research Ethics Committee at Peninsula Health; Executive Member of the Nursing Section, World Association Disaster and Emergency Medicine; and Associate Editor, *BMC Nursing* and on the *International Emergency Nursing* Editorial Board.

Madrean Schober, PhD, MSN, RN, ANP, FAANP

President, Schober Global Healthcare Consulting, International Healthcare Consultants, Indiana, USA

Madrean Schober is President of Schober Global Healthcare Consulting. She is a nurse practitioner, educator, writer, lecturer, and consultant with an aim to promote insightful healthcare services to diverse populations, which includes strategic planning for improved access to all. Her consultancy experience extends to over 40 countries in the process of developing advanced practice nursing roles with expertise in healthcare policy, curriculum design, and program development.

Nicola J Stock, RN, MPhil, MSc, BSc, PGDip, PGCert

After completing nurse training with the British Army, Nicola Stock worked in various locations throughout the world, but predominantly in the UK. Her experience and post-registration in the UK were in orthopedics. Whilst studying for a BSc (Hons) in Military Nursing Studies with the University of Portsmouth, she developed a greater interest in healthcare law and clinical ethics as drivers to promote standards of patient care, following up her degree with a PGDip in Healthcare Ethics from King's College London and an MPhil in Medical Law from the University of Glasgow. With a conviction that education was another key to the delivery of good patient care, during this time Nicola also qualified as a Practice Educator and spent 10 years working between Birmingham City University and military deployments, before leaving the army in 2011. Since then she has continued to work as a sessional lecturer and in clinical practice, dividing her time between the UK and an oil and gas project in the Middle East.

Christine de Vries de Winter, MScN, RN

Head of Department Nursing Studies, Faculty Health, Behavior and Society, University of Applied Science Arnhem en Nijmegen, The Netherlands

Christine de Vries de Winter studied nursing in Leiden and nurse science at the University of Antwerp, together with management and leadership at the TIAS School for Business and Society. As national chair of the Master in Education for Advanced Nursing Practice, she was closely involved in the development of advanced nursing roles in The Netherlands, one of the few European countries to develop full advanced practice roles during the early part of the twenty-first century.

Helen White, MEd, PGDip Clin. Onc., PG Cert L&T in HE, BSc (Hons) Radiotherapy

Head of Department of Radiography, Birmingham City University, UK

Helen White has worked in radiography education for over 15 years, teaching across clinical and academic components of a variety of healthcare programs at undergraduate and postgraduate levels of academic study. She is currently working with postgraduate students studying leadership and advanced practice, and works with clinical service leaders to promote advanced and consultant practice opportunities. Helen is a Visitor for the Health and Care Professions Council, offering expert advice and contributing to decision-making processes on whether educational programs meet the Council's standards. She is a member of the College of Radiographers' Approval and Accreditation Board and the Radiotherapy Advisory Group, which reports to the College's UK Council on issues relating to therapeutic radiography, including career development pathways. She is also an experienced assessor for the professional body the College of Radiographers.

Nick White, MSc Radiography, BSC (Hons) Human Anatomy, BSC (Hons) Radiotherapy, BA Open

Clinical tutor, Radiotherapy Department, University Hospitals Birmingham, and Senior Lecturer, Department of Radiography, Birmingham City University, UK

Nick White has a dual role as clinical tutor and senior lecturer. He has worked in radiography education for 15 years, teaching on undergraduate and postgraduate courses in radiography and the health professions. He is an experienced lecturer in advanced practice and leadership, and is module leader for post-registration radiographers studying leadership within programs which support development as advanced and consultant practitioners. He is a Senior Fellow of the Higher Education Academy, this award being received in recognition of his innovative approach to healthcare education, including MSc supervision, the use of skills simulation, and the involvement of students as academic partners. Nick is an experienced course assessor for the College of Radiographers. His current research includes the development and delivery of approaches to the teaching of palliative and end-of-life care within healthcare programs, and how this is implemented within clinical practice.

INTRODUCTION

Advanced practice is an evolving field of healthcare in which experienced nurses and members of allied health professions undergo further preparation to improve health, prevent disease, and provide treatment and care for patients in a wide range of settings. Their enhanced expertise enables advanced practitioners to address inequalities in access to healthcare, particularly for people who are marginalized and socially excluded. Tackling what may be entrenched disadvantage requires a willingness to try new approaches to ensure that health services are designed and provided in ways that meet the needs of local populations. Advanced practitioners are, therefore, pioneers of new forms of practice that may not only increase the availability of healthcare, but also provide it in ways that are experienced by patients as appropriate and meaningful. This last point is important because, whilst care and caring are universal phenomena, the actions, values, and beliefs that underpin them vary considerably between and within social groups. Thus, care and caring require a deep engagement with people in order to understand what is important to them and a flexible, adaptable approach to professional practice.

The development of advanced practice challenges established ideas about professional roles. It forms part of the global reconceptualization of the current and future healthcare workforce as being at the forefront of meeting Sustainable Development Goals to ensure "equitable access to health workers within strengthened health systems" by 2030 (United Nations 2015; World Health Organization [WHO] 2016, p. 3). Nurses in particular form the largest part of any healthcare workforce and have the potential to make a considerable difference, particularly in underserved areas. Members of allied health professions also have potential which could be more widely used. Utilizing this potential places non-medical health professionals at the forefront in the global plan to reduce significantly the complex factors that affect health: changing needs, finance, quality, new technology, workforce preparation, gender, deployment, and accessibility, urban versus rural settings, and health policies (WHO 2014). In this context, advanced practitioners have the expertise to make a significant contribution to the achievement of the Sustainable Development Goals.

i.1 The Aims of this Book

Advanced practitioners are now an established part of healthcare workforces, in many countries, as a level of practice beyond initial registration. Advanced practitioners are clinical experts whose main activity is the provision of direct patient care in their specialty. They practice autonomously in many settings, particularly those in which they deliver complete episodes of care and treatment. Their work in direct care is complemented by a set of generic competences which inform their ability to challenge professional boundaries and pioneer innovations.

The aims of this book are to consider the following:

- The contribution of diverse advanced practice roles, in different countries, professions, and care settings.
- The influence of health policy and professional organizations on the conceptualization and development of advanced practice.
- The dynamic interface between medicine and advanced nursing practice.
- Legal and ethical issues in advanced practice.
- The preparation of advanced practitioners and assessment of their competence.
- Meeting healthcare needs in a diverse society and the role of the advanced practitioner in tackling discrimination.
- The future of advanced practice 2018–2030.

i.2 Key Features of This New Edition

Each chapter in this book begins with an introductory panel which highlights the key issues and objectives. Interaction with the text is facilitated through short exercises which are set within the text and can be undertaken individually or in a group discussion. Each chapter also contains a case study through which different aspects of advanced practice are examined, with particular reference to the

- Country in which the case study takes place.
- Profession of the advanced practitioner.
- Context of care and treatment.
- Dependency and acuity of the patient.

At the end of each chapter there are:

- Key questions which provide a basis for further debate and investigation.
- A glossary of terminology.

This book is divided into four sections.

Part 1: Five chapters focus on the diverse nature of advanced practice at an international level and introduce a number of issues that are further explored later in the book. Chapter 1 focuses on the conceptualization of advanced practice in relation to *competence* and *variation*. The specific areas of competence in advanced practice are well rehearsed in the literature, as is the belief that preparation for the role should be at Master's level. However, as this chapter points out, the term "Master's level" is open to interpretation, which raises potential concerns about whether all advanced practitioners are equipped to practice at the same level. Competence, it is argued, is not enough; advanced practitioners must also demonstrate *capability* to cope effectively with unpredictable situations and adapt practice accordingly. Variation is discussed through the medium of a case study which demonstrates how advanced practice has developed in different ways in each of the four countries that make up the UK, and provides insight into factors that will continue to have an impact over the next decade.

This concept of variation leads into the following four chapters. Chapter 2 presents a broad overview of the global development of advanced nursing practice and the disparate issues that shape it. Chapters 3, 4, and 5 offer detailed accounts of advanced practice in the Netherlands, Australia, and the UK. Each account gives a different perspective, which reflects variation in the nature and stage of development and provides insight into local needs and issues. Despite the differences, there are similarities in practice which are illustrated through the case studies: direct patient care, holistic patient assessment based on a body systems approach, and the management of long-term conditions. There are also some similarities in the issues faced in every country: acceptance by medical staff, determining the impact of advanced practice, and the influence of health policies.

Part 2: Three chapters focus on advanced practice in *allied health professional* roles. This is a development that seems only have occurred in the UK, and that has expanded considerably since the last edition of this book. The chapters demonstrate the diverse and multifaceted advanced roles that are developing in allied health professions and their potential on a global scale with regard to the achievement of the Sustainable Development Goals (United Nations 2015).

Part 3: Four chapters examine particular aspects of advanced practice in the clinical setting and focus particularly on *nursing*. Chapter 9 presents an updated account of the *prescribing* regulations for non-medical practitioners in the UK: nurses, pharmacists, optometrists, and some allied health professionals. Whilst this is a country-specific example of one approach to regulation, it also takes the reader through the principles of good prescribing, which are applicable in any setting and are illustrated in the case study. That is followed by a discussion of the systematic and detailed *assessment* performed by an advanced clinical nurse practitioner in Chapter 10. This is based around a case study which takes the reader through a complete episode of care, beginning with meeting the patient and progressing to history taking and the physical examination, using simple tools that can be memorized as mnemonics. This process informs the formulation of a differential diagnosis and the choice of subsequent interventions. This case study also raises issues about the nature of advanced practice, and whether it is an extension of a professional role or a means of plugging gaps in services because of a shortage of doctors.

Chapter 11 takes up this point by examining the advanced nurse practitioner's role in relation to critical care, an environment in which patients are seriously ill and require support with two or more vital systems. This is an intellectually and ethically challenging context, and we are indebted to Dr. Pat James of Birmingham City University for clarifying some aspects of the physiology of acute respiratory distress syndrome. This chapter discusses two important issues in relation to advanced critical care practice and advanced practice more generally. The first is the *process of developing new professional roles*, which may, over time, lead to the establishment of a new profession. That raises questions about whether it is absolutely necessary to have a background in an already established health profession, or whether direct entry to, for example, advanced critical care practitioner roles might be possible as part of workforce transformation. The second is the *relationship between advanced practice and medicine*, particularly in fields such as critical care, where there is a certain amount of overlap between medical and nursing roles.

Chapter 12 examines the *interface between advanced nursing practice and medicine* more closely within the context of general practice. The pressures facing general practitioners have created opportunities for advanced nurses to develop new skills, plug gaps in services, and develop new approaches to care. Here again, a close alignment with medicine is evident through collaboration between the Royal Colleges of Nursing and General Practitioners, which culminated in the publication of specific competences for advanced nurses in general practice. This is a positive sign that doctors and advanced nurses can work together, and provides balance to the image that medical practitioners are inevitably hostile. However, doctors do have to be confident that advanced practitioners are competent in providing treatment and care. Variations in the level of preparation undertaken by advanced practitioners can cause some unease among doctors, and may also affect what the advanced nurse can achieve.

Part 4: This part looks beyond competence in direct patient care to examine the *wider role of advanced practitioners*. Modern healthcare is very complex. It requires the ability to make decisions not only about what is possible, but also about what is appropriate. The increasing range of new technologies creates many exciting possibilities, but this must not be allowed to obscure the needs and wishes of individual patients. An ethical working environment is one in which day-to-day practice is conducted in an open, respectful manner among professionals and between patients and professionals. As clinical and professional *leaders*, advanced practitioners must be able to play a leading role in developing and sustaining this environment. *Ethical practice* is not limited to direct patient care, but applies to all aspects of their work, so that patients, relatives, and staff are treated equally, irrespective of any individual distinguishing characteristics. Thus, ethical practice also informs the advanced practitioner's ability to identify and investigate what needs to change and why, to challenge accepted ways of doings things, and to lead others toward new and better patient care. All of these raise issues about *preparation* of advanced practitioners and the *methods used to determine proficiency*.

The final chapter brings the book to a close with a reflection on the issues raised and how advanced practice may develop in future as a vital part of health services.

Paula McGee
Chris Inman

References

United Nations (2015) Transforming our world. The 2030 agenda for sustainable development. https://sustainabledevelopment.un.org (accessed January 14, 2019).

World Health Organization (2014). *A Universal Truth: No Health without a Workforce*. Geneva: WHO.

World Health Organization (2016). *Global Strategy on Human Resources for Health: Workforce 2030*. Geneva: WHO.

PART 1

Advanced Practice as a Global Phenomenon

CHAPTER 1

The Conceptualization of Advanced Practice

Paula McGee and Chris Inman
Birmingham City University, Birmingham, UK

Key Issues
- Concepts of "competence" and "capability"
- Critical practice
- Collaborative practice
- Factors in pioneering innovations
- Master's level preparation of advanced practitioners

LEARNING OBJECTIVES

By the end of this chapter you will be able to:

- Explain the global context in which advanced practice has developed.
- Critically examine the concepts of "competence" and "capability" in relation to advanced practice.
- Critically discuss the concept of "critical practice" in relation to advanced practice.

1.1 Introduction

Healthcare has never been as good as it is now, in the early twenty-first century. New knowledge, technology, and the expertise of doctors, nurses, and allied health professionals (AHPs) now make it possible to prevent many diseases, cure others, and alleviate the suffering caused by factors that we cannot yet overcome. The world is now a much better place for human beings than it was, for example, in 1800 (Rosling et al. 2018). As a result, human beings can now lead healthier, more productive, and longer lives than their forebears, providing that they are able to access good-quality services, which meet their needs and which they experience as acceptable. Unfortunately, this is not always the case,

Advanced Practice in Healthcare: Dynamic Developments in Nursing and Allied Health Professions, Fourth Edition. Edited by Paula McGee and Chris Inman.
© 2019 John Wiley & Sons Ltd. Published 2019 by John Wiley & Sons Ltd.

because these advances and advantages are not evenly distributed within or between countries. Escalating costs, poverty, geography, conflict, violence, malnutrition, and lack of basic infrastructure such as electricity and roads are among the many factors that delay, prevent, or even reverse the equitable distribution of healthcare. As a result "many of the 7 billion people who inhabit our planet are trapped in health conditions of a century earlier" (Frenk et al. 2010, p. 7).

Alongside this situation is an increase in communicable diseases. These include viral infections for which there is, as yet, no cure or vaccine: Ebola, Zika, Marburg, and the Lassa virus. The incidence of preventable communicable diseases, such as measles, is rising among unvaccinated populations, including those previously protected by immunization programs; in Europe, 31 deaths from measles were reported in July 2018 (European Centre for Disease Prevention and Control 2018). The influence of the anti vaccination movement is one of the many factors that have affected the uptake of vaccination. Gonorrhea, syphilis, and other sexually transmitted infections are also increasing, particularly among young people (Public Health England 2018a). Even diseases for which cures are available remain highly prevalent. Each year, viral, parasitic, and bacterial diarrheal diseases due to poor sanitation and lack of clean drinking water account for over half a million deaths among children aged under 5 (WHO 2017). The incidence of tuberculosis is declining, but not fast enough to meet Sustainable Development Goal 3; the multi-drug-resistant strain of tuberculosis is a major threat to health (United Nations 2015).

Noncommunicable diseases, often associated with increasing affluence and lifestyle, are also increasing in prevalence. Obesity, smoking, alcohol and other substance abuse, lack of exercise, and eating insufficient fruit and vegetables all contribute to the development of disease. An estimated 451 million adults have diabetes, usually Type 2, and many more may be undiagnosed (International Diabetes Federation 2018). Cancer, heart disease, stroke, and respiratory diseases are among the leading causes of death worldwide. Approximately one in four adults and an increasing number of children will suffer from some form of mental illness at least once during the course of their lives. Lack of education and understanding about mental illness can prevent individuals from seeking help and lead some to suicide.

Populations are also changing as large numbers of people seek better economic or social opportunities elsewhere. Some 68.5 million people have become refugees, seeking to escape violence and persecution outside their own countries, and many are displaced within their own nations (United Nations High Commission for Refugees 2018). Their health needs are often complex and multifaceted: untreated long-term conditions such as diabetes and asthma, injuries sustained as a result of conflict or torture, sexual abuse, pregnancy, and mental health problems arising from these and other health issues.

It is in this context that advanced nursing practice has gradually developed from the work of individual practitioners in rural areas of the USA into a movement that now spans many different countries, societies, and cultures across five continents. Advanced nurse practitioners have shown that, given suitable preparation, they are competent to meet everyday healthcare needs, reduce pressures on hospital services, and develop local solutions to specific health challenges. In doing so, they have also revealed the previously untapped creative potential of nurses to innovate and improve the accessibility and acceptability of health service delivery and care, particularly to members of underserved groups. Local and country-specific needs have been at the forefront of these developments and, consequently, there is considerable variation in advanced nursing practice roles, work activities, preparation, and regulation (Schober and Affara 2006). In comparison to nursing, the development and impact of advanced practice in allied health professions is less well documented and there is no evidence of a global movement. The UK appears to be one of the few countries that has invested in advanced allied health practitioners; preparation is at the same level as that of advanced nurses. Given the inequitable distribution of health services and care, we argue that advanced allied health professionals have untapped potential to provide accessible, affordable and appropriate care to patients in many parts of the world (WHO 2014).

This chapter examines two issues in advanced practice: *competence* and *variation*. It begins with a discussion about competence. There are numerous ideas about this and lists of what advanced practitioners should be competent in, and usually these are examined separately. This discussion differs by emphasizing their interrelatedness under three broad topics: *professional maturity, challenging professional boundaries*, and *pioneering innovations*. It also builds on ideas about advanced practice developed through the last two editions of this book, our own research, one author's (PM) experience as a consultant nurse in National Health Service (NHS) Trusts, and, as educationalists, our many years' experience in preparing nurses and AHPs to become advanced practitioners.

The second discussion is based around a case study about the four countries in the UK. This highlights variation in the development of advanced practice. It introduces the concept of *capability* in advanced practice; this is discussed here with reference to the difference between "capability" and "competence." The discussion brings the chapter to a close by highlighting how lack of clarity about *Master's-level* preparation for advanced practice and local issues, for example, changes in initial nurse education may have implications for this level of practice.

1.2 Competence

Competence, as a personal, educational, and professional attribute, is a central feature of the discourse about advanced practice. There appears to be a general agreement that competence in the provision of treatment and care directly to patients is the essential criterion for all advanced practice roles (Department of Health 2010; Hamric 2014; Manley 1998; McGee 2009; International Council of Nurses [ICN] 2008; Royal College of Nursing [RCN] 2018a). Health professionals who do not engage in practice cannot be advanced practitioners. As clinical experts, advanced practitioners are professionally mature. They work collaboratively, across professional boundaries, as clinical and professional leaders; provide education for patients, families, carers, and fellow professionals; and pioneer new, evidence-based approaches to care. Thus, competence in direct patient care is complemented and enhanced by competence in other domains and the integration of additional skills through which advanced practitioners can broaden their sphere of influence (Hamric 2014). Leadership, educating others, research skills, collaborative working, and ethical reasoning are regarded as generic competences for all advanced practice roles (Department of Health 2010; Hamric 2014; Manley 1998; McGee 2009; International Council of Nurses 2008; RCN 2018a). These are complemented by specialty-specific competences, which receive rather less attention in the advanced practice literature. In addition, individual theorists have added other competences, for example acting as a consultant for others is a domain for Hamric (2014) but not the RCN (2018a). Some of this may be due to the ways in which competences are described: the RCN's (2018a) standards for advanced nursing practice leave room for broad interpretation, whereas Hamric's (2014) descriptions are more detailed. However, as advanced practice has evolved, we question if it is necessary to consider whether new generic competences are needed (Table 1.1).

TABLE **1.1**

Additional areas of competence for advanced practice.

Competence	Examples of attributes of competence to include
Interpersonal skills	Ability to communicate effectively with: • A wide range of people at different levels in the organization and outside. • Patients, families and carers, and different age groups. Ability to adapt different communication styles, broker communication between parties, manage and resolve conflict. Effectively manage situations in which patients and professionals do not share a common language.
Computer and information technology	Familiarity with and ability to use a variety of packages, conduct internet searches, contribute to the development of online research for patients and families. Ability to advise and guide patients in using the internet to learn about/manage their health problems.
Promoting equality and diversity	Identifying and acting on organizational, professional, and individual factors that help/hinder appropriate, accessible, and acceptable care and treatment. Developing and sharing accurate and up-to-date knowledge about diverse individuals and communities with other health professionals. Developing own and others' practice to provide care and treatment for diverse individuals and communities. Recognizing and tackling discrimination.
Legal issues	Familiarity with relevant legal issues in treatment and care as they relate to specific fields of advanced practice.
Policy issues	Understanding of current national health policy and how this is made, as well as the implications of this for the organization and for the treatment and care of patients. Ability to apply understanding of policy to advocate for and bring about change.

1.2.1 Professional Maturity

Direct patient care is a performance art requiring the integration of knowledge and skill that go well beyond those needed for usual professional practice. Advanced practitioners, particularly those who provide complete episodes of care and treatment, need to be able to listen attentively and respectfully to patients' explanations of their health problems and respond in ways that are meaningful. Listening is an active skill that is difficult to learn, mainly because it is taken for granted. People assume that they know how to listen, that they are listening to what is being said to them, but, if questioned afterward, they may remember very little. True listening means being open to the experiences of another person and being attuned to their preferred communication style, language, and emotional expression. It requires empathy and compassion in order to recognize and respond to another's difficulties and suffering (Papadopoulos 2018). Listening means paying full attention to what another person is saying, rather than thinking about what one is going to say in return or the information that one has to record (Covey 2006). Listening properly is hard work, because concentrating on what another person is saying can be very tiring. However, it is through paying full attention and synthesizing the information gained with clinical knowledge that the advanced practitioner is able to identify an individual patient's particular needs. Inherent in this process is *critical practice*, which facilitates ethical decision making about the best course of action to be taken (Brechin 2000). Personalized interventions can then be selected from a wide range of clinical and technical skills and developed through broad experience with members of diverse populations (Tracy 2014). Their outcome can be evaluated in the light of the individual's response.

Critical practice (see Exercise 1.1) is an "open minded, reflective appraisal that takes account of different perspectives, experiences and assumptions" that is essential in dealing with the unpredictable and changing nature of individual patients' health problems (Brechin 2000, p. 26). It is also essential to advanced practice. Critical practice begins with analysis of a patient's needs and progresses to *critical reflection*, which synthesizes different forms of knowledge to create practical knowledge, "knowledge that accrues over time in the practice of an applied discipline" and is not acquired through formal teaching or reading (Benner 1984, p. 1). Critical reflection provides the reasoning which, in turn, informs *critical action*, the decisions and actions taken. This is mastery of practice, "an active synthesis of skill, an art of practice which goes beyond established boundaries" (Schön 1983, p. 19).

EXERCISE 1.1

Select an episode of care from your own practice. To what extent did/ might critical practice inform your actions?

Developing and sustaining mastery in practice depend first on the preparation of the advanced practitioner. There is no international agreement about the educational level of courses preparing nurses to become advanced practitioners. The ICN (2008, p. 20) originally stated that "there is a growing global acceptance that this education should be set at Master's level," but this has now softened to "educational preparation at advanced level" (ICN 2018). The terminology used invites a broad interpretation of educational level, and consequently courses and preparation can vary in length and standard. For example, in the UK the framework for advanced clinical practice requires successful completion of a Master's-level course which addresses the key theoretical and practical elements; this could be a full Master's degree or a graduate diploma. Alternatively, aspiring advanced practitioners may undertake "a formal accredited work-based programme" or "submit a portfolio of evidence or work-based learning," which will be assessed through "a process of accrediting or recognising prior formal or informal learning and experience" (NHS Health Education England 2017, pp. 16–17). Unfortunately, the shelf life of "informal learning and experience" is not stated.

In contrast, in the USA, the American Association of Colleges of Nursing (AACN) has reported on the development of doctoral-level programs. These are justified if there is a need for higher-level study that goes well beyond that required for Master's level, and the "challenge will be to identify, using an evidence-based approach, the curricular standards associated with both master's and doctoral APN education and provide for a seamless interface between educational programs" (AACN 2004, p. 12). Variations in the level of preparation of advanced practitioners must, therefore, be a matter of concern. If the level, content, and quality of preparation differ, then there may be inequalities in the knowledge and competence of advanced practitioners produced via diverse routes. This may also undermine acceptance of advanced practice by medical and other colleagues, and may even prevent career progression. These issues are not addressed in current advanced practice research. However, it is also important to acknowledge that broad statements about "Master's level" may be advantageous in countries that do not have the resources to fund higher-level study. Sending their health professionals abroad for Master's degrees creates a temporary loss of experienced, capable practitioners who may not return. In addition, individual practitioners, even in wealthy countries, may not be able to meet the cost or find the opportunity to become advanced practitioners.

1.2.2 Challenging Professional Boundaries

Health professions have tended to develop in response to either the needs of underserved populations, such as those requiring physical rehabilitation, or technological advances, for example the use of radiation. Each grew to occupy a specific niche within health services, providing treatment and care at the discretion of the patient's doctor, who was regarded as having overall control and responsibility. Thus, the doctor could decide to refer a patient for physiotherapy, but if that therapist thought that the patient would benefit from help with speech problems, the physiotherapist could only recommend this to the doctor, who could then choose whether to act on the suggestion.

The complexity of modern healthcare means that this system, in which all decisions can only be made and initiated by the doctor, is no longer viable. What is needed is "interprofessional and transprofessional education that breaks down professional silos while enhancing collaborative and non-hierarchical relationships in effective teams" (Frenk et al. 2010, p. 6). This will not be easy to achieve. Medicine is a very diverse field with multiple specialities in which traditional responsibility for all aspects of patient treatment have lain with doctors. In this context, there are challenges to be faced in gaining full acceptance of advanced practitioners' expertise. However, it must also be recognized that no profession can encompass all the expertise needed to treat and care for patients. In all health professions, technological and clinical advances have not only brought changes to professional practice, but also contributed to an increase in the amount and level of post-qualifying education required to specialize. There is also no doubt that the cost of healthcare continues to rise. In the UK, spending on the NHS is expected to be around £126.269 billion in the 2018/19 financial year, but this may not be enough to meet demand (NHS Confederation 2017). NHS England (2014, p. 5) has predicted a shortfall of "nearly £30 million a year by 2020/21." Consequently, funders and providers are challenged to use resources, including staff, more economically and to find the best value for money, which includes allowing professionals to practice in more efficient and effective ways. Referring every decision to a single professional who has the absolute power of veto is potentially wasteful in terms of certain types of decision. It creates a cumbersome system that can work to patients' disadvantage, and can undermine other professionals, especially if their expertise is ignored or overridden.

Patients' needs and expectations are changing as their lifespans increase (see Chapter 12). Global life expectancy increased by five and a half years during the first 16 years of the twenty-first century, which means that the number of adults aged over 65 is rising (Office for National Statistics 2017; WHO 2018). Members of this age group are likely to have more than one long-term condition as well as the problems that arise with the process of aging. Younger people with long-term conditions from which earlier generations died can now lead longer lives. These changes call for new approaches to patient care. Patients with multiple and complex needs are currently treated by a similar number of professionals who have specialized in one area. This system can place considerable demands on patients as they attend multiple appointments to receive advice and treatment from different people; they struggle to make sense of everything they have been told and balance what may seem like conflicting ideas. In this context, being a patient is like having a full-time job.

Modern healthcare and professional education have not kept pace with these changes. What is needed is a different approach, and it is here that advanced practitioners can effect change by applying their expertise, and interpersonal competence in particular, in working across professional boundaries and acting as a care coordinator for patients. Care coordination is a vital role. Advanced practitioners can act as lynchpins for patients with complex needs, streamlining their care, advocating on their behalf, and improving their quality of life. People are more than the various illnesses or conditions that affect them. What they need is not always more specialized services, but the equivalent of a "one-stop shop" where the majority of their needs can receive attention from generalists who are skilled in tackling an individual's multiple health problems and who can call on specialists when necessary.

Advanced practitioners could lead the way in developing such an approach by collaborating with fellow professionals. *Collaboration* is "a dynamic, interpersonal process in which two or more individuals make a commitment to each other to interact authentically and constructively to solve problems and learn from each other to accomplish identified goals, purposes or outcomes" (Hanson and Spross 2005, p. 34; see Exercise 1.2). It is a process based on the sharing of power between individuals and/or groups, who respect each other as equals and who value and trust one another's professional expertise. It also requires a willingness to consider different points of view and new ideas without being obstructive or insisting that one's own opinion must prevail. Reasons for collaboration in patient care include more timely, better-coordinated treatment, improvements in patient safety (Hsueh and Dorcy 2016), and better management of long-term conditions (Kutzleb et al. 2015).

EXERCISE 1.2

As an advanced practitioner, who do you collaborate with and why?

To what extent does your collaboration match the definition provided by Hanson and Spross?

However, collaboration, especially across professional boundaries, may involve conflict. Advanced practitioners need to be able to manage this effectively and ensure transparency in decision making based on sound knowledge of patients, the best evidence available, and the ethical issues inherent in the situation. Ethical issues may arise if there is tension between what is possible, what a patient wants, and the costs in terms of resources, finance, time, and likely outcomes. The various parties involved in collaboration may struggle to understand each other and communicate effectively. Nursing in particular has a long history of clarifying and rephrasing what has been said to facilitate understanding between professionals and patients. Advanced practitioners may find that they have to do the same in brokering conflict between colleagues.

Collaborative skills enable the advanced practitioner to develop networks that extend across the healthcare organization and externally into local, national, or international settings. These networks provide a wide range of personal contacts, at differing levels and "know-how" about how systems in the organization really work, and how to make things happen. It is often through networks that opportunities arise for collaborative working on specific issues and a deeper understanding of diverse professional perspectives. Here, collaboration overlaps with leadership to create and maintain the advanced practitioner's sphere of influence. However, networks have to be nurtured and sustained. Connections with others depend on good interpersonal skills and commitment to genuine working relationships, in which people feel valued rather than used as means to an end.

1.2.3 Pioneering Innovation

As a leader, the advanced practitioner uses research skills to evaluate current practice to determine what is going well, what needs to be improved or changed, and how this may be achieved. Ethical reasoning informs consideration of both what is happening and what should happen, together with a willingness to challenge the way things are done. Good interpersonal skills enable the advanced practitioner to communicate effectively about the need for change and actively involve others in developing and enhancing patient care. The advanced practitioner's collaborative networks connect people and resources to involve them in a new venture. These include people both inside and outside the immediate working environment, because innovation may require support from managers in charge of resources, senior personnel responsible for the organization as a whole, and ancillary staff who provide services. Thus, the first point about pioneering innovation is that it brings together several competences: research, leadership, collaboration, ethics, and expertise in clinical practice; the second is the importance of involving the right people.

Patients and their families or carers should be involved at every stage in the development of innovation. In the UK this is a requirement set out in the Health and Social Care Act 2012, which states that patients have the right to be involved in all decisions about their care. There are several ways in which patients, families, and carers are currently involved in making their voices heard in the NHS: the Friends and Family Test, surveys, and patient-reported outcome measures. These methods usually involve the use of questionnaires given to patients. Methods aimed at the more active involvement of patients, families, and carers, for example patient groups, require careful planning to make clear the nature of the project and ensure a broad spectrum of opinion. In some instances, training may be necessary to ensure that people feel able to voice their opinions and understand the processes through which innovation develops. Funding may also be needed to cover travel expenses.

Innovation may have implications beyond the immediate working environment. Consequently, managers and senior personnel in the organization must be involved, because they are responsible for ensuring that the innovation is clearly thought out in terms of the anticipated benefits, costs, and any potential difficulties. They must also ensure that those involved achieve the competences required for the performance of their new activities. Policies and procedures must be formulated to address practice standards and monitor performance.

Thus, innovation requires a wide range of people with different perspectives and priorities. The leader's task is to focus their energies on the achievement of the new venture by devoting an equal amount of time to each of six activities: gathering information about what is proposed, identifying the ways in which the proposal might work in the setting concerned, examining the value and benefits of what is proposed, expressing feelings, looking honestly at what may go wrong, and identifying the management issues involved (De Bono 1991). In this way the proposed development can be examined from multiple perspectives; everyone has a chance to contribute, but no single point of view is allowed to dominate until all the angles have been considered.

Research skills inform the leader's activities through rigorous evaluation of the current situation in order to justify to everyone why a particular innovation is needed, what it will involve, and whether it is successful. Evaluation is therefore a continuous process of inquiry that informs each stage of development. *Critical practice* facilitates evaluation through *critical analysis* of current treatment and care and *critical appraisal* of evidence drawn from a variety of sources. Good-quality research, particularly meta-analyses and systematic reviews, is among the best sources of evidence, but it may still be necessary to conduct a wider search, particularly if the subject is not widely addressed. *Critical reflection* assists in clarifying the aims of an evaluation and the nature and analysis of the evidence required. *Critical action* relates to the outcomes of evaluation in terms of both the impact on practice and patient care and the presentation of the outcomes to the different groups involved: patients, managers, colleagues, and senior personnel (Brechin 2000).

Research skills also enable the advanced practitioner to identify and pursue aspects of practice that require deeper investigation, either through leading a project or working collaboratively as a team member alongside other researchers. Alternatively, the advanced practitioner may act as a resource by coaching and guiding less experienced colleagues, enabling them to develop research skills and complete their own projects.

Professional maturity, challenging professional boundaries, and pioneering innovation all require the integration of direct care with a range of other competences. Some of these are generic and generally accepted: leadership, ethics, research skills, working collaboratively, and educating others. Interpersonal competence is crucial to success in relation to each one. Without it, treatment and care are exercises in technical skill and clinical expertise, but the real nature of helping patients lies in the way in which that help is given, and interpersonal skills are the channel through which that nature is made explicit.

Interpersonal competence is addressed as part of generic competences. For example, in discussing guiding and coaching, Spross and Babine (2014, p. 195) state that interpersonal competence enables advanced practitioners to "establish therapeutic caring relationships." The problem with subsuming such an important area under another competence is that its central role throughout all aspects of advanced practice may receive less attention. For this reason, we argue here that interpersonal competence should be a competence in its own right (Table 1.1).

1.3 Variations in Advanced Practice

The UK consists of four separate countries, which vary in terms of population size, geography, and economy. Scotland, Wales, and Northern Ireland have their own national assemblies devolved from a central government based in England. Devolved powers include responsibility for the NHS. The preparation and practice of health professionals are required to meet standards set by UK national bodies such as the Nursing and Midwifery Council. The title of "advanced practitioner" is not protected and there is no additional regulation for advanced practice roles. Consequently, "advanced practitioner" may be included in some job titles, but this does not guarantee that the postholder has successfully completed the expected Master's-level preparation.

Initial work on advanced practice began in the 1990s and was undertaken by nurses. It is documented in earlier editions of this book. An account of contemporary developments and sources of influence is available in chapter 5. The discussion presented here focuses on developments in each country since 2007. Recent developments in England are presented last, because these raise a number of contentious issues.

1.3.1 Scotland

The definition of advanced nursing practice issued by the ICN (2008) was broadly accepted. In 2007, NHS Education for Scotland identified four main themes for advanced nursing practice: advanced clinical/professional practice, facilitating learning, leadership/management, and research. These were launched as part of the Advanced Practice Toolkit, an online repository of resources which continues to support the development of advanced practice (www.advancedpractice.scot.nhs.uk). This repository is wide ranging and includes examples of good practice as well as resources for the assessment of competence and activity analysis. Whilst many items in the repository reflect advanced nursing practice, they are not exclusive and can be used to apply to advanced AHP roles. The four themes are now accepted across the UK as the *four pillars* of this level of practice (RCN 2018a).

1.3.2 Wales

Wales has pursued a slightly different path in developing advanced practice based around the four pillars developed in Scotland. From the outset, the Welsh strategy incorporated both advanced nurses and AHPs to create a framework for advanced practice that was "applicable across all areas of practice and include staff working in clinical, education, management and leadership roles," which required Master's-level preparation and an integrated approach to workforce planning (National Leadership and Innovation Agency for Healthcare [NLIAH] 2010, p. 4). Here, the four pillars have been adapted to meet the demands of two roles. Clinical practice forms the core of both, but the leadership and management pillars are less pronounced in roles that carry an emphasis on research and education; this situation is reversed in roles that require greater leadership and management responsibility. This demonstrates that the four pillars can be combined in different ways depending on the individual's particular post, (see Exercise 1.3) and the flexibility this affords is now reflected in the RCN's credentialing criteria (RCN 2018b).

EXERCISE 1.3

What combination of the four pillars best reflects your role as an advanced practitioner?

1.3.3 Northern Ireland

Northern Ireland was the last of the four countries to introduce advanced practice. Its new framework is based around the four pillars and the work undertaken in Scotland, Wales, and England. Direct clinical practice is still the core pillar, and it is the level and scope that differentiate the advanced nurse practitioner from other nurses. The other three pillars are combined in a slightly different way: leadership and collaborative practice, education and learning, research and evidence-based practice. Advanced practitioners are expected to demonstrate "highly developed assessment, diagnostic, analytical and clinical judgement skills" that enable them to practice autonomously (Department of Health, Social Services and Public Safety [DHSSPS] 2016, p. 4). This framework is for nursing only and, as yet, there do not appear to be any plans to extend it to include AHPs. However, the current strategy is committed to developing AHP roles (DHSSPS 2012).

1.3.4 England

Advanced nursing practice was previously defined as a level of practice "beyond that of first level registration," the main features of which are "clinical/direct care practice; leadership and collaborative practice; improving quality and developing practice; and developing self and others" (Department of Health 2010, p. 5). Nurses working at this level were described as autonomous practitioners and were "able to apply knowledge and skills to a broad range of clinically and professionally challenging and complex situations" (Department of Health 2010, p. 7). The new framework for advanced clinical practice extends these ideas in line with Scotland and Wales, to include AHPs. Thus, in three UK countries, advanced practice has now expanded beyond nursing to incorporate AHPs and provided opportunities for them to use their expertise in new ways.

Like their advanced nurse practitioner counterparts, appropriately prepared AHPs are able to use their skills to provide complete episodes of treatment and care, promote health, and pioneer new approaches to practice.

The advanced clinical practice framework introduces capability alongside the four pillars and the concept of competence (NHS Health Education England 2017; see Exercise 1.4). The idea of capability originates in economic theory and is concerned principally with people's freedom and opportunities to achieve quality of life (Sen 1999). It is concerned with what someone can do in the context or situation in which they find themselves. Capability has attracted quite a lot of attention in other fields such as human resources, but there is very little reference to its application in advanced practice or healthcare generally (O'Connell et al. 2014).

EXERCISE 1.4

How would you define:
- Competence?
- Capability?

Capability is "a combination of skills, knowledge, values and self-esteem which enables individuals to handle change" and "the ability to formulate and devise solutions in unfamiliar situations" (O'Connell et al. 2014, p. 2731). It is a step beyond competence, which is focused on knowledge and skill acquisition measured against standards. Competence is essential in ensuring the performance of practice at the required level, but it does not take account of the unique situation of each patient or the context in which treatment and care are delivered. The real world is a volatile and, at times, chaotic place. The capable practitioner is able to cope with this complexity, work within it, and still find solutions that bring some form of partial or complete resolution. Thus, the introduction of capability in relation to the four pillars "is intended to convey the extent to which health and care professionals working at the level of advanced clinical practice can adapt to change, generate new knowledge and apply it in different ways to formulate and problem solve within a context of complexity and uncertainty" (NHS Health Education England 2017, p. 6). The four pillars constitute the "core capabilities" which are then to be applied to the "knowledge, skills and behaviours relevant to the health and care professional's setting and job role" and "may be manifested/demonstrated in different ways depending on the profession, role, population group, setting and sector in which an individual is practising" (NHS Health Education England 2017, p. 6).

Alongside this framework is the introduction of two other factors which have the potential to have an impact on advanced practice. First, there are new standards for initial nurse education issued by the Nursing and Midwifery Council (2018). These are presented as seven platforms and include some procedures that, until recently, have been considered part of advanced nursing practice. The level of practice expected may not be the same as for advanced practice, but this development does raise some awkward questions about work activities. Advanced practitioners have taken on some of the activities previously performed only by doctors; now professional nursing practice is undertaking work that was part of advanced practice. This suggests that assistant practitioners may have to adopt more aspects of professional practice, with possible consequences for patient care.

The second factor is the introduction of NHS apprenticeships, which provide employer-based training for individuals seeking health-related careers. Apprentices are employees who undergo training whilst at work that is complemented by day or block release at a college or university; those successfully completing the end-point assessment receive qualifications or certificates of competence. Initially apprenticeships focused mainly on assistant practitioner roles, but they have now been extended to undergraduate nursing and to advanced clinical practice for both nurses and AHPs. The new Master's-level apprenticeships will "allow employers to train new and existing staff in advanced clinical practice," and training will take 36 months (NHS Employers 2018). The scheme forms a major part of NHS workforce transformation, which is aimed at developing staff to meet the anticipated needs of patients over the next 10 years by improving and expanding knowledge and skills and increasing staff retention (Public Health England 2018b). It may well prove attractive, particularly to those who wish to avoid the high costs of student loans or whose personal circumstances favor part-time learning. It can also be seen as an attempt to address the decline in recruitment which has occurred following the replacement of bursaries for students. The ensuing 2016–2018 shortfall in nursing alone is estimated to be in the region of 16 580, which, when combined with the number of nurses eligible for retirement and current vacancies, represents a near catastrophic loss of nursing expertise (RCN 2018c). However, the apprenticeship scheme also raises a number of concerns about the preparation of advanced practitioners, particularly with regard to the meaning of "Master's level" and whether there are likely to be advanced practitioners with differing levels of qualification.

1.4 Conclusion

Advanced practice continues to develop in the context of multiple changes as countries seek to find the best ways of applying their resources to meet the needs of patients, combat escalating diseases, and contain costs. In doing so, they have opened up new possibilities for nurses and AHPs to expand their contributions to treatment and care through advanced practice. This development has necessitated a strong focus on competence but, in the UK at least, it seems that this is no longer enough: the practitioner's capability to perform in diverse contexts and under pressure is also becoming important. It is certainly something that other countries may wish to consider because, in the context of healthcare, change has never been as fast as it is now, but it will never again be as slow.

Key Questions

1. What aspects of your work as an advanced practitioner do you think could or should be part of usual professional practice in your field? Give reasons.
2. Is a full Master's degree essential for all advanced practitioners? Give reasons.

3. As an advanced practitioner in your field:
   a. What competences are required and why?
   b. What capabilities are required and why?

Glossary

Collaboration: a term with two meanings in the advanced practice literature:

- The interpersonal processes described in this chapter.
- The requirement in many US states for advanced practitioners to have a signed contract regarding collaboration with a doctor.

Department of Health and Social Care (DHSC; https://www.gov.uk/government/organisations/department-of-health-and-social-care): a government department responsible for "strategic leadership and funding" of health and social care in England. **NHS Scotland, NHS Wales**, and the **Department of Health, Social Services and Public Safety (DHSSPS) in** Northern Ireland are responsible for the health service in their respective countries

DHSC oversees several bodies, including:

- **NHS England** (www.england.nhs.uk), which is responsible for the health service in England.
- **NHS Healthcare Education England (HEE**; www.hee.nhs.uk), which is a government-funded body that works across England to deliver education to the healthcare workforce.
- **Public Health England** (https://www.gov.uk/government/organisations/public-health-england), which is responsible for all issues relating to public health including health promotion, tackling health inequalities, and health security.

Friends and Family Test (www.england.nhs.uk/fft): a measurement of patient satisfaction. Patients are asked if they would recommend the service, treatment, and care they have received to members of their family and their friends. Data are published monthly. NHS staff are also surveyed on an annual basis.

Nursing and Midwifery Council (www.nmc.org.uk): the professional regulator for nurses and midwives in the UK.

Patient-reported outcome measure: a measurement of patients' health-related quality of life, experiences of treatment, symptom management, or some other health-related issue. Data are gathered directly from patients, usually through a questionnaire, and are unmediated by the views of professionals.

Royal College of Nursing (www.rcn.org.uk): a trade union and professional body for nurses and healthcare assistants in the UK.

UK: the United Kingdom of Great Britain and Northern Ireland, consisting of four countries. The overall population is just over 66 million. England has the largest population (55.6 million) and is the location of central government. The DHSC provides policy and leadership for health and social care in England through NHS England. Scotland (5.4 million), Wales (3.1 million), and Northern Ireland (1.8 million) have devolved responsibility for healthcare (Office for National Statistics 2018).

References

American Association of Colleges of Nursing (2004). Position statement on the practice doctorate in nursing. https://www.aacnnursing.org/Portals/42/News/Position-Statements/DNP.pdf (accessed January 7, 2019).

Benner, P. (1984). *From Novice to Expert: Excellence and Power in Clinical Nursing Practice*. Menlo Park, California: Addison Wesley.

Brechin, A. (2000). Introducing critical practice. Chapter 2. In: *Critical Practice in Health and Social Care* (ed. A. Brechin, H. Brown and M. Eby), 25–47. Buckingham: Oxford University Press.

Covey, S. (2006). *The 8th Habit. From Effectiveness to Greatness*. London: Simon and Schuster.

De Bono, E. (1991). *The Five-Day Course in Thinking*. London: Penguin.

Department of Health (2010). *Advanced Level Nursing: A Position Statement*. London: Department of Health.

Department of Health and Social Services and Public Safety (2012). *Improving Health and Well-Being Through Positive Partnerships. A Strategy for the Allied Health Professions in Northern Ireland 2012–17*. Belfast: DHSSP.

Department of Health and Social Services and Public Safety (2016). *Advanced Nursing Practice Framework. Supporting Advanced Nursing Practice in Health and Social Care Trusts*. Belfast: Northern Ireland Practice and Education Council for Nursing.

European Centre for Disease Prevention and Control (2018). Communicable disease threat report, 8–14 July 2018, week 28. https://ecdc.europa.eu/en/publications-data/communicable-disease-threats-report-8-14-july-2018-week-28 (accessed January 7, 2019).

Frenk, J., Chen, L., Bhutta, Z.A. et al. (2010). Health professionals for a new century: transforming education to strengthen health systems in an interdependent world. *The Lancet* 376 (9756): 1923–1958.

Hamric, A. (2014). A definition of advanced practice nursing. Chapter 3. In: *Advanced Practice Nursing. An Integrative Approach*, 5e (ed. A. Hamric, C. Hanson, M. Tracy and E. O'Grady), 67–85. St Louis: Elsevier Saunders.

Hanson, C. and Spross, J. (2005). Collaboration. Chapter 10. In: *Advanced Nursing Practice. An Integrative Approach*, 3e (ed. A. Hamric, J. Spross and C. Hanson), 341–378. St Louis: Elsevier Saunders.

Hsueh, M. and Dorcy, K. (2016). Improving transitions of care with an advanced practice nurse: a pilot study. *Clinical Journal of Oncology Nursing* 20 (3): 240–243.

International Council of Nurses (2008). *The Scope of Practice, Standards and Competencies of the Advanced Practice Nurse*. Geneva: ICN.

International Council of Nurses (2018). Nurse practitioner/advanced nursing practitioner network definition and characteristics of the role. https://international.aanp.org/Practice/APNRoles (accessed January 7, 2019).

International Diabetes Federation (2018). IDF Diabetes Atlas 2017. http://www.diabetesatlas.org (accessed January 7, 2019).

Kutzleb, J., Rigolosi, R., Fruhschien, A. et al. (2015). Nurse practitioner care model: meeting the health care challenges with a collaborative team. *Nursing Economics* 33 (6): 297–305.

McGee, P. (2009). The conceptualisation of advanced practice. Chapter 4. In: *Advanced Practice in Nursing and the Allied Health Professions*, 3e (ed. P. McGee), 43–55. Oxford: Wiley Blackwell.

Manley, K. (1998). A conceptual framework for advanced practice: an action research project operationalising an advanced practitioners/consultant nurse role. Chapter 8. In: *Advanced Nursing Practice* (ed. G. Rolfe and P. Fulbrook), 118–135. Oxford: Butterworth-Heinemann.

National Health Service Health Education England (2017). Multi-professional framework for England. https://www.hee.nhs.uk/our-work/advanced-clinical-practice/multi-professional-framework (accessed January 7, 2019).

National Leadership and Innovation Agency for Healthcare (2010). Framework for Advanced Nursing, Midwifery and Allied Health Professional Practice in Wales. Llanharan, NLIAH. https://www.wales.nhs.uk/sitesplus/documents/829/NLIAH%20Advanced%20Practice%20Framework.pdf (accessed January 7, 2019).

NHS Confederation (2017). NHS statistics, facts and figures. https://www.nhsconfed.org/resources/key-statistics-on-the-nhs (accessed January 7, 2019).

NHS Employers (2018). Advanced clinical practitioner apprenticeship approved. https://www.nhsemployers.org/news/2018/04/advanced-clinical-practioner-apprenticeship-approved (accessed January 7, 2019).

NHS England (2014). Five Year Forward View. https://www.england.nhs.uk/wp-content/uploads/2014/10/5yfv-web.pdf (accessed January 7, 2019).

Nursing and Midwifery Council (2018). *Future Nurse: Standards of Proficiency for Registered Nurses*. London: Nursing and Midwifery Council.

O'Connell, J., Gardner, G., and Coyer, F. (2014). Beyond competencies: using a capability framework in developing practice standards for advanced practice nursing. *Journal of Advanced Practice* 70 (12): 2728–2735.

Office for National Statistics (2017). Overview of the UK population: July 2017. https://www.ons.gov.uk/peoplepopulationandcommunity/populationandmigration/populationestimates/articles/overviewoftheukpopulation/july2017 (accessed January 19, 2019).

Office for National Statistics (2018). Population estimates: June 2018. https://www.ons.gov.uk/peoplepopulationandcommunity/populationandmigration/populationestimates (accessed January 7, 2019).

Papadopoulos, I. (2018). *Culturally Competent Compassion. A Guide for Healthcare Students and Practitioners*. Abingdon: Routledge.

Public Health England (2018a). Sexually transmitted infections and screening for chlamydia in England, 2017. *Health Protection Report* 12 (20). London: Public Health England.

Public Health England (2018b). Facing the Facts, Shaping the Future. A draft health and care workforce strategy for England to 2027. For consultation. London: Public Health England.

Rosling, H., Rosling, A. and Rosling, O. (2018) *Factfulness: Ten reasons we're wrong about the world - and why things are better than you think*. London, Sceptre.

Royal College of Nursing (2018a). *Advanced Level Nursing Practice: Introduction*. London: Royal College of Nursing.

Royal College of Nursing (2018b). *RCN Credentialing for Advanced Level Nursing Practice. Handbook for Applicants*. London: Royal College of Nursing.

Royal College of Nursing (2018c). Ministers must look again at student funding, the RCN says, as nursing degree applications fall further. https://www.rcn.org.uk/news-and-events/news/removing-the-student-nurse-bursary-has-been-a-disaster (accessed January 7, 2019).

Schober, M. and Affara, F. (2006). *International Council of Nurses, Advanced Nursing Practice*. Oxford: Blackwell Science.

Schön, D. (1983). *The Reflective Practitioner. How Professionals Think in Action*. London: Avebury.

Sen, A. (1999). *Development as Freedom*. Oxford: Oxford University Press.

Spross, J. and Babine, R. (2014). Guidance and coaching. Chapter 8. In: *Advanced Practice Nursing. An Integrative Approach*, 5e (ed. A. Hamric, C. Hanson, M. Tracy and E. O'Grady), 183–212. St Louis: Elsevier Saunders.

Tracy, M. (2014). Direct clinical practice. Chapter 7. In: *Advanced Practice Nursing. An Integrative Approach*, 5e (ed. A. Hamric, C. Hanson, M. Tracy and E. O'Grady), 147–182. St Louis: Elsevier Saunders.

United Nations High Commission for Refugees (2018). *Global Trends. Forced Displacement in 2017*. Geneva: United Nations.

United Nations (2015). Transforming Our World. The 2030 Agenda for Sustainable Development. https://sustainabledevelopment.un.org/post2015/transformingourworld/publication (accessed January 7, 2019).

World Health Organization (2014) A Universal Truth: No Health Without a Workforce. https://www.who.int (accessed 9 May, 2019).

World Health Organization (2017). Diarrhoeal disease. https://www.who.int/news-room/fact-sheets/detail/diarrhoeal-disease (accessed January 7, 2019).

World Health Organization (2018). Global Health Observatory (GHO) data: life expectancy. https://www.who.int/gho/mortality_burden_disease/life_tables/situation_trends/en/ (accessed January 7, 2019).

CHAPTER 2

An International Perspective of Advanced Nursing Practice

Madrean Schober

Schober Global Healthcare Consulting, Indiana, USA

Key Issues

- The concept of advanced nursing practice (ANP) from a global perspective
- The extent of the international presence of ANP
- The challenges for development and implementation of ANP
- The potential future of ANP worldwide

LEARNING OBJECTIVES

By the end of this chapter you will be able to:

- Provide an international definition and characteristics for the advanced practice nurse (APN).
- Identify drivers for the growing presence of APNs worldwide.
- Describe the influence of international organizations in advanced nursing practice (ANP) development.
- Compare country and regional illustrations of APN practice.
- Specify controversial issues confronted with ANP development.

Advanced Practice in Healthcare: Dynamic Developments in Nursing and Allied Health Professions,
Fourth Edition. Edited by Paula McGee and Chris Inman.
© 2019 John Wiley & Sons Ltd. Published 2019 by John Wiley & Sons Ltd.

2.1 Introduction: Overview of Advanced Nursing Practice

The introduction of the concept of advanced nursing practice (ANP) and associated interest in advanced practice nursing (APN) roles has resulted in a dynamic and evolving global phenomenon. This rapidly emerging field is a vibrant contemporary development in nursing, capturing not only the attention of nurses and other healthcare professionals, but also key decision makers and healthcare planners as they face issues of healthcare reform and provision of healthcare services. New initiatives that include the integration of innovative models of practice and a healthcare workforce skill mix have increased the visibility of nursing roles and highlighted the importance of nursing's contribution to the provision of healthcare services worldwide.

This chapter aims to identify drivers contributing to the global interest in advanced clinical nursing initiatives. The role international organizations play as new schemes are considered is highlighted. The official position of the International Council of Nurses (ICN) on the definition and characteristics for APN roles is provided. In addition, this chapter comments on controversial issues arising and challenges faced with the integration of APNs into healthcare systems. Regional and country illustrations are used to draw attention to the realities of integration of these nurses into the healthcare workforce. The chapter concludes with speculation on future directions for advancement in nursing practice.

2.2 Advanced Nursing Practice Defined: An International Position

The ICN regards clear definitions as an essential part of identifying and introducing a new nursing role (Styles and Affara 1997). Definitions are key to distinguishing who a healthcare worker is and providing boundaries for practice. Role definitions can be viewed as a brief method to convey what services to expect from a specific healthcare provider and under what conditions these services will be offered (Schober and Affara 2006).

To contribute to a common understanding and guide ANP development internationally, ICN, through the expertise of its Nurse Practitioner (NP)/Advanced Practice Nursing Network (APNN), developed a definition and characteristics of NP and APN roles. These guidelines reflect the official position of ICN and are meant to represent current and potential roles worldwide. The intent and purpose is to promote an exchange of ideas that lead to development that is responsive to the needs of a region or country (Table 2.1).

2.2.1 Characteristics

The characteristics of ANP refer to educational preparation (Table 2.2), the nature of practice (Table 2.3), and regulatory mechanisms recommended to be in place to support and identify the APN (Table 2.4).

Regional and national approaches to shaping a definition and characteristics include the use of APN or ANP as an all-inclusive term for all APNs. In the USA, by using the label *Advanced Practice Registered Nurse* (APRN), this approach includes clinical nurse specialists (CNSs), NPs, nurse anesthetists, and nurse

TABLE 2.1

Definition of an advanced practice nurse (APN).

"A Nurse Practitioner/Advanced Practice Nurse is a registered nurse who has acquired the expert knowledge base, complex decision-making skills and clinical competences for expanded practice, the characteristics of which are shaped by the context and/or country in which she/he is credentialed to practice. A Master's degree is recommended for entry level."

Source: International Council of Nurses (2008), p. 29. Reproduced by permission.

TABLE 2.2

Educational preparation for an advanced practice nurse.

- Educational preparation at an advanced level.
- Formal recognition of educational programs preparing nurse practitioners/ advanced nursing practice roles as accredited or approved.
- Formal system of licensure, registration, certification, and credentialing.

Source: International Council of Nurses (2008), p. 29. Reproduced by permission.

TABLE 2.3

The nature of advanced practice.

- Integrates research, education, practice, and management.
- High degree of professional autonomy and independent practice.
- Case management/own caseload.
- Advanced health assessment skills, decision-making skills, and diagnostic reasoning skills.
- Recognized advanced clinical competences.
- Provision of consultant services to health providers.
- Plans, implements, and evaluates programs.
- Recognized first point of contact for clients.

Source: International Council of Nurses (2008), p. 29. Reproduced by permission.

TABLE 2.4

Regulatory mechanisms.

- Right to diagnose.
- Authority to prescribe medication.
- Authority to prescribe treatment.
- Authority to refer clients to other professionals.
- Authority to admit patients to hospital.
- Legislation to confer and protect the title "Nurse Practitioner/Advanced Practice Nurse."
- Legislation or some other form of regulatory mechanism specific to advanced practice nurses.
- Officially recognized titles for nurses working in advanced practice roles.

Source: International Council of Nurses (2008), p. 29. Reproduced by permission.

midwives (NCSBN 2008). In Canada, ANP is an umbrella term encompassing NPs and CNSs (CNA 2008). The parameters for developing terminology, a role definition, and scope of practice for the APN include the work setting, specialty knowledge, patient population, level of education, available resources, nursing/ healthcare culture, and professional standards (personal communication, R. Goodyear, July 26, 2017). All these issues must be considered when drafting documents and developing the foundation for an ANP initiative.

2.2.2 Assumptions

Key assumptions are implied when referring to the nurse prepared at the post-basic generalist level who is subsequently recognized as an APN. Fundamental components supportive of ANP should be found wherever nursing exists and thus provide the foundation for the development of advanced levels of clinical practice. The assumptions in Table 2.5 provide a basis for international deliberation and discussion.

In addition, the ICN position emphasizes that "The degree of judgment, skill, knowledge and accountability increases between the preparation of nurse generalists and that of the APN. This added breadth and depth of practice is achieved through additional education and experiences in clinical practice; however, the core does not change and remains the context of nursing" (ICN 2008, p. 9).

These assumptions and the ICN position describe, in general terms, the APN as an integral part of the healthcare workforce, able to confront the challenges of changing population healthcare needs.

2.2.3 Country Issues that Shape Development

The possibility of introducing and developing the APN role rests on the fundamental level of a country's nursing practice and access to an adequate level of appropriate education. The questions in Table 2.6 provide guidance on exploring the concept of ANP. The maturity and professional status of nursing

---

TABLE 2.5

Assumptions about advanced practice.

All advanced practice nurses:
- Are practitioners of nursing providing safe and competent patient care.
- Have their foundation in registered generalist nurse education.
- Have roles which require formal education beyond the preparation of the generalist nurse.
- Have roles of increased levels of competence that are measurable.
- Have competences which address the ethical, legal, care-giving, and professional development of the advanced practice role.
- Have competences and standards which are periodically reviewed for maintaining currency in practice.
- Are influenced by the global, social, political, economic, and technological milieu.

Source: International Council of Nurses (ICN) (2008), p. 11. Reproduced by permission.

> **TABLE 2.6**
>
> **Country issues that shape the development of advanced practice.**
>
> - What is the nurses' perspective of advancement and advanced nursing practice?
> - What does advancement or professional progression for nursing mean within the country?
> - Is there a career structure for promotion that could support the integration of advanced practice nurses?
> - Is there an official place for the advanced practice nurse within the healthcare system with well-defined job descriptions and a career pathway commensurate with their qualifications and capabilities?
> - Are the key components of advanced nursing practice acknowledged and addressed?
>
> *Source:* Schober (2016), p. 5. Reprinted by permission from Springer.

in a country or region will influence its ability to introduce and successfully implement a sustainable ANP initiative.

2.3 Drivers and Motivation

The emergence of ANP has caught international attention as healthcare planners respond to the increasingly diverse needs of the world's populations (Buchan et al. 2013; Delemaire and LaFortune 2010; Sastra-Fullana et al. 2014; Schober 2016). There is increasing acknowledgment that nurses in advanced clinical roles should be educated, recognized, and authorized to practice to their full potential. This section identifies incentives and motivators that contribute to the consideration and introduction of ANP schemes.

The potential for considering the concept of ANP is shaped by country or regional context (De Geest et al. 2008; Delemaire and LaFortune 2010; Schober 2016). Four main themes are identified as providing momentum for launching a new initiative:

- An identified healthcare need for service provision.
- An answer to skill mix and healthcare workforce planning.
- A desire for the advancement of nursing roles to enhance professional development.
- Public demand for improved access to healthcare services and delivery.

No single starting point is viewed as pivotal when launching a successful and sustainable ANP scheme. The sensitive nature of the milieu underpinning ANP development warrants advanced assessment of the specific setting(s) in which the APN will practice, along with consideration of a framework as a guide (Schober 2017). Motivation alone does not describe the complexities involved in proceeding to integrate APNs into a healthcare system. The factors listed in Table 2.7, along with identified drivers, provide a foundation for launching the ANP concept. It is important to keep in mind that success in one region or country provides a point of reference to consider, but is not necessarily transferable to another setting (consider Exercise 2.1). Country and regional illustrations provided later in this chapter offer exemplars of the variance in developmental processes.

> **TABLE 2.7**
>
> **Drivers for the development of advanced practice roles.**
>
> - An identified need for advanced practice nurse (APN) roles, frequently based on population needs for healthcare services.
> - Strong education programs for the generalist nurse that provide a robust foundation to pursue advanced education.
> - Flexible and pragmatic education alternatives that not only educate competent APNs, but offer options to bridge the gaps in nursing education when a country is in a transitional stage in program development.
> - Clinical career pathways for professional progression.
> - Available APN models and effective mentorship.
> - Presence of effective, influential nursing leadership at the governmental, ministry of health, regulatory agency, and health department levels.
> - Access to international consultant expertise that is continuous and sustainable.
> - Ability of agencies and organizations to work together when coordinating integration of APNs in the healthcare workforce.
>
> *Source:* Schober (2016), p. 10). Reprinted by permission from Springer.

EXERCISE 2.1

What drivers have influenced the heightened interest in promoting ANP in your country?

2.4 Influence of International Organizations

International organizations have a beneficial influence in promoting efforts that support the launching of the ANP concept. The authority of and endorsement by international entities have the potential to convince key decision makers of the benefits of APNs as healthcare providers. When the idea is viewed as part of global advancement for nursing, this degree of support presents an increased level of credibility to proceed with a proposal or project. The following sections illustrate how international influence can make a difference.

2.4.1 International Council of Nurses

ICN is a federation of more than 130 national nursing associations representing more than 16 million nurses worldwide. Founded in 1899, ICN is the world's first and widest-reaching international organization for health professionals. Operated by nurses and leading nursing internationally, ICN works to ensure quality care for all, advance sound health policies globally, promote the advancement of nursing knowledge, and foster the presence worldwide of a respected nursing profession. The networks and international linkages of ICN with national, regional, and international nursing and non-nursing organizations build positive relationships supportive of the advancement of nursing (www.icn.ch).

ICN began to note the emergence of ANP in 1994 and continued to follow its growth globally. In 2000, ICN launched its NP/APN Network (NP/APNN) in order to provide organizational support for new developments in the field of ANP. The aim of NP/APNN is to act as a resource for nursing and healthcare communities by disseminating information and facilitating a research agenda. Its aim is enhanced by biennial international conferences, biannual news bulletins, and periodic postings on the network's website: www.icn-apnetwork.org.

Through the expertise of its network members in 2002, ICN developed international guidelines for ANP (ICN 2008) and continues to review the relevance of its official organizational position relevant to this nursing field. The decision of ICN to take an official position on APN roles provides a benchmark from which member countries and others can use and adapt pertinent information when proceeding with developmental schemes (Tables 2.1–2.4).

ICN also actively represents nursing in such global arenas as the World Health Organization's governing body, the World Health Assembly, and provides representation to other international organizations to ensure that nursing is visible in discussions of effective and quality healthcare. At the 2017 Congress in Barcelona, Spain, ICN announced the formation of a Global Alliance, with its NP/APNN providing the prototype for the advancement of nursing within a new organizational model. The ICN Global Alliance will provide for an expansion of resources to enhance the representation of nursing worldwide. The development of this concept is a work in progress. As of the beginning of 2019, there was no update on plans for the Global Alliance.

2.4.2 International Federation of Nurse Anesthetists

Eleven countries with specific nurse anesthesia education founded the International Federation of Nurse Anesthetists (IFNA) in 1989. As of the beginning of 2019, IFNA has 43 country members and is an affiliate member of ICN. This international organization is dedicated to the advancement of global education and practice standards which will advance the art and science of anesthesiology, and thereby support and enhance quality anesthesia care worldwide. IFNA establishes and maintains effective cooperation with institutions that have a professional interest in nurse anesthesia (http://ifna.site)

Over the years, IFNA has assisted countries with developing nurse anesthesia in areas such as curriculum development and redevelopment. In addition, an international accreditation program for nurse anesthesia has been developed, along with a framework and guidelines for a continuous professional development program. Not only is IFNA an affiliate member of ICN, it also participates in the World Health Organization (WHO) Global Initiative for Essential and Emergency Surgical Care, and liaises with the World Federation of Societies of Anesthesiologists and the European Society of Anesthesiology. Furthermore, IFNA encourages its member countries to develop relationships with other professional healthcare organizations, and assists member countries with policy and practice information for the promotion of nurse anesthesia (personal communication, J. Rowles, IFNA President, June 15, 2017).

2.4.3 World Health Organization (WHO)

As an agency of the United Nations, WHO works to further international cooperation aimed at improving healthcare worldwide. Its emphasis is not specific to nursing, but can influence the extent of attention given to nursing professionals and their provision of healthcare services. The organization works with an array of partners at the global, regional, and country levels in efforts to strengthen nursing and midwifery services, including ANP.

Activities linked to WHO occur more directly under the guidance of regional offices, and for nursing under the auspices of Regional Directors of Nursing. For example, in 2001 the WHO Regional Nursing Director for the Eastern Mediterranean Region (EMRO) took a proactive position to promote exploration and support for ANP in the region (WHO EMRO 2001). Representatives of 14 member nations gathered in Pakistan to discuss ANP and nurse prescribing. An action plan and strategies were developed. Following this meeting and with support from the EMRO regional office in Cairo, Egypt, the Kingdom of Bahrain and the Sultanate of Oman continued to investigate the possibility of ANP in their respective countries. As of January 2019, Oman has six NPs, all educated in the USA, working in various settings in the country. Pakistan continues to explore and develop the concept, however the APN role has yet to be fully implemented (site visits by the author in 2016 and 2017).

When effective, international organizations provide the capacity to strengthen support for ANP by facilitating discussion forums, workshops, conferences, sharing information through publications, and providing consultancy expertise. Resources and support from the international community can incentivize key decision makers to consider the integration of ANP in healthcare systems.

2.5 Regional and Country Profiles of Advanced Nursing Practice

2.5.1 Regional Development

Countries in a geographic region have commonalties that can be utilized to assess the environment in order to progress with an ANP scheme. Regional efforts can emerge with the support of organizations such as WHO. Interest in WHO EMRO was introduced in the previous section. The following section portrays developments in Latin America within the Pan American Health Organization (PAHO).

2.5.2 Latin America/Pan American Health Organization

Members of PAHO, the Americas' regional office of WHO, in 2013 passed Resolution "CD52.R13 Human Resources for Health: Increasing Access to Qualified Health Workers in Primary Healthcare-Based Health Systems" (Schober 2016). This resolution advocated education and implementation of APNs as a key strategy in addressing primary healthcare (PHC) system development and access to services. The impetus emerged from interest and subsequent lobbying by nursing organizations, leaders in nursing education, and health ministries from across the region.

In an effort to progress with this agenda, a summit was convened in 2015 by PAHO/WHO and the Collaborating Centre in Primary Healthcare and Human Resources at McMaster University in Canada (Schober 2016). Participants from the region representing health ministries, nursing associations, and nursing schools concentrated on the possibilities of implementing APN roles in different countries and developed relevant priorities. A plan that included one-year and three-year steps toward implementation was established. In addition, the summit promoted greater collaboration between nursing leaders and institutions in North America and those in Latin America and the Caribbean.

Outcomes of the summit included a subsequent conference in Bogota, Colombia in 2016 to support ANP in Colombia, and launching of a Master's degree Nurse Practitioner in Adult Acute Care program in Chile in collaboration with Johns Hopkins University in the USA. In November 2015, Brazil, with support from PAHO, discussed and prepared a document for the Ministry of Health (MOH) defining the APN scope of practice, with a follow-up seminar in 2016 to increase the visibility of their discussions. Follow-up meetings, built on priorities identified in 2015, proceeded to identify APN competences and curriculum development. Challenges identified by PAHO include:

- Lack of recognition of the role of nurses in the healthcare system.
- Lack of postgraduate nursing education.
- Change to health system policies that enable APNs to practice to their full potential (Schober 2016).

Instrumental in ANP development has not only been regional support, but also shared experiences of APN implementation from Canada, the USA, and other countries. These experiences provide insights to support strong policies for effective APN implementation in the PAHO region.

2.5.3 **Sub-Saharan Africa**

Postgraduate nursing programs that produce specialist and advanced practice nurses are rare in most sub-Saharan countries (Munjanja et al. 2005; Uys and Middleton 2011). Whilst Malawi has introduced postgraduate programs, progress in other sub-Saharan countries has been slow, limiting advancement beyond basic nursing education for the majority of the nurses on the continent.

Due to the lack of medical doctors in Southern Africa, particularly in rural/semi-rural settings where the majority of populations live, nurses are traditionally trained in health assessment, pharmacology, diagnosis, and treatment at preregistration diploma or degree level. Most nurses in these areas also have prescribing authority on qualification, albeit within their scope of practice and usually limited. This may be part of the reason why the registration and regulation of advanced practice remain variable across the continent and, at times, are not recognized at the level they deserve. The success seen in the management of human immunodeficiency virus (HIV) has been attributed to the role played by specialist nurses and midwives in this specialty in the region. In particular, there has been an increase in pediatric HIV-trained specialist nurses who are autonomously managing pediatric antiretroviral treatment (ART), a domain previously held by medical doctors only.

The University of Namibia, for example, offers a Postgraduate Diploma in Clinical Nursing Science, Health Assessment, Treatment, and Care, with its content similar to that offered in some universities in the UK for ANP/ACP courses. Other specialist nursing courses offered and registrable with the Health

Professions Council of Namibia at the same level include anesthetics, trauma nursing science, and oncology. Specialist midwives (midwifery and neonatology), critical care specialist nurses, and mental health specialist nurses all hold Master's degrees and these are registrable specialties (Health Professions Council of Namibia 2008).

It should also be noted that there are variations in the background of clinical officers (COs) in Southern Africa. Whilst some countries, for example Zimbabwe, require background and experience as a qualified nurse and midwife prior to training in the model, other countries, such as South Africa and Kenya, have separate courses with a minimum of three years' training, not necessarily requiring a nursing qualification as a prerequisite. A clinical officer from an African perspective has more authority, including signing off medical sick notes, and preparing and signing off postmortem examination reports and death certificates. Usually they are part of the medical team in tertiary hospitals and may be lead clinicians in district or rural health hospitals. Therefore, in some countries in Africa, nurses may choose to take this route in advancing practice instead of enrolling in nursing-related postgraduate courses.

There are additional initiatives within the region, such as the African Federation for Emergency Medicine (AFEM), which led to the development of the continental emergency nursing curriculum (Scott and Brysiewicz 2016) to establish emergency care as a specialty. The creation of an Afrocentric interprofessional education (IPE) organization, Africa Interprofessional Education Network (AfrIPEN), will also be integral in the training of an advanced practice workforce in its establishment of IPE and collaborative practice. In Zimbabwe, for instance, advanced practice is developing in a similar way to in the UK, with this level of practice inclusive of registered professionals from nursing as well as allied health professionals such as radiographers. It is hoped that other international initiatives such as the United Nations' (UN 2015) 2030 Agenda for Sustainable Development will also pave the way for further developments in advanced practice within the region as governments attempt to implement this plan.

In an attempt to strengthen PHC, the College of Primary Health Care Physicians of Zimbabwe has developed a four-year curriculum for the family medicine Master's degree (MMed; CPCPZ 2014), due to commence in 2018. This is one of the few medical specialties developing in the country. Previously doctors would provide general practice training without any accredited further training. Nursing leaders and academics hope that this medical development will provide a baseline for the development of the family nurse practitioner (FNP) role at master's level, a role currently only well established in Botswana in the Southern African Development Community region (personal communication, S. Sibanda, November 26, 2017).

2.6 Country-specific Initiatives

The country-specific initiatives described in this section reveal the complexities of introducing ANP into the healthcare workforce. The diversity in which these nursing roles become part of the provision of healthcare services is sensitive to the nursing, healthcare, and consumer cultures of the country in which the concept develops. The following country profiles provide illustrations of development, but are not intended to represent the entirety of the international expansion of ANP. After reading them, you may want to consider Exercise 2.2.

2.6.1 **Canada**

Two ANP roles are identified in Canada: NP and CNS (CNA 2008). Nurses are regulated at the provincial and territorial levels. A national framework to promote a common understanding of ANP in Canada was developed in 1999, with key elements revised in 2002 (CNA 2008) and core competences for NPs revised in 2010 (CNA 2010). The Canadian Nurses Association provides professional leadership for ANP advancement.

Currently, the NP is the only advanced role with additional professional regulation and title protection beyond the generalist nurse. Significant progress on the evolution of the NP occurred following the Canadian Nurse Practitioner Initiative (CNPI), launched in 2004 (CNA 2016). CNPI supported coordination and expansion of the scope of practice across all jurisdictions, along with a pan-Canadian title description, a common role description, and adequate liability coverage. In addition, key stakeholders considered standardization of master's-level education as significant to the success of the NP role. A 10-year retrospective of the CNPI (CNA 2016) confirmed progress for NPs; however, it considered the role to be consistently underused despite the demonstrated benefit to the Canadian healthcare system.

The CNS provides health system support throughout Canada. Despite the fact that the CNS has been present for the past four decades, the title is still not protected and there is a lack of consensus on role definition and education. Discussion continues as to the core competences of the CNS. In spite of this disparity, the professional and policy environment in Canada is receptive to integrating ANP roles into the healthcare system (Schober 2016).

2.6.2 **Jamaica**

In July 2017, the island of Jamaica celebrated 40 years of APNs providing healthcare services. Even though NPs, midwives, and nurse anesthetists have a presence in the country's healthcare system, it continues to be an uphill struggle to obtain appropriate professional regulation and prescriptive authority to support the roles. Discussions on the expanded role of the nurse in Jamaica began in 1972. Twenty-five experienced nurses entered the first NP program in Jamaica in 1977. The program was established as a cooperative effort involving personnel from the MOH (Ministry of Health), University of West Indies (UWI), and PROJECT Hope. The first group of NPs began practice in 1978. In 2002, the program became fully university based at the UWI and was upgraded to master's level. Desiring improved NP representation, especially for legislative issues, the Jamaica Association of NPs (JANP) was formed in 2009 and became an affiliate member of the American Association of Nurse Practitioners (AANP) in 2013 (personal communication, H. McGrath, President JANP, July 4, 2017).

2.6.3 **The Netherlands**

The Netherlands has 20 years' experience developing the Dutch interpretation of ANP. The Dutch title is "nurse specialist." The ANP idea was conceived as a task reallocation scheme within the Dutch healthcare system, in response to a projected shortage of physicians. The education consists of a program that combines apprenticeships in a healthcare facility and vocational education at a university. Support by the Dutch government has contributed to progress in the country, as exemplified by the provision of grants for salary compensation and payment for training on hospital wards.

In 2009, legislation was developed to guarantee the quality of education and practice for ANP. Regulations included title protection, required accreditation for education programs, and criteria for the credentialing of APNs based on a chosen practice specialty. A total of 2750 APNs had been educated and registered in the Netherlands as of 2016. In the current healthcare environment, they are no longer seen only as substitutes for physicians, but also as a presence that enhances quality and access to services (Schober 2016).

2.6.4 **Singapore**

Formal and informal discussions among nursing leaders and key stakeholders provided the conceptual beginnings for ANP in Singapore. A nursing task force recommended a nurse clinician role to keep highly skilled nurses in clinical practice (Lim 2005). Historically, Singapore was losing highly skilled nurses to management and education career tracks for promotion and remuneration. Impetus for the APN role is attributed to a request by nursing leaders for a career path for clinical advancement.

A hybrid model based on blending of the CNS and NP roles in the USA formed the basis for the APN role. The first academic program was introduced in 2003 at the National University of Singapore at master's level under the auspices of the Yong Loo Lin School of Medicine. The use of the title "advanced practice nurse" is protected in law. Additional regulations include a role definition, scope of practice, and competences. The path to successful integration has included significant confusion over what the APN can do that is different from the generalist nurse or nurse clinicians who hold positions as care managers. As of 2016, there were 197 identified APNs, mainly employed in the public sector (MOH 2016). Although the numbers are small, the APN initiative continues to progress, with a transformative effect on the provision of healthcare in Singapore.

> **EXERCISE 2.2**
>
> Compare and contrast the development in one of the countries described in this chapter with development in the country in which you are currently working.

2.7 International Collaboration for a New Initiative

When exploring the concept and framework for ANP, the question arises as to what the starting point is for a new initiative and what factors need to be taken into consideration. Launching a new scheme is multifaceted and all too often key decision makers underestimate the complexities of launching a sustainable initiative. The following exemplar offers a description of factors that were addressed in the early stages of development in Lithuania.

| CASE STUDY | **Advanced Nursing Practice in Lithuania** |

The Lithuanian University of Health Sciences (LUHS) partnered with a US university in 2013 to introduce the NP role. In 2014, the Health Care Minister of the Republic of Lithuania appointed a special work group to review the feasibility of developing an ANP program. Findings from the study indicated that (i) higher education was capable of preparing highly qualified NPs, but the legal basis did not allow for the implementation of wider competences in practice; (ii) the rapidly developing healthcare system could not react resourcefully to changing patient needs because of the long preparation for physicians; (iii) the shortage of nursing specialists affected access to healthcare and increased inequalities between urban and rural areas; and (iv) the need for nursing services in the home was not being satisfied. The Health Care Minister and MOH (Minister of Health) approved the concept of ANP and confirmed the APN role as part of the direction of nursing through 2025.

LUHS is an academic health center with a medical school and hospital, so resources for some advanced nursing courses were already established. Faculty used US guidelines to develop a two-year, four-semester, full-time NP curriculum, with consultation from their US partner. During 2015, LUHS University Senate approved the ANP program, with accreditation through the Ministry of Education and Research. The first cohort of 13 students enrolled in September 2015 in primary care, emergency care, or anesthesia and intensive care specialties. Clinical rotations began in 2016 with physician preceptors. In 2017, the MOH approved legislation for ANP competences and functions. The first students graduated in June 2017.

To apply for the ANP program in Lithuania, a candidate must have achieved a Bachelor of Science degree in nursing. A Master of Science degree is awarded to the student on successful completion of the program. A second cohort of students started the program in September 2016 for graduation in June 2018. A third cohort began the program in 2017, with expectations to graduate in June 2019. Because there are no NP role models in Lithuania, lack of knowledge about ANP and the NP role and acceptance from stakeholders have created challenges. LUHS continues to address legal issues of title, licensure, regulation, certification, and credentialing, scope of practice, and compensation or appropriate salaries. These efforts have meant astutely pursuing legislative actions while also planning the ANP curriculum. Implementation of the role has been problematic, as physicians are hesitant, even though the Minister of Health for the Republic of Lithuania has issued approval of the title and role of Advanced Practice Nurse (personal communication, J.A. Newland and A. Blazecieviene, December 5, 2017).

1. In your field of practice, what factors would managers have to consider in planning a new ANP service?

2. What is a role model? Who has influenced you as a role model? What qualities do they possess? How did the person help you?

3. Are you a role model for others in your workplace?

2.8 Controversial Issues

Characteristics and assumptions that shape the nature of APN practice are identified earlier in this chapter. Identifying these attributes portrays this level of nursing to other healthcare professionals, decision makers, and the public. This is especially significant when issues arise that are controversial in promoting this change in the concept of what nurses and specifically APNs do. The next section considers key controversial questions that might arise.

2.8.1 **Prescriptive Authority**

When considering launching an ANP initiative, the debate focuses on changes in the boundaries of nursing practice. Prescriptive authority for nurses, especially for APNs, fuels animated debate. Critics assert that nurses simply do not have the knowledge to prescribe medicines and therapeutic interventions correctly. Even though the focus is on the appropriateness of prescriptive authority for APNs, inquiry into the realities of this allegation reveals that nurses are already safely prescribing in various capacities, but outside a legal framework and without appropriate education consistent with current practice (Ball 2009). In addition, prescriptive authority would seem to be a prerequisite for some APN roles, especially in primary care settings.

Even though prescriptive authority is a controversial issue, there is an identified increase in the number of countries where nurses have various levels of regulatory authority to prescribe medicines (Ball 2009; Kouwen and van den Brink 2014; Schober 2017). Nurse prescribing varies from country to country and is not necessarily linked to ANP, but can be associated with general nursing practice in specific settings. Ball (2009, p. 67) suggests that the question is not "Can nurses prescribe?" but "To what extent is nurse prescribing established?"

The way in which nurse prescribing evolves can be shaped by the motivation to identify this as a component in APN practice within country-contextual development of the ANP concept. The exact nature varies significantly, from circumstances where nurses prescribe independently to situations where prescriptive authority is restricted under close supervision of a physician (Ball 2009; Schober 2017). Nurse prescribing may not succeed if efforts lack a supportive infrastructure or an identified motivation to include this feature of clinical practice. On the other hand, efforts toward healthcare reform and/or healthcare crises can be the stimulus needed to include prescribing in the scope of practice.

2.8.2 **Making an Initial Diagnosis**

Conversation on a scope of practice that includes the APN making an initial diagnosis is sensitive to country context. Making a diagnostic decision can be viewed as educated decision making by a healthcare provider with and on behalf of a patient or family. This issue reaches heightened importance in primary care settings and in situations where the APN is the sole healthcare professional. In some settings and countries, the scope of practice can be excessively restricted when the ability to make a diagnostic decision is relevant only to medicine. It is the opinion of this author that use of a common diagnostic language and decision making is one way to attain consistency in the provision of healthcare services (Schober 2016).

2.8.3 **Hospital Privileges**

In many parts of the world, admission to and discharge from a healthcare facility are associated with physician responsibility. This policy has the potential to compromise the delivery of effective healthcare. The concept of hospital privileges began with the method of awarding status to physicians who had successfully satisfied a screening process (Buppert 2015). Based on hospital and institution policy, a healthcare professional has full access to the records of the patients they admit, as well as decision-making authority over management and discharge.

For the APN, obtaining hospital privileges provides practice authority for specific care within a designated institution. Privileges are usually established based on license, education, experience, and identified competence. Even though this issue is not usually a top priority when launching an ANP initiative, in an era of healthcare reform decision makers should be encouraged to see this option as advantageous for APN practice and the populations they care for.

2.8.4 Professional Regulation, Legislation, and Credentialing

Professional regulation is the legitimate and appropriate means – governmental, professional, private, and individual – whereby order, identity, consistency, and control are brought to the profession. The profession and its members are defined; the scope of practice is determined; standards of education and ethical and competent practice are set; and systems of accountability are established (ICN 2005). Professional regulation for ANP consists of standards and policies that recognize the APN and officially credential APNs for their identified position in the healthcare workforce (Hanson 2014). The significance of having appropriate regulatory mechanisms in place is to support APNs to the full potential of their practice.

2.8.5 Maintaining Competence

Maintenance of professional competence is a continuous process of documenting professional accomplishments and activities. Mandatory demonstration of competence maintenance is often a requirement for relicensure and ongoing credentialing for APNs. Criteria for maintaining competence are generally linked to the APN scope of practice and/or practice setting, identified competences, and certification/licensure requirements. In addition to verification that the APN is currently in clinical practice, there can be a range of choices considered acceptable for competence maintenance. The range of choices could include participation in or conduct of research, writing for publication, mentoring APN students, clinical teaching, in-service education, structured interactive activities, and leadership actions.

The timeline for verification of competence maintenance (commonly every five to eight years), documentation of accomplishments, and audit is usually determined by professional credentialing bodies/authorities. Some type of standardization of competence assessment and reassessment is thought to be essential to ensuring APN credibility and legitimacy.

2.9 Challenges

Integrating APNs into the healthcare workforce is a dynamic process characterized by change, alterations in service delivery, and progress toward a new period in nursing practice. The following sections discuss the importance of role clarity, issues that arise among other healthcare professionals, and acceptance by the public when the view of nursing represents a variance in the provision of healthcare services.

2.9.1 Lack of Role Clarity

A topic that dominates the international literature attempting to describe ANP and that impedes implementation of APNs is lack of role clarity relevant to roles and functions within healthcare systems. It is vital that the APN is recognized by healthcare planners and other professionals as a distinct category of nurse, with a specific description of skills and competences to identify them as legitimate members of the healthcare workforce.

Unfortunately, there is a lack of international consensus on labeling and defining APNs in actual practice. In a survey of 32 countries conducted by Pulcini et al. (2010), 13 titles were identified that are used worldwide to identify ANP. Often titles and definitions of practice are used interchangeably when attempting to describe the nature of practice for an APN. The literature indicates that when little distinction is made in identifying ANP and APN roles from other extended or specialized levels of nursing practice, development proceeds in an ad hoc manner (DiCenso et al. 2010; Donald et al. 2010; East et al. 2014). As a result, lack of role clarity is viewed as posing major barriers to role integration and recognizable professional positions within healthcare systems.

2.9.2 Interaction with Health Professionals

A change in the definition and scope of practice for nurses has impacts on an entire healthcare structure and, subsequently, interaction among all professionals providing care. The most written-about interactions, those that cause the most conflict, appear to be rooted in relationships between APNs and other nurses, with physicians, and to a lesser degree with pharmacists. In a scope of practice where duties cross over or overlap with another professional's scope, attempts to block or sabotage the APN can become heated.

Nurses voice concern that the new advanced practice roles are not really nursing and follow too closely a medical model approach to healthcare, consequently leaving behind the core principles of nursing education. The reality is that, in the development and implementation of ANP, concepts representative of medical and nursing scopes of practice do overlap, thus raising concerns among APNs themselves as to how their roles are viewed in the healthcare structure. In addition, Roodbol (2005) cites reported beliefs that APNs lack a respectful attitude to nurses who competently function in other nursing capacities, thus contributing to dissension among nurses expected to work together. In this study, nurses did not share the physician's view of a positive identity for ANP, and conversely the APNs felt conflict about role expectations. On the one hand, the NP is expected to be a nurse; on the other hand, the scope of practice overlaps with medical practice.

Physicians are often placed in a position of authority and supervision over other healthcare professionals as designated gatekeepers for healthcare services. When the scope of practice for the APN overlaps areas of jurisdiction traditionally claimed by physicians, the competence or authority of a nurse to function in an advanced capacity is challenged. On the other hand, a physician who understands the value of advanced nursing roles is often the pivotal, most supportive champion.

At the beginning of a new initiative, time and again other professionals do not comprehend the educational background, scope of practice, or regulations underpinning advanced practice, and thus either do not understand or misunderstand the competences and capabilities of a nurse in this role. These misunderstandings, if left unexplained, can lead to fragmented care and gaps in service delivery, unless they are addressed clearly and openly. In effect, a cautious renegotiation of professional boundaries within healthcare structures and settings is beneficial in acknowledging variations in service delivery, to better ensure that providers and the public are aware of the benefits of a new model of service delivery.

2.9.3 Public Acceptance

A systematic review of the literature conducted from 1990 to 2008 (Newhouse et al. 2011) not only found a high level of evidence that APNs provide safe and effective care, but also confirmed equivalent levels of patient satisfaction. Research further indicates that education of the public regarding the function of APNs and related healthcare services is crucial. Bryant-Lukosius et al. (2004) identify six factors that influence the promotion of APN services to the public (Table 2.8).

The failure of the public to understand who the APN is introduces a barrier to the full development and implementation of ANP. In an era of healthcare reform, the complexities of bringing clarity to who should or will provide healthcare is pivotal. Consumers of healthcare services deserve to have a fundamental understanding of their choices.

2.9.4 Future Directions

Nursing is in a position to develop beneficial and innovative alternatives for the provision of healthcare services worldwide. APNs are in a position to play a decisive role in promoting strategies for the development of an optimal healthcare workforce.

TABLE 2.8

Six factors that influence the promotion of advanced practice nurse (APN) services to the public.

- Confusion about APN terminology.
- Failure to clearly define roles.
- Overemphasis on replacing or supporting physicians.
- Underutilization of all spheres of APN practice.
- Failure to address contextual factors that can undermine APN practice.
- Limited utilization of an evidence-based approach to development, implementation, and evaluation.

Source: Bryant-Lukosius et al. (2004).

In countries where nursing is in its infancy, capacity building and transitioning from current levels of practice, competence, and education to advanced levels will take well-thought-out consideration to meet a minimal standard for practice, whilst taking care to avoid dampening enthusiasm for new roles. Balancing cost-effective options appropriate to populations, and requesting and requiring the necessary services, will increasingly have an impact on choices for APN services. An adequate supply of qualified educators is central to ensuring that practitioners competently develop the skills necessary for practice. Appropriate legislation and credentialing are pivotal to ensure that an APN can practice at the level to which they are educated.

2.10 Conclusion

A proactive voice on behalf of nursing is pivotal in order to demonstrate the value and diversity of ANP. Nurses will be obliged to attain the outlook, knowledge, and skills to respond and adapt to current and future healthcare needs. Healthcare planners, key decision makers, and other professionals are in a position to determine what strategies will best move the world's healthcare agenda forward. Nursing advocacy, strong leadership, and a sound evidence base will aid decision makers in their choice of options that facilitate the provision of innovative, cost-effective, high-quality advanced nursing services.

Key Questions

1. What are the arguments for and against prescribing by APNs in your country?
2. What steps can you take to maintain your competence as an APN?

3. Should APNs in your country have admitting and discharge privileges?

Glossary

Accreditation: a process of review and approval by which an institution, program, or specific service is granted time-limited recognition of having met established standards.

Advanced nursing practice: the field of nursing that requires a higher level of practice from that of the post-basic generalist nurse, based on an advanced level of critical thinking, decision making, and increased accountability in clinical practice.

Advanced practice nurse: a registered nurse who is credentialed, licensed, and registered to function at a level consistent with a country's definition of ANP.

Competence: the effective application of a combination of knowledge, skill, and judgment by an individual in practice/job performance.

Continued competence: the ongoing ability to practice capably in a designated role.

Credentialing: a term used to indicate that an individual, institution, or program has met established standards, as set by a governmental or nongovernmental entity.

Professional regulation: the legitimate processes by which identity and consistency are brought to a profession.

Scope of practice: the range of functions, responsibilities, and activities a registered/licensed professional is educated for, competent in, and authorized to perform. It defines the accountability and limits of practice.

References

Ball, J. (2009). *Implementing Nurse Prescribing*. Geneva: International Council of Nurses.

Bryant-Lukosius, D., DiCenso, A., Browne, G., and Pinelli, J. (2004). Advanced practice nursing roles: development, implementation and evaluation. *Journal of Advanced Nursing* 48 (5): 530–540.

Buchan, J., Temido, M., Fronteira, I. et al. (2013). Nurses in advanced roles: a review of acceptability in Portugal. *Revista Latino-Americana de Enfermagem* 21 (Spec.): 38–46.

Buppert, C. (ed.) (2015). *Nurse Practitioner's Business Practice and Legal Guide*, 5e. Burlington, MA: Jones & Bartlett Learning.

Canadian Nurses Association (CNA) (2008). *Advanced Nursing Practice: A National Framework*. Ottawa: CNA.

Canadian Nurses Association (CNA) (2010). *Canadian Nurse Practitioner Core Competency Framework*. Ottawa: CNA.

Canadian Nurses Association (CNA) (2016). *The Canadian Nurse Practitioner Initiative: A 10-Year Retrospective*. Ottawa: CNA.

College of Primary Care Physicians of Zimbabwe (2014) Concept Note for development of MMed Family Medicine in Zimbabwe. http://cpcpz.co.zw/downloads/concept-note-version-5.doc (accessed January 7, 2019).

De Geest, S., Moons, P., Callens, B. et al. (2008). Introducing advanced practice nursing/nurse practitioners in healthcare systems: a framework for reflection and analysis. *Swiss Medical Weekly* 138 (43–44): 621–628.

Delemaire, M., LaFortune, G. (2010). Nurses in advanced roles: A description and evaluation of experiences in 12 OECD countries. OECD Health Working Papers, No. 54. Paris: OECD Publishing, doi: https://doi.org/10.1787/5kmbrcfms5g7-en

DiCenso, A., Bryant-Lukosius, D., Bourgeault, I. et al. (2010). *Clinical Nurse Specialists and Nurse Practitioners in Canada: A Decision Support Synthesis*. Ottawa: Canadian Health Services Research Foundation.

Donald, F., Bryant-Lukosius, D., Martin-Misener, R. et al. (2010). Clinical nurse specialists and nurse practitioners: title confusion and lack of role clarity. *Canadian Journal of Nursing Leadership* 23(Spec.: 189–210.

East, L.A., Arudo, J., Loefler, M., and Evans, C.M. (2014). Exploring the potential for advanced nursing practice development in Kenya: a qualitative study. *BMC Nursing* 13: 33.

Hanson, C.M. (2014). Understanding regulatory, legal and credentialing requirements. In: *Advanced Practice Nursing: An Integrative Approach*, 5e (ed. A.B. Hamric, C.M. Hanson, M.F. Tracy and E.T. O'Grady), 557–578. St. Louis: Elsevier Saunders.

Health Professions Council of Namibia (2008). Education and registration. http://www.hpcna.com/index.php/councils/15-councils/allied-health-professions-council-of-namibia/47-education-and-registration (accessed January 7, 2019).

International Council of Nurses (ICN) (2005). *ICN regulatory terminology*. Geneva: ICN.

International Council of Nurses (ICN) (2008). *The Scope of Practice, Standards and Competencies of the Advanced Practice Nurse*, ICN Regulation Series. Geneva: ICN.

Kouwen, A.J., van den Brink, G.T.W.J. (2014). Task reallocation and cost prices: Research of obstacles concerning substitution. Report from Radboud University Medical Center to the Dutch Ministry of Health, Welfare and Sport.

Lim, D. (2005). Developing professional nursing in Singapore: a case for change. *Singapore Nursing Journal* 32: 34–47.

Ministry of Health Singapore (MOH) (2016). Health Manpower. https://www.moh.gov.sg/resources-statistics/singapore-health-facts/health-manpower (accessed January 7, 2019).

Munjanja, O.K., Kibuka, S., and Dovlo, D. (2005). *The Nursing Workforce in Sub-Saharan Africa*, Issue paper 7. Geneva: International Council of Nurses https://www.ghdonline.org/uploads/The_nursing_workforce_in_sub-Saharan_Africa.pdf (accessed December 4, 2017).

National Council of State Boards of Nursing (NCSBN) (2008). Consensus model for APRN regulation: Licensure, accreditation, certification and education. https://www.ncsbn.org/aprn-consensus.htm (accessed January 7, 2019).

Newhouse, R.P., Stanik-Hunt, J., White, K.M. et al. (2011). Advanced practice outcomes 1990–2008: a systematic review. *Nursing Economics* 29 (5): 1–21.

Pulcini, J., Jelic, M., Gul, R., and Loke, A.Y. (2010). An international survey on advanced practice nursing education, practice and regulation. *Journal of Nursing Scholarship* 42 (1): 31–39.

Roodbol, P. (2005). Studies, toll roads and song track: role definition between nursing and doctors. Doctoral thesis, University of Groningen.

Sastra-Fullana, P., De Pedro-Gomez, J.E., Bennasar-Veny, M. et al. (2014). Competency frameworks for advanced practice nursing: a literature review. *International Nursing Review* 61 (4): 534–542.

Schober, M. (2016). *Introduction to Advanced Nursing Practice: An International Focus*. Cham, Switzerland: Springer International.

Schober, M. (2017). *Strategic Planning for Advanced Nursing Practice*. Cham, Switzerland: Springer International.

Schober, M. and Affara, F. (2006). *Advanced Nursing Practice*. Oxford: Blackwell.

Scott, P. and Brysiewicz, P. (2016). African emergency nursing curriculum: development of a curriculum model. *International Emergency Nursing* 27: 60–63.

Styles, M.M. and Affara, F.A. (1997). *ICN on Regulation: Towards a 21st Century Model*. Geneva: International Council of Nurses.

United Nations (2015). Transforming our world: the 2030 Agenda for Sustainable Development. https://sustainabledevelopment.un.org/post2015/transformingourworld (accessed December 5, 2017).

Uys, L. and Middleton, L. (2011). Internationalising university schools of nursing in South Africa through a community of practice. *International Nursing Review* 58: 115–122.

World Health Organization-Eastern Mediterranean Regional Office (WHO-EMRO) (2001). Fifth Meeting of the Regional Advisory Panel on Nursing and Consultation on Advanced Practice Nursing and Nurse Prescribing: Implications for Regulation, Nursing Education and Practice in the Eastern Mediterranean Region. WHO-EM/NUR/348/E/L. Cairo: WHO-EMRO.

CHAPTER 3

Development of Advanced Practice Nursing Roles in the Netherlands

Christine de Vries de Winter

HAN University of Applied Sciences, Arnhem and Nijmegen, The Netherlands

Key Issues
- The development of advanced nursing practice in the Netherlands
- The regulation of advanced nursing practice
- Current issues in advanced nursing practice

LEARNING OUTCOMES

By the end of this chapter you will be able to:
- Briefly outline the Dutch healthcare system.
- Critically discuss the Dutch approach to the establishment of advanced nursing practice.
- Critically examine the challenges in maintaining and further developing advanced nursing practice in the Netherlands.

3.1 Introduction

In common with many countries, the Netherlands has experienced a number of changes that have challenged health services. These include increasing numbers of older adults and people with long-term conditions, the impact on health

Advanced Practice in Healthcare: Dynamic Developments in Nursing and Allied Health Professions,
Fourth Edition. Edited by Paula McGee and Chris Inman.
© 2019 John Wiley & Sons Ltd. Published 2019 by John Wiley & Sons Ltd.

of global travel, the need to combat the spread of communicable diseases, coupled with the rising expectations of consumers. These have all served to create a need for new ways of working and the development of new roles in healthcare. This chapter presents an account of the Netherlands' development of advanced nursing practice roles to meet the needs of patients in both community and hospital settings. It begins with a brief overview of the Dutch healthcare system, as a background to the explanation of the main impetus for the introduction of advanced nursing practice. This is followed by an account of the introduction of regulation for advanced nurse practitioners, and the chapter closes with consideration of a number of current issues. It should be noted here that many different titles are used to refer to advanced nursing practice in the Netherlands. Examples include advanced practice, advanced nurse practice, advanced practice nurse, Master's in advanced nursing practice, nurse practitioner, and specialist practitioner. This chapter uses only three: *advanced nursing practice, advanced nurse practitioner,* and *nurse practitioner.*

3.2 The Dutch Healthcare System

Healthcare in the Netherlands is characterized by the principle that adequate care should be accessible to everyone. In 2006, an insurance system based on risk equalization was introduced. This involves a compulsory insurance package available to all citizens at affordable cost, without the need for the insured to be assessed for risk by insurance companies. Prior to 2006, there were separate public and private systems, with short-term health insurance which was implemented by nonprofit health funds, and financed by premiums taken at source from salaries. People earning less than a certain threshold qualified for the public insurance system. However, anyone with an income above that threshold was obliged to have private insurance instead. People who had previously accessed the old system sometimes viewed its demise with regret, as the new system provided health insurance companies with increased control over terms, conditions, and services. Nevertheless, the new insurance system has been cited as an example of an efficient, universally accessible system that has successfully integrated a strong competitive market component (Boot 2013). This is despite the fact that, together with Denmark and Sweden, the Netherlands has one of the most expensive care systems in Europe and one in which costs continue to escalate (OECD Health Data, https://data.oecd.org). Nevertheless, these care systems score well in terms of quality of care and customer friendliness. The Netherlands has 48 different quality indicators, including information provision, quality of hospital care, accessibility, and drug use, suggesting the best care system in Europe (Björnberg 2018).

Healthcare in the Netherlands has three echelons of care relating to physical and mental health. The first and largest echelon comprises community-based general practitioners (GPs), allied healthcare practitioners, and nurses. The second echelon is hospital based; patients are referred, by GPs, to hospital services for assessment, or may self-refer in order to access emergency services. The third echelon is referral to specialist services in academic centers of excellence. Advanced practitioners contribute significantly to all three echelons, with individual practitioners developing expertise in a wide range of settings, including strategic leadership roles in nursing homes and advanced roles in general practice and hospital-based specialties.

3.3 Development of Advanced Nursing Practice in the Netherlands

Courses in advanced practice commenced in 1996 in response to an anticipated shortage of doctors, particularly GPs. Additional factors included the need to:

- Provide opportunities for nurses to further develop their skills in patient care.
- Encourage experienced nurses to remain in clinical practice rather than transfer into education or management to further their careers.

The development of advanced practice was supported by Dr. E. Borst (1932–2014), one of the former Ministers of Public Health, and the Council for Public Health and Health Care, now amalgamated into the Council for Health and Society as a way of reducing costs in healthcare. Academic nurse leaders from three Universities of Applied Sciences in Utrecht, Groningen, and Arnhem–Nijmegen prepared a Master's curriculum for training and educating advanced practice nurses, and the first students graduated in 2000. In 2004, the Dutch government provided structural funding for the training of nurse practitioners. This funding is divided into two payments for each student: one for the university to cover fees, and the other for medical specialists. The introduction of structural funding helped enormously to engage support from doctors to assist nurses in their training program for the advanced nursing practice role. During their training, student advanced nurse practitioners continue to be employed by their healthcare institution and receive a salary; usually this is the same as in their role as a nurse. Once qualified, they are paid as advanced nurse practitioners.

In 2009, the Dutch government approved advanced practice in five specialties. Four of these specialties related to physical care provided by the advanced nurse practitioners: *acute care, chronic care, preventive care,* and *intensive care.* The fifth specialty was *mental healthcare,* in which the advanced nurse practitioner was required to integrate aspects of prevention, treatment, emergency treatment, counseling, and support of patients with mental illnesses. In order to contribute to the acceptance and recognition of these new professionals, advanced nurse practitioners in these specialties were to have the title *Verpleegkundig Specialist* (nursing specialist), which was similar to that used for Dutch physicians: *Medisch Specialist* (medical specialist). The five specialties were further subdivided based on care needs and regardless of the organizational setting. The emphasis here was on preventing, treating, supervising, and/or supporting individuals by focusing on one or more of the following populations: children and adolescents, adults, elderly people, forensic psychiatry, and addiction care (V&VN/VS, https://venvnvs.nl/venvnvs/over-de-verpleegkundig-specialist). This systematic approach to identifying specific specialties was intended to clarify the advanced practitioners' area of knowledge and expertise, and thus reassure patients and other care givers about these new professionals. However, evaluation of this approach demonstrated that the five designated specialties did not match what was happening in practice (Platform Zorgmasters, www.platformzorgmasters.nl). Consequently, in 2017, advice prepared for the Ministry argued for simplification and a division into two main categories: *general healthcare* and *mental healthcare* (https://venvnvs.nl/venvnvs/information-in-english).

Now that you are aware of how the Dutch system works, consider Exercise 3.1.

EXERCISE 3.1

Compare and contrast the Dutch approach with the development of advanced practice in your field.

What role has your nursing organization played in the development of advanced practice?

3.4 Regulation of Advanced Practice

The Individual Healthcare Professions Act (1997) authorizes the regulation of healthcare professions through the BIG register (https://english.bigregister.nl). The Act covers all health professions, but divides them into different categories. Nursing is categorized under Article 3, along with medicine, dentistry, midwifery, pharmacy, psychotherapy, physical therapy, and health psychology. In order to practice, members of these professions must be registered with the BIG register, which also provides professional regulation, discipline, and protection of professional titles. Registration authorizes members of the eight professions to carry out *reserved procedures*; that is to say, those which may be performed only by healthcare providers. Examples of these procedures include performing surgery, prescribing prescription drugs, specialist injections, catheterization, and endoscopy procedures. In addition to BIG registration, five professions are recognized as having specialties: nursing, medicine, dentistry, health psychology, and pharmacy (https://english.bigregister.nl). Specialists must be registered with the specialist registration committee of their respective profession, which notifies the BIG register. The Registration Committee Specialisms Nursing (RSV) (https://vsregister.venvn.nl) fulfills this role for advanced nurse practitioners, thus distinguishing them from other nurses; the protected title is *Nurse Practitioner*. Specialist registration allows the advanced nurse practitioner to practice autonomously, as an expert in a specific field, to perform reserved procedures, and to refer patients directly to and receive referrals directly from other health professionals. Specialist registration requires the advanced nurse practitioner to be proactive in pursuing professional development in order to continue registration as a nurse practitioner.

In relation to registration, think about Exercise 3.2.

EXERCISE 3.2

What are the advantages and disadvantages of registration for advanced practitioners?

3.5 Preparation of Advanced Nurse Practitioners

The Dutch national curriculum for advanced nurse practitioner education is based on the Canadian Medical Education Directions for Specialists (CanMEDS; Royal College of Canada 2005 and 2015, http://www.royalcollege.ca/rcsite/canmeds-e). This is similar to the curriculum for medical training in the

Netherlands, and thus contributes to a degree of acceptance of advanced nursing roles. The CanMEDS framework has seven roles, each of which is clearly defined and is linked with advanced nursing practice roles (Table 3.1). A competent advanced nurse practitioner seamlessly integrates the competences of all

---

TABLE 3.1

Examples of learning objectives linked to the seven CanMEDS roles.

CanMEDS domain	Explanation	Advanced nursing roles
Clinical expert	Synthesis of all the other domains into excellent patient care.	Integration of cure and care by practising autonomously within the advanced practitioner's own field of expertise. Offering complex, evidence-based specialist nursing care and protocol-based medical care. Promoting continuity and quality of nursing care and medical treatment. Supporting the patient's ability to improve self-management and improve their quality of life.
Communicator	Forming effective communication with patients in order to ensure that they are informed about all aspects of their health issues and care.	Effective oral, written, or electronic transfer communication across the care chain.
Collaborator	Working effectively with other health professionals to deliver high-quality care.	Awareness of own professional limitations. Referring patients to other healthcare providers in compliance with legislation and regulations, thus ensuring continuity of care. Ensuring patient safety through effective collaboration with other healthcare professionals.
Organizer/leader	Contributing to clear goals and taking responsibility for the delivery of high-quality care	Providing clinical and professional leadership to support others (junior colleagues) and positively influence care and organizational outcomes. Redesigning services based on care needs and taking account of factors such as cost, continuity, quality, service, and speed to achieve a lasting improvement. Developing and updating professional knowledge and skills.
Health advocate	Acting on behalf of those unable to do so for themselves.	Recognizing factors that threaten patients and/or specific groups and making policy proposals in the field of prevention.
Scholar	Being commited to lifelong learning	Applying expertise and critical ability expressed in the assessment of new knowledge, research results, and new procedures.Promoting the development and deepening of scientific expertise through practical research and innovative projects.
Professional	Being committed to ethical practice and behavior.	Ethical practice and behavior that promote patients' autonomy and self-determination.

Source: Summarized from Canadian Medical Education Directions for Specialists (CanMEDS), Royal College of Physicians and Surgeons of Canada (http://www.royalcollege.ca/rcsite/canmeds-e).
Based on the Dutch general competences profile of advanced practice nursing (V&VN Algemeen besluit 2016).

seven of the CanMEDS roles. Almost all the nursing, medical, and paramedic courses use this framework, thus providing some degree of standardization across professional groups.

All entrants to advanced nurse practitioner education have already undertaken a four-year Bachelor's degree program in order to qualify as nurses and completed a number of years in post-qualified practice. Consequently, advanced nurse practitioner education is at Master's level and in line with the Dutch Qualification Framework (NLQF) level 7. The Master's degree is a mandatory requirement for entry to the specialist register. Each university must be approved by the RSV to provide this degree, but there is some flexibility in the system which allows each institution to develop its own education program based on the CanMEDS framework. Thus, there is some variation between courses, for example in terms of assessment methods. Courses take two years to complete and require 1680 hours of study per year.

In all courses the generic content focuses on clinical reasoning, nursing leadership, nursing research, pharmacotherapy, ethical issues, and care provided through interprofessional cooperation. The emphasis is on developing an inquiring attitude in which the student not only accepts the professional reality as a given, but critically asks questions. The important Dutch skill *het onderzoekend vermogen* is best translated as "the capacity for critical and analytic inquiry," and is the basis for finding and appraising the best available evidence and applying this in practice. Critical and analytic skills also inform the identification of questions emerging from practice, the conception and conduct of practice-oriented research, and lifelong learning.

Theoretical elements are studied alongside periods of practice, which take up about two-thirds of the total course. Generic competences agreed by all universities must be applied by students to their own practice and specialty. This means that all students must be employed in healthcare practice and settings before they begin the course. Moreover, these settings must provide the conditions required for the delivery and support of the relevant education program. Supervision and practice-based teaching are, preferably, supported by a medical specialist and a nurse practitioner; that is to say, a practitioner who is recognized by the RSV. There are two reasons for this dual supervision. First, in the early years of advanced nurse practitioner education, there were not enough nurse practitioners available and so doctors provided supervision. Second, it is acknowledged that there are overlaps between the medical and advanced nursing roles, for example with regard to the performance of reserved procedures. Reflective learning encourages students to engage in a process in which experiences, including the student's own performance, are reviewed in terms of their potential to provide a basis for learning; new knowledge, abilities, attitudes, and skills can then be identified, tested, and incorporated into earlier learning (Kolb 1984).

In this light, consider Exercise 3.3.

EXERCISE 3.3

Choose one aspect of practice-based learning that student advanced nurse practitioners in your field must achieve.

What competences does this aspect require?

How are these assessed and by whom?

3.6 Issues in Advanced Practice in the Netherlands

Dutch issues relating to advanced nursing practice are generally similar to global challenges, as identified by Kleinpell et al. (2014), but in the Netherlands predominantly relate to lack of understanding of the advanced nursing practice role, variable respect for the nursing profession, the dominance of the medical profession, and issues related to credentialing. Thus, although the regulatory barriers are solved, some institutional and cultural barriers need to be overcome.

It became imperative to address this situation and demonstrate the added value that advanced nursing practice could bring to healthcare. Consequently, the Ministry of Health, Welfare and Sport commissioned a national study to evaluate the effect on healthcare of granting independent authorization of reserved procedures to nurse practitioners and physicians' assistants (PAs; De Bruijn-Geraets et al. 2014). The research was supported by the Dutch nurses' associations. Surveys of nurse practitioners, patients, physicians, and PAs aimed to examine a range of factors such as safety, workload, patient-centered care, and costs. These were complemented by focus groups and interviews to clarify factors that helped or hindered nurse practitioners and PAs. Data were collected longitudinally for two and a half years in total, but several aspects of the work were reported during that period. For example, investigation into the deployment of nurse practitioners and PAs with regard to independence to perform reserved procedures such as endoscopies, elective cardioversion, and defibrillation was completed in 2015 (De Bruijn-Geraets et al. 2016, 2018). The conclusion of this partial research was that:

- Conditions for quality and safety had been met.
- Many nurse practitioners and PAs made use of the possibilities created by the amendment to perform cardioversions, defibrillations, and endoscopies independently.

It is possible that these opportunities are not yet being used to the full. However, when they are, there is the potential for greater efficiency in care delivery and cost savings, although there were insufficient data to make recommendations about this aspect. There was also a lack of data about the relative costs of nurse practitioners and PAs, because the computer system did not allow them to record that they initiated treatment. Consequently, several branches of the research are continuing at the request of V&VN/VS and the Dutch Professional Association of PAs (NAPA). The quality of care, patient satisfaction, and the development of the profession were also evaluated (De Bruijn-Geraets et al. 2014, 2016). Findings suggested that the focus on the development of medical skills was evolving and developing depending on the practice setting and practitioner's specialty. Patient-centered care has recently become central in order to bridge the gap between physician and patient. Educationalists describe APN as working "on the edge of cure and care" due to the dynamic changes that have taken place and are confirmed in the research findings (De Bruijn-Geraets et al. 2014). Aspects of the research reports can be found on Platform Zorgmasters, a national website (https://platformzorgmasters.nl).

3.7 Education

Finally, there have been some concerns about the educational preparation for advanced practice. The Dutch qualification framework for higher education is similar to that in many other countries in providing Bachelor's, Master's, and PhD degrees which correspond with levels 6, 7, and 8 of the European Credit Transfer System, which describes qualifications in terms of generic competences and learning outcomes. One challenge in the recent past for Dutch science universities, not research universities, offering Master's courses in advanced nursing practice was that the Master's level was not recognized internationally as an equivalent award. This led some Dutch graduates to complete an internationally recognized MSc in England, thus provoking considerable controversy within higher education, especially for Dutch research universities. This issue has only recently been resolved through changes in policy. In 2015, the Ministry of Education, Culture and Science (OC&W) changed the degree qualification for advanced nursing practice from a Master's in Advanced Nursing Practice (MANP) to a Master of Science (MSc); this change came into effect on September 1, 2015 and the MANP degrees were discontinued. The introduction of the MSc degree and associated title brought the Netherlands into line with higher education internationally.

3.8 The Future of Advanced Nursing Practice: Innovation in Healthcare and Education

Allowing nurse practitioners to perform reserved procedures should lead to more efficient and better-quality care delivery, because routine procedures are taken care of and medical specialists have more time for patients with complex needs. Wallenburg et al. (2015) found that nurse practitioners and PAs were deployed in four different ways:

- As members of medical teams.
- In specific parts of the care pathway.
- In specific units such as nurse-led clinics or outpatient clinics.
- As independent therapists.

The findings suggest that the two roles were treated in quite similar ways. Practitioners had to demonstrate knowledge and expertise in practice, and build personal contacts and trust with medical specialists before working more independently. There was frequent consultation between medical specialists and nurse practitioners or PAs. This occurred in both formal moments, allowing discussion of patients such as during the transfer, but also informally, during lunch and by telephone. Thus, through frequent consultation, nurse practitioners or PAs could conduct low-threshold consultations regarding patients' specific details, and the specialist could remain informed of patient care and work performed by nurse practitioners or PAs. Trust and teamwork were central to the success of both these roles.

Nurse practitioners also have a role to play in the Dutch government's vision for affordable and accessible healthcare in 2030. This is based on two assumptions:

- Health is the ability to adapt and self-manage social, physical, and emotional challenges and not a "state of complete well-being" (Huber et al. 2011), as the World Health Organization's (www.who.int) 1948 definition of health assumes.
- Treatment and care should be patient centered, provided initially by generalists, and take account of individual circumstances, age, and additional factors such as personal preferences.

In this context, nurse practitioners are seen as having a particular role in promoting and educating patients about self-management. This aspect of nursing has so far received little attention in care in the Netherlands, because of the traditional strong focus on treatment and doing for patients what they cannot do for themselves. Self-management could benefit by being promoted in the country. More attention to self-management requires expert professionals who, together with the patient and care givers, look at how to effectively deal with the effects of illness and daily life limitations. Nurse practitioners could play an important role in shifting the focus to what patients can do for themselves. This is illustrated in the following case study.

CASE STUDY

Mr. Janssen, aged 71, was a retired mechanical engineer who enjoyed gardening and working in the orchard on his farm. He was married and had two adult children. Mr. Janssen was referred, by his GP, to the cardiology outpatient heart failure clinic because of shortness of breath and reduced exercise tolerance. This multidisciplinary setting provided access to medical specialists, nurse practitioners, and other professionals such as social workers and psychologists.

Ten years earlier, Mr. Janssen experienced an acute pre-wall infarction requiring rescue percutaneous coronary intervention. Two years earlier, he had coronary artery by-pass surgery, since when he had atrial fibrillation.

Before you read on, consider Exercise 3.4.

EXERCISE 3.4

What specific factors would you look out for in assessing Mr. Janssen?

Examination in the outpatient clinic showed that he was breathless when walking but not at rest. His echocardiogram revealed a left ventricular ejection fraction (LVEF) of 20%, with severe dilatation of the left atrium. His electrocardiogram (ECG) showed atrial fibrillation with a frequency of 100 beats per minute and a QRS of 125 milliseconds. A diagnosis of heart failure based on New York Heart Association (NYHA) 11 classification system was made.

The nurse practitioner then instituted a treatment plan based on the European Society of Cardiology Guidelines on Acute and Chronic Heart Failure (https://www.escardio.org/Guidelines/Clinical-Practice-Guidelines, 2016). The aim was to enable Mr. Janssen to engage in managing his condition by providing a range of interventions and advice:

- Reviewing and prescribing heart failure medication based on his renal function and ECG: metoprolol 150 mg, fosinopril 40 mg. Spironolactone and furosemide were added to manage edema.
- Information and guidance for Mr. Janssen and his wife about:
  - Taking a sodium-restricted diet of no more than 2000 mg daily and fluid intake of 1500–2000 ml daily.

- The symptoms of heart failure, weight monitoring, and the self-management of dyspnea.
- The symptoms of progression in heart failure and when to seek medical help.

Following the visit to the outpatient clinic, Mr. Janssen's health improved, he felt well, and was able to work in his garden and orchard again.

Now consider Exercise 3.5.

EXERCISE 3.5

What aspects of the advanced nurse practitioner role are evident here?

Unfortunately, after five months, Mr. Janssen's condition worsened. He contacted the nurse practitioner directly to say that he had gained 2 kg in weight and his exercise tolerance was severely reduced. He reported that could no longer manage his orchard. He had to ask his wife to do more and more jobs for him. He found this very difficult to deal with and said he felt like an old man. The nurse practitioner was able to offer an appointment on the same day.

Assessment showed that Mr. Janssen's dyspnea had increased and that he had orthopnea. He had not had any recent illnesses and did not have chest pain. He had adhered to the nurse practitioner's prescribed medication and previous advice about diet and fluid, but his appetite had decreased. Physical examination showed crepitus in both lungs, ankle edema, and an increase in waist circumference. His diagnosis was upgraded to NYHA 111.

The nurse practitioner increased the furosemide to 80 mg for five days and, after consultation with the cardiologist, replaced the fosinopril with valsartan, a drug suitable only for a specific patient group within heart failure, and which could only be prescribed after consultation with the cardiologist. The implantable cardiac defibrillator (ICD) was upgraded with cardiac synchronization therapy to improve heart rhythm.

Mr. Janssen improved slightly, but was not very satisfied. After a few weeks the work in the orchard was getting heavier, despite spreading his activities throughout the day. The nurse practitioner then began to focus more on helping him to cope with and manage his limitations to try to improve his quality of life, and discussed his prognosis with the multidisciplinary team in the clinic.

Finally for this case study, review Exercise 3.6.

EXERCISE 3.6

At what point would you, as an advanced practitioner, consider palliative care for Mr. Janssen and why?

Which guidelines would you follow and why?

3.9 Conclusion

The development of advanced nursing practice in the Netherlands demonstrates some important steps, particularly with regard to the need for close cooperation between many stakeholders and legal embedding of the nurse practitioner role. Government, professional associations, healthcare professionals, and education professionals have to work together collaboratively to tackle the challenges in their field and time frame. This requires deepening understanding of each other's profession, learning to speak each other's language, and really wanting to understand one another, because it concerns an interest across professions, namely good patient care. At this moment (2018), the Netherlands is facing a large capacity problem. Estimates indicate a shortage of 100 000 healthcare professionals in 2021. The advanced practitioners will be able to show that they can contribute to good patient care like no other and thus increase acceptance of their role.

Key Questions

1. How can advanced practitioners actively influence the policy agenda in order to promote broader acceptance by other health professionals, doctors, and policy makers of advanced roles?

2. When asked, how do you approach an explanation of the advanced practice role for your practice setting?
3. To what extent could interprofessional education with medical staff would be beneficial or problematic for advanced practitioners?

Glossary

BIG register (https://english.bigregister.nl): a register of health professionals licensed to practice in the Netherlands.

Canadian Medical Education Directions for Specialists (CanMEDS; Royal College of Canada 2005 and 2015, www.royalcollege.ca/rcsite/canmeds-e): a framework for the education of medical students in Canada that provides educational and practice standards.

Council for Public Health and Society (Raad voor Volksgezondheid en Samenleving, RVS; https://www.raadrvs.nl): an independent body which provides strategic advice on health policy to the Dutch government.

Dutch Professional Nurse Practitioner Organization (http://venvnvs.nl/venvnvs/information-in-english): the professional organization for nurse practitioners in the Netherlands.

Dutch Qualification Framework (www.nvao.com): a framework linked to and compatible with the European qualification framework for the European Higher Education Area.

New York Heart Association (NYHA; www.heart.org): classification of heart failure. There are four classifications based around the degree of limitations in physical activity experienced by the patient and medical assessment.

Physicians' assistant (PA): a role introduced in the Netherlands in 2000 to provide medical care under the supervision of a qualified doctor. The Dutch Professional Association of Physicians Assistants (www.napa.nl/english) is the professional organization.

Platform Zorgmasters (http://www.platformzorgmasters.nl/categories/engelstalig): a Dutch digital knowledge platform with articles about nurse practitioner and PA developments and research.

Registration Committee Specialisms Nursing (RSV; https://vsregister.venvn.nl/Over-het-register/Registratiecommissie-Specialismen-Verpleegkunde): maintains a register of advanced nurse practitioners and protects the title of Nurse Practitioner.

Acknowledgment

The case study was contributed by Patricia Ann Ninaber MANP, Nurse Practitioner, Rijnstate Hospital Arnhem, Netherlands.

References

Björnberg A. (2018). Euro Health Consumer Index 2017. Marseillan: Health Consumer Powerhouse. https://healthpowerhouse.com/media/EHCI-2017/EHCI-2017-report.pdf (accessed January 19, 2019).

Boot, J.M.D. (2013). *De Nederlandse Gezondheidszorg*. Uitgever: Bohn Stafleu van Loghum.

De Bruijn-Gerraerts, D.P., van Eijk-Hustings, Y.J.L., and Vrijhoef, H.J.M. (2014). Evaluating newly acquired authority of nurse practitioners and physician assistants for reserved medical procedures in the Netherlands: a study protocol. *Journal of Advanced Nursing* 70 (11): 2673–2682.

De Bruijn-Gerraerts, D.P., Bessems-Beks M.C.M., van Eijk-Hustings, Y.J.L., Vrijhoef, H.J.M. (2016). VoorBIGhouden, Eindrapportage Evaluatieonderzoek Art. 36a Wet BIG met betrekking tot de inzet van de Verpleegkundig Specialist en de Physician Assistant. Maastricht: Maastricht UMC+, Patiënt & Zorg.

De Bruijn-Gerraerts, D.P., van Eijk-Hustings, Y.J.L., Bessems-Beks, M.C.M. et al. (2018). National mixed methods evaluation of the effects of removing legal barriers to full practice authority of Dutch nurse practitioners and physician assistants. *BMJ Open* 8 (6): e019962.

Huber, M., Knottnerus, J.A., Green, L. et al. (2011). How should we define health? *British Medical Journal* 343 (4163): 235–237.

Kleinpell, R., Scanlon, A., Hibbert, D. et al. (2014). Addressing issues impacting advanced nursing practice worldwide. *OJIN: Online Journal of Issues in Nursing* 19 (2): Manuscript 5.

Kolb, D. (1984). *Experiential Learning: Experience as the Source of Learning and Development.* Upper Saddle River, NJ: Prentice-Hall.

Wallenburg, I., Janssen, M., and de Bont, A. (2015). Taakherschikking: zelf regisseren. *De Verpleegkd Specialist* 10 (4): 4–7. https://doi.org/10.1007/s40884-015-0047-8.

Advanced Practice in Nursing and Midwifery: The Contribution to Healthcare in Australia

Grainne Lowe[1] and Virginia Plummer[2]

[1]*Deakin University, Geelong, Victoria, Australia*
[2]*Monash University and Peninsula Health, Frankston, Victoria, Australia*

Key Issues
- The development of advanced practice in Australia
- The role and professional status of the nurse practitioner
- Unique advanced roles for populations in remote and rural areas

LEARNING OBJECTIVES

By the end of this chapter you will be able to:

- Examine the development of a differential diagnosis.
- Critically discuss barriers to advanced practice in Australia.
- Describe the unique advanced roles developed in Australia.

4.1 Introduction

Nurses practice in a broad range of clinical and nonclinical roles and specialty areas, making a unique contribution to the health of communities worldwide. Health needs are diverse and nurses "are often the first and sometimes the only health professional that people see and the quality of their initial assessment,

Advanced Practice in Healthcare: Dynamic Developments in Nursing and Allied Health Professions,
Fourth Edition. Edited by Paula McGee and Chris Inman.
© 2019 John Wiley & Sons Ltd. Published 2019 by John Wiley & Sons Ltd.

care and treatment is vital" (All-Party Parliamentary Group on Global Health [APPG] 2016, p. 3). The changing global context is having impacts on health and other national priorities, and health services are shifting focus from in-hospital to community care, disease prevention, and health promotion. There is a greater emphasis on access, safety and quality of care, technology, and the labor market. These changes present opportunities and challenges for advanced nurses but, at present, many are limited from working to the full level of their competence (APPG 2016). The future of advanced nurses' contribution to health involves both understanding the power of nursing and the provision of political and practical support for advanced practice nurses willing to develop new roles (Foley and Bryce 2014; Hughes 2017). Nurses in established and emerging advanced practice will require significant organizational and political support, although many come from a range of international historical beginnings (Dunphy et al. 2009). This chapter presents examples of advanced nursing and midwifery practice, together with their contribution to healthcare in Australia. It begins with an overview of the development of this level of nursing, how it is currently defined and legally protected, and then highlights some of the current issues. A case study helps to demonstrate the standards required for advanced practice through a series of practical steps and exercises. The chapter then moves on to discuss current issues in advanced practice in Australia, with particular reference to the roles and settings in which practitioners work. It closes with a brief discussion about advanced practice in midwifery in Australia.

4.2 Advanced Practice in Australia

In Australia, the total expenditure on health has grown each year, from approximately AU$95 billion in 2003–2004 to AU$155 billion in 2013–2014, growing faster than gross domestic product (GDP; AIHW 2016). Nurses comprise the largest health professional group in Australia (Health Workforce Australia 2014). Unlike other healthcare professionals, the ratio of nurses to population across various geographic locations remains fairly stable and is between 3.2 times (city) to 6.2 times (very remote) the number of medical practitioner numbers (Table 4.1). The statistics on Australia's health workforce reveal a declining number of medical graduates choosing primary care as their preferred option (Health Workforce Australia 2012a) and workforce planning reports predict a shortfall of 123 000 by 2030 (Health Workforce Australia 2014). The range of

TABLE 4.1

Nurses and medical practitioner numbers by geographic location.

Area	Nurses/Midwives (n)	Medical practitioners (n)
Major city	220 698	70 073
Inner regional	54 856	12 035
Outer regional	24 657	5134
Remote	4002	828
Very remote	2224	359

Source: Data from Australian Bureau of Statistics 2014, http://www.abs.gov.au/ausstats/abs@.nsf/mf/4819.0

strategies needed to cope with this deficit include advanced practice nurses, who are regarded as essential to the development of contemporary and future healthcare models.

Work on this issue began with an attempt to recognize nurses already working in expanded roles, particularly in rural and remote areas, with lobbying to change policies to enable increased scope of practice. New South Wales (NSW) was the first state to implement the nurse practitioner (NP) model of care, with the first NP authorized to practice in 2000. This was the result of a long journey beginning in 1990, when the first NP committee was formed. Following the convening of this committee, discussions led to the formation of a steering committee, followed by pilot projects in 1994. The authorization process was finally formalized in 1999, paving the way for the first endorsement in 2000. Following the lead of NSW, a significant number of pilot studies, evaluation studies, and pre-implementation studies were conducted across Australian jurisdictions, all testifying to the positive benefits of NPs to improve the delivery of healthcare (ACT DoH 2002; O'Connell and Gardner 2012; Queensland Health 2003; WA DoH 2003; Victorian DHS 2000).

The NP is now defined as "an advanced practice nurse endorsed by the NMBA who has direct clinical contact and practises within their scope under the legislatively protected title 'nurse practitioner' under the National Law" (Nursing and Midwifery Board of Australia [NMBA] 2016). When endorsed, there is an expectation that NPs understand and vary their scope of practice from that of a registered nurse and comprehend the ways in which the changes affect their responsibility and accountability for practice. The role itself is described as *advanced practice nursing* (APN) and is distinguished from other advanced roles due to the addition of legislative functions and the regulatory requirements necessary for NP endorsement (NMBA 2017). The NP role and title are protected by legislation. Nationally, registration with the NMBA as an endorsed NP is a requirement to practice in this role. This strategic decision has ensured more clarity of definition of NP roles and provided a basis for more meaningful evaluation. A Master's degree is a requirement for endorsement as a NP in Australia. When an individual obtains an Australian Nursing and Midwifery Accreditation Council (ANMAC) approved Master's degree, an application is then forwarded to the NMBA, the registering body for the nursing profession, which sits within the Australian Health Practitioner's Registration Authority (AHPRA).

Advanced nursing practice is also recognized by the NMBA and is defined as "a continuum along which nurses develop their professional knowledge, clinical reasoning and judgement, skills and behaviours to higher levels of capability (that is recognisable). Nurses practicing at an advanced level incorporate professional leadership, education and research into their clinically based practice. Their practice is effective and safe. They work within a generalist or specialist context and they are responsible and accountable in managing people who have complex health care requirements" (NMBA 2017). The NMBA recognizes that advanced nursing practice is not a role, but a level of practice within a specific context. Other than for the NP role, there is no educational requirement stipulated for advanced nursing practice.

Until recently, there was a poor understanding of how many advanced practice nurses were working in Australia, what their title meant (Gardner et al. 2017), what they did, and how they were making a difference. A study by Gardner et al. (2017) was undertaken to identify Australian nursing workforce practice patterns according to title. NPs and APNs were two clusters identified in all states and territories except the Northern Territory (NT), where the title of NT Registered Nurse equated to clinical advanced practice in remote and isolated locations. The latest figures indicate that there are approximately 1745 NPs endorsed to practice in a variety of specialties nationally (NMBA 2018). There are no figures on the number of nurses working in positions leading them toward endorsement. In comparison to the international position, the number of NPs is small relative to population, making up approximately 0.1% of the nursing workforce, but, whilst slow, the growth is consistent. Increasing awareness of the potential to improve patient outcomes will raise the profile and value of NPs, resulting in increasing numbers.

Whilst the NP title is protected, there are numerous unprotected advanced nurse practitioner titles across Australia. Indeed, a recent study reported more than 70 titles, with a suggestion that many nursing positions were developed in response to an individual or setting need, rather than strategic organizational planning (Gardner et al. 2017). Within these contexts, the advanced nurse practitioner's worth and added value to the healthcare system remains understated. The difficulty lies in the inability to clearly define the significant contribution of roles which are haphazardly named and lack a consistent position description. These findings indicate the need for greater clarity and consistency.

CASE STUDY

The NP standards framework is underpinned by four domains: clinical, education, research, and leadership (NMBA 2017). These domains, often referred to as pillars, provide an approach to the case as outlined below. The scenario could take place at a metropolitan emergency department, a rural or remote urgent care center, or a community primary care setting. The information guiding critical thinking and practice should be adaptable to almost any environment/case.

The integration of the NMBA Standards for practice are evident in the various steps undertaken throughout the case study. Gathering information through advanced assessment facilitates the identification of differential diagnoses and aligns with the first pillar. Planning the most appropriate care, including the patient, family, carers, and other healthcare team clinicians in a collaborative relationship aligns with the second pillar. Prescribing therapeutic interventions and evaluating outcomes align with pillars three and four. Enmeshed within the critical thinking and planning of patient care are the necessary domains of education, research, and leadership. The NP provides clear education about the plan so that the patient understands their role in the process; the NP uses up-to-date evidence to inform best practice; and the NP provides leadership of the care required and of the team involved

in care. The case study also reflects what the NP adds to the healthcare team. What differentiates the NP from other advanced practice roles, such as clinical nurse specialist (CNS), is that the NP assesses diagnoses and treats a patient with an undifferentiated condition or illness; diagnostic reasoning is necessary to determine the specific interventions required.

Karen was a 56-year-old woman who was complaining of a painful left thumb. She reported that she had been in a car accident the day before and that her thumb was "giving a bit of grief today," particularly when trying to use her left hand. Karen was awake, alert, and answering questions appropriately. She walked independently to the assessment area. Her gait was normal; she showed no obvious distress on movement or evidence of injury/illness.

Before reading on, consider Exercise 4.1.

EXERCISE 4.1

What observations would you make? What information do you require at this stage?

Karen lived alone and had two grown children who lived some distance away in another state. She worked full time as a primary school music teacher. Her workplace was a 20-minute drive from her residence.

HISTORY

The injury occurred on the previous day, when there had been a motor vehicle accident. An ambulance was not called; the drivers shared respective details and both left the scene without further action. There was no past medical history of note. Karen was normally healthy and well. She had eaten a light breakfast at 0700 and had finished a 375 ml bottle of water prior to attending the clinic. Therefore, her fasting status was food

four hours, fluids one hour. Karen was left hand dominant and the painful left thumb was having an impact on her normal routine, which included playing the guitar.

Karen stated she had an allergy to penicillin. She was unaware of what happened, but her mother told her she "gets a rash."

Her only current medication was the oral contraceptive pill.

FOCUSED ASSESSMENT

Her left thumb was swollen and bruised, with increasing pain on palpation. There were no open wounds and there was no evidence of dislocation. The neurovascular examination was normal, with intact sensory and motor function, although the latter was altered with a decreased range of movement at the first metacarpal joint and grip, and the opposition of the thumb was reduced.

Before reading on, consider Exercise 4.2.

> ### EXERCISE 4.2
>
> How would you assess Karen's thumb? What structures would you examine/test?

At this point, a number of differential diagnoses were hypothesized:

- Soft tissue bruising of the left thumb/hand
- Sprain/strain of the thumb/hand
- Gamekeeper's thumb/skier's thumb (ulnar collateral ligament injury)
- Fracture
- Dislocation

Clinical reasoning processes were utilized to determine the next course of action. An X-ray would be needed to determine the presence of a fracture. Suspicion of a gamekeeper's thumb injury would require an ultrasound to

determine if the ulnar-collateral ligament of the thumb was intact.

Further questioning about how the hand injury occurred revealed more details about the accident. Karen was driving a car which was hit at approximately 60 km/h by a medium-sized removal truck. There was cabin penetration to both vehicles. This additional information changed the differential diagnoses, because it indicated the possibility of higher-level trauma, which required a more thorough physical examination.

Think about Exercises 4.3 and 4.4 before reading on.

> ### EXERCISE 4.3
>
> What guidelines would you use to conduct a spinal assessment? What information would you be looking for?
>
> What actions would you take and why if you discovered:
>
> - abdominal pain?
> - decreased air entry on one side of the thorax?

> ### EXERCISE 4.4
>
> What guidelines would you use to conduct a neurological assessment? What information would you be looking for?

HEAD-TO-TOE EXAMINATION

Inspection and palpation of the head: no obvious wounds, bruising or deformity. No headache.

Cervical neck examination: inspection and gentle palpation revealed normal alignment, no obvious

bruising or swelling, with mid-line tenderness at C3–4. Karen was measured and fitted with a collar to immobilize and protect the cervical spine until the situation was clarified.

Chest assessment including inspection, palpation, auscultation, and percussion: no obvious rib injuries, lung expansion was normal on both sides. Air entry was good on auscultation.

Abdominal assessment using inspection, ausculta-tion, palpation, and percussion techniques: no evidence of bruising or mass, the abdomen was soft and non-tender, with bowel sounds evident in all quadrants.

Full neurological examination including a cranial nerve assessment: this was normal.

A *full musculo-skeletal examination to exclude other non-life threatening injuries:* other than injuries already identified, the assessment was normal.

OUTCOME

The new information indicated the need for an X-ray of the left thumb and a computed tomogra-phy (CT) scan of Karen's cervical spine to exclude a more serious neck injury. The results showed:

- Normal alignment of the proximal and distal phalanges of the left thumb.
- Normal alignment of the first metacarpal.

- No obvious fracture, but particular note was taken of the base of the proximal phalanx to exclude an avulsion fracture, making a damaged ulnar-collateral ligament the more likely diagnosis.
- Normal alignment of the cervical vertebra with no obvious fracture.

MANAGEMENT STRATEGIES

Before you read on, think about Exercise 4.5.

> **EXERCISE 4.5**
>
> What are your prescribing options?

Management strategies included:

i. Analgesia advice – written and oral with regard to:
  - How to manage pain associated with the injury.
  - Regular analgesia in the initial management period to maintain comfort: – a combination of paracetamol, a non-opioid analgesic, and ibuprofen, a non-steroidal anti-inflammatory drug (Therapeutic Guidelines 2017).

ii. A thumb spica immobilizer was fitted to Karen's left thumb. Whilst the X-ray ruled out a fracture, an ulnar-collateral ligament injury could not be excluded at this stage. To improve the long-term outcome, an immobilizing splint was used whilst Karen awaited further review and examination by a specialist to determine the extent of injury and whether she required surgery.

iii. A referral for an ultrasound of the left hand to determine the presence of ulnar-collateral ligament injury.

iv. Before discharge, the neurovascular status of her thumb was checked to ensure that the splint fitted well and that her pain was ade-quately controlled. Advice was given about nonpharmacological pain relief techniques, for example positioning and relaxation.

The management plan was discussed with Karen to ensure she understood the information she had received and the need for follow-up.

4.3 Current Issues in Advanced Practice in Australia

NPs now function in a variety of settings, such as primary care, acute care, specialty medical services, and community care (Centre for International Economics [CIE] 2013; Willis et al. 2009). The numbers of NPs have increased in response to identified gaps in service delivery. Indeed, Parry et al. (2015) identify NPs as able to fill the gaps in communities of deprivation evidenced in rural and remote regions of Australia. They describe the overuse of emergency departments in areas with low ratios of GPs. Whilst the recognition and increasing numbers of NPs in the Australian context appear to be lagging behind other countries, it should be acknowledged that their growth in Australia continues to be exponential. To put this into perspective, the role was first endorsed in Australia in 2000. The number of endorsed NPs based on December 2013 figures was 1000, a figure which grew to over 1745 in the September 2018 figures (NMBA 2018).

Evidence continues to mount in support of NP roles, particularly in terms of the maintenance of quality care, effective patient management, and improved access (Kelly et al. 2017; Jennings et al. 2015). Although some improvements have been made, it is evident that NPs continue to function against resistance to their full scope of practice. Persistent barriers, both nationally and internationally, frustrate attempts by organizations and private practitioners to adequately integrate the NP role (Carter et al. 2015; Gardner and Duffield 2013; Lowe et al. 2013).

There are a number of legislative barriers which restrict the full potential of NP roles. One of the frustrating factors for many NPs is the inequity of access to the Medicare Benefits Schedule (MBS), which creates difficulty in relation to the financial viability of the NP role, both in the public and private healthcare sectors. The barriers encountered hinder attempts to improve service delivery through the extension of NP roles as key personnel for future workforce planning (White 2012). Furthermore, the limited financial viability resulting from the restricted access to MBS impedes the financial viability of the NP role, making it an unattractive option not only for healthcare managers (Considine and Fielding 2010), but also for the individual NP (Lowe et al. 2013).

Opposition from the medical profession and a lack of progressive government policies have hampered this reform to healthcare provision (Considine and Fielding 2010). A lack of clarity around role function preparation and scope of practice creates additional barriers, frustrating attempts by organizations to adequately integrate the NP role (Li et al. 2013). These barriers also limit the ability of the NP to set up in independent practice, which in turn limits the ability to create services where they can be most beneficial, such as in rural and remote communities, complex and chronic healthcare, mental health services, and aged care.

Despite these realities, more robust political support is required to extend the number and location of NP roles. In the future, in newly defined problem areas where demand far outweighs supply, the need for NPs is set to increase (Lauder et al. 2003). Indeed, workforce planning for the future relies on the removal of the barriers which currently impede working to full scope of practice (Health Workforce Australia 2012b).

4.3.1 **Nurse-led Clinics**

A number of nurse-led clinics are operational across Australia. There is evidence of positive outcomes resulting from such clinics in a variety of specialty areas, including Parkinson's disease, chronic kidney disease, cardiac failure, antenatal asthma management, and hepatic diseases. These clinics are of particular significance in Australia's more rural and remote geographic locations. In some cases, the clinic is NP led/supported, but with a team of nurses skilled in the specialty area and able to assist in the provision of holistic, timely, and accessible care. These clinics provide good examples of the best utilization of nursing skill mix and are collaborative, team based, and patient centered rather than hierarchical in their approach.

4.3.2 **Clinical Nurse Consultants**

With the introduction of new nursing roles to improve healthcare efficiency, it is important that the public, other healthcare providers, and indeed nurses themselves have an understanding of the various nursing roles in terms which are meaningful (Gardner et al. 2007; Rosenfeld et al. 2003). In order for nursing to have an impact on the provision of health services, a clear understanding of their practice is imperative (Donald et al. 2010).

As advanced practice proliferates, discussions about clarity, definition, and regulation remain, creating confusion for those in management or policy positions (Griffiths 2006). There is difficulty in disseminating knowledge of roles and functions, when due attention is not paid to the provision of consistent titles. Consistency and the protection of titles to maintain professionalism and to ensure public safety and confidence are important considerations (Christofis 2001).

Whilst the clinical nurse consultant (CNC) and CNS titles are often used interchangeably, they are acknowledged as having differing definitions and levels of skill, depending on which Australian state or territory the role is enacted in (Gardner et al. 2017). Indeed, haphazard and ineffective approaches to advanced practice do little to promote and regulate the nursing profession and its outcomes, thereby creating confusion about clinical practice.

Professional accountability for nursing roles is paramount to prevent APN roles becoming defined by what other health professionals, such as physicians, do not *want* to do, or aspects of care they feel too busy to do (Bailey et al. 2006). It is counterproductive to progress advanced nursing roles defined by what is undesirable by other healthcare professionals, or what is directed by nonclinical managers or individual nurse clinicians, whose approach may be misguided (Bailey et al. 2006; Bryant-Lukosius et al. 2004; Klein 2008; van Soeren and Micevski, 2001).

It has been reported that even in the beginning stages of CNC and CNS role development, the process was haphazard and often the positions emerged so hastily to satisfy and retain experienced nurses that role ambiguity and role conflict eventuated (Appel and Malcolm 2002). Whilst the NP role gained legislative protection, other advanced nurse practitioner roles are regulated under a comprehensive industrial agreement (Roche et al. 2013). As previously noted, there has been a more scattered approach to the development of APN roles across Australia, which provides challenges when evaluating the roles or articulating their true value.

With that history in mind, Baldwin et al. (2013) report that the CNC role was implemented in NSW in 2000, and that five years' full-time post-registration equivalent experience was required, together with a post-registration qualification, to be appointed to the role. Whilst Baldwin et al. (2013) provide insight into the role and function of the CNC in one hospital setting, what is lacking is the distinction of these roles across boundaries. The authors also acknowledge a lack of consistency from a national perspective. Roche et al. (2013) report on CNC roles within a large tertiary hospital. They conclude that there is not a clear distinction for the three grades of CNC role outlined in the award structure. The roles and functions of the 56 CNC positions within the organization do not provide clear evidence of all of the domains of practice established by the regulatory body, the Public Hospitals Nurses' Award (NSW Department of Health).

Rural and isolated practice endorsed registered nurses (RIPERN) in Victoria are equivalent to rural and isolated practice registered nurses (RIPRN) in Queensland. The RIPERN/RIPRN nurse was introduced to address the issue of access to healthcare in rural and remote areas in some Australian jurisdictions. The specifics of the role are that they are registered nurses who have undertaken a recognized (RIPERN/RIPRN) course. On completion of a Board-approved course of study, the RIPERN/RIPRN can apply to the Board for an endorsement to supply and administer limited medications according to a protocol. Other states have different protocols for medication prescribing by nurses in rural and isolated practice (NMBA 2018).

4.3.3 Remote Area Nursing

The most complex areas of nursing and midwifery practice are those are in rural, remote, and isolated areas of Australia. Living and working in these communities includes challenges of isolation, distance, extremes of weather, limited access to medical and allied health services, equipment, and supplies, together with a higher burden of disease than that experienced in metropolitan Australia (Coyle et al. 2010). According to the Australia Health Report 2016 (AIHW 2017), "Australians living in rural and remote areas tend to have shorter lives, higher levels of disease and injury and poorer access to and use of health services compared to people living in metropolitan areas. Poorer health outcomes in rural and remote areas may be due to a range of factors, including a level of disadvantage related to education and employment opportunities, income and access to health services. They may also have more occupational and physical risk, more tobacco and alcohol misuse. Higher death rates and poorer health outcomes outside major cities, especially in remote areas, also reflect the higher proportion of the population in those areas who are Aboriginal or Torres Strait Islander Australians."

The workload for nurses in these settings is clearly very high and involves high non-nursing work, for example driving ambulances and repairing equipment. Primary care is prioritized before primary healthcare (Coyle et al. 2010). Therefore, the range of skills is also high, including a focus on communication where English is the second or third language or dialect spoken among indigenous communities. Nurses are frequently on call 24 hours per day and 7 days per week. There are differing levels of nursing practice evident in rural and remote communities, including general registered nurses and midwives, advanced nursing practice roles, and nurse practitioners (Coyle et al. 2010).

There has been agreement between states and territories (Queensland, South Australia, Northern Territories, and Western Australia) on the role and, whilst completion of a Rural and Isolated Practice (Scheduled Medicines) Registered Nurse course is required in some states, other states and territories have *standing orders* in place. These are legal, written instructions for an authorized person to administer medicines in situations that require prompt action and are based on a standard procedure (Department of Health 2006). This advanced practice role and the following example of endorsed midwives include endorsement as part of their practice to supply medications which have been prescribed by a medical practitioner or by standing orders of the Chief Health Officer of the state or territory, in areas appropriate to the scope of practice of the nurse or midwife. This is different from the practice of the NP, who is endorsed to prescribe medication.

4.4 Advanced Practice in Midwifery

Internationally, there are various points of view on advanced practice in midwifery and a useful debate continues in some settings. In New Zealand, midwives are considered to be at their full scope of practice from graduation, and advanced practice in midwifery is not a consideration (Smith et al. 2010). It could be argued that this position would create difficulties for the development of midwifery practice. Furthermore, advanced practice in Wales is defined by the midwife reaching a level of competence rather than professional boundaries (National Leadership and Innovation Agency for Healthcare (NLIA) 2010). The view is that advanced practice is a "'level of practice' rather than a specific role and it is not exclusively characterized by the clinical domain but may also include those working in research, education, management/leadership roles" (NLIA 2010, p. 10), a view shared by the NMBA. Further examples come from Africa, where there are advanced scope of practice roles such as obstetric surgery in Mozambique and nurse-owned clinics to ensure access (APPG 2016).

However, mixed views remain in Australian midwifery. The Australian College of Midwives (ANMC) considers it important to educate midwives to the "full scope of practice" and in the last decade has reviewed midwifery national education standards and national accreditation, and participated in a new national registration scheme (ANMC 2009). Medicare-eligible midwives, now known as endorsed midwives, in Australia provide antenatal, intrapartum, and postnatal care working in collaboration with a specified medical practitioner, providing Medicare-rebatable services, in assessment, pathology, diagnostic services, and referrals to obstetricians and pediatricians up to six weeks postpartum. These midwives are prepared with a Master's degree and must meet the eligibility requirements of the NMBA. The endorsed midwife in Australia may be in private practice or employed by a hospital, and the role is underpinned by experience, competence, continuity of care, and unhindered practice. Midwives are practicing in interdisciplinary ways and are not a substitution for other professions (Smith et al. 2010). All midwives should be supported in gaining experience and postgraduate education.

4.5 Conclusion

In Australia, there is a critical need for further policy changes to enable full integration of NP roles to the full scope of practice. Once the NP role has been well entrenched into the system, there is scope for other APN positions to develop and work at the top of their competence level. Currently, the barriers to practice remain and reduce the capacity of the NP in particular to adequately fill the gaps which have been previously reported. Positive outcomes resulting from nurse-led clinics in a variety of specialty areas will ensure a significant improvement in patient outcomes, and will have distinctly positive implications in Australia's more rural and remote geographic locations. Engaging organizational executives, politicians, community members, and other professional groups is essential to make sure that the ultimate potential of all nursing roles is realized. This is a global concern and provides a challenge to address for nurses generally, and nursing leaders in particular.

Key Questions

1. What barriers to advanced practice occur in your field of practice? How do these compare with those in the Australian context?
2. In your country, are advanced practitioners and nurse consultants the same or different? If there are differences, what are they?
3. Are there local populations in your area that might require specialized advanced nursing roles? How might these be developed?

Glossary

Clinical nurse consultant: a registered nurse with a role similar to that of the CNS in some states of Australia, and also similar to the role of CNS in the UK and USA. However, CNC is a distinct role in Victoria, with higher levels of academic preparation and experience, and CNCs are regarded as experts in their field.

Clinical nurse specialist: a registered nurse prepared beyond the level of a generalist nurse and authorized to practice as a specialist with advanced expertise in a branch of the nursing field. Specialist practice includes clinical, teaching, administration, research, and consultant roles.

Endorsement of nurses and midwives: identifies those practitioners who have additional qualifications (NMBA, www.nursingmidwiferyboard.gov.au).

Gamekeeper's thumb: an injury to the ulnacollateral ligament.

Medicare (www.humanservices.gov.au/individuals/medicare): a publicly funded healthcare insurance scheme for Australian citizens.

Nursing and Midwifery Board of Australia (www.nursingmidwiferyboard.gov.au): the regulatory body for nurses and midwives.

Pharmaceutical Benefits Scheme (www.pbs.gov.au): a government-funded scheme through which various medications are subsidized for Australian citizens.

Remote area nurse: a registered nurse who has undertaken a recognized RIPERN/RIPRN or equivalent course to practice in areas which are typically rural or remote, with a low density of population, and without a permanent medical practitioner.

Rural and isolated practice endorsed registered nurses (RIPERN/RIPRN): registered nurses who have been endorsed by the Nursing and Midwifery Board of Australia to obtain, supply, and administer scheduled medicines, following completion of a Board-approved course

References

All-Party Parliamentary Group on Global Health (APPG) (2016). *Triple Impact: How Developing Nursing will Improve Health, Promote Gender Equality and Support Economic Growth.* London: APPG.

Australian Capital Territory Department of Health (2002). The ACT Nurse Practitioner Project: Final report of the steering committee. ACT Government, Canberra.

Australian Institute of Health and Welfare. (2016). Australia's health system. https://www.aihw.gov.au/reports/australias-health/australias-health-2016/contents/health-system (accessed January 19, 2019).

Australian Institute of Health and Welfare (2017). Australia Health 2016 Report. https://www.aihw.gov.au/reports/australias-health/australias-health-2016/contents/summary (accessed January 19, 2019).

Australian Nursing and Midwifery Council (2009). *Accreditation of nursing and midwifery courses – a national project undertaken by the Australian Nursing and Midwifery Council 2009.* Canberra: ANMC.

Appel, A. and Malcolm, P. (2002). The triumph and continuing struggle of nurse practitioners in New South Wales, Australia. *Clinical Nurse Specialist* 16 (4): 203–210.

Australian Bureau of Statistics (2014). Australian Social Trends, April 2013. http://www.abs.gov.au/AUSSTATS/abs@.nsf/Lookup/4102.0Main+Features20April+2013 (accessed January 7, 2019).

Bailey, P., Jones, L., and Way, D. (2006). Family physician/nurse practitioner: stories of collaboration. *Journal of Advanced Nursing* 53 (4): 381–391.

Baldwin, R., Duffield, C., Fry, M. et al. (2013). The role and function of clinical nurse consultants, an Australian advanced practice role: a descriptive exploratory cohort study. *International Journal of Nursing Studies* 50: 326–334.

Bryant-Lukosius, D., DiCenso, A., Browne, G., and Pinelli, J. (2004). Advanced practice nursing roles: development, implementation and evaluation. *Journal of Advanced Nursing* 48 (5): 519–529.

Carter, M., Owen-Williams, E., and Della, P. (2015). Meeting Australia's emerging primary care needs by nurse practitioners. *Journal for Nurse Practitioners* 11 (6): 647–652.

Centre for International Economics (2013). *Responsive patient centred care: The economic value and potential of Nurse Practitioners in Australia.* Canberra: Centre for International Economics.

Christofis, L. (2001). Nurse practitioners: an exploration of the issues surrounding their role in Australian emergency departments. *Australasian Emergency Nursing Journal* 4 (2): 15–20.

Considine, J. and Fielding, K. (2010). Sustainable workforce reform: case study of Victorian nurse practitioner roles. *Australian Health Review* 34: 297–303.

Coyle, M., Al-Motlaq, M., Mills, J. et al. (2010). An integrative review of the role of registered nurses in remote and isolated practice. *Australian Health Review* 34: 239–245.

Department of Health (2006). Guiding Principle 11 - Standing orders. http://www.health.gov.au/internet/publications/publishing.nsf/Content/nmp-guide-medmgt-jul06-contents~nmp-guide-medmgt-jul06-guidepr11 (accessed January 17, 2018).

Department of Human Services Victoria (2000). *The Victorian Nurse Practitioner Project: Final report of the taskforce.* Melbourne: Department of Human Services Victoria.

Donald, F., Bryant-Lukosius, D., Martin-Misener, R. et al. (2010). Clinical nurse specialists and nurse practitioners: title confusion and lack of role clarity. *Nursing Leadership* 23 ((Spec.)): 189–210.

Dunphy, L.M., Smith, N.K., and Quinn Younkin, E. (2009). Advanced practice nursing: doing what has to be done – radicals, renegades and rebels. In: *Advanced Practice Nursing: Essentials for Role Development*, 2e (ed. L.A. Joel), Chapter 1. Philadelphia: F.A. Davis.

Foley, E. & Bryce, J (2014). Is it advanced or extended practice? Australian Nursing and Midwifery Federation. http://anmf.org.au/pages/professional-july-2014 (accessed January 7, 2019).

Gardner, G., Chang, A., and Duffield, C. (2007). Making nursing work: breaking through the role confusion of advanced practice nursing. *Journal of Advanced Nursing* 57 (4): 382–391.

Gardner, G. and Duffield, C. (2013). Advanced practice nursing: the missing link. *Nursing Review* 11: 19–20.

Gardner, G., Duffield, C., Doubrovsky, A., and Adams, M. (2016). Identifying advanced practice: a national survey of a nursing workforce. *International Journal of Nursing Studies* 55: 60–70.

Gardner, G., Duffield, C., Doubrovsky, A. et al. (2017). The structure of nursing: a national examination of titles and practice profiles. *International Nursing Review* 64 (2): 233–241.

Griffiths, H. (2006). Advanced nursing practice: enter the nurse practitioner. *Nursing BC* 38 (2): 12–16.

Health Workforce Australia (2012a). *Australia's Health Workforce Series Doctors in Focus*. Adelaide: Health Workforce Australia.

Health Workforce Australia (2012b). *Health Workforce 2025 – Doctors, Nurses and Midwives – Volume 1*. Adelaide: Health Workforce Australia.

Health Workforce Australia (2014). Australia's Future Health Workforce – Nurses. Detailed report August 2014, Australian Government. Adelaide: Health Workforce Australia.

Hughes, F. ONZM – Former Chief Executive Officer, International Council of Nurses, Keynote Address Advanced Nursing Practice Policy Summit, Australian College of Nursing. Canberra, 20 April 2017.

Jennings, N., Clifford, S., Fox, A. et al. (2015). The impact of nurse practitioner services on cost, quality of care, satisfaction and waiting times in the emergency department: a systematic review. *International Journal of Nursing Studies* 52 (1): 421–435.

Kelly, J., Garvey, D., Biro, M., and Lee, S. (2017). Managing medical service delivery gaps in a socially disadvantaged rural community: a nurse practitioner led clinic. *Australian Journal of Advanced Nursing* 34 (4): 42–49.

Klein, T. (2008). Credentialing the nurse practitioner in your workplace: evaluating scope for safe practice. *Nursing Administration Quarterly* 32 (4): 273–278.

Lauder, W., Sharkey, S., and Reel, S. (2003). The development of family health nurses and family nurse practitioners in remote and rural Australia. *Australian Family Physician* 32 (9): 750–752.

Li, J., Westbrook, J., Callen, J. et al. (2013). The impact of nurse practitioners on care delivery in the emergency department: a multiple perspectives qualitative study. *BMC Health Services Research* 13: 356. http://www.biomedcentral.com/1472-6963/13/356.

Lowe, G., Plummer, V., and Boyd, L. (2013). Nurse practitioner roles in Australian healthcare settings. *Nursing Management* 20 (2): 28–35.

National Leadership and Innovation Agency for Healthcare (2010). *Framework for Advanced Nursing, Midwifery and Allied Health Professional Practice in Wales*. Llanharan: NLIAH.

Nursing and Midwifery Board of Australia (2017). Nurse and midwife registrant data: 2017. http://www.nursingmidwiferyboard.gov.au/About/Statistics.aspx (accessed January 7, 2019).

Nursing and Midwifery Board of Australia (2018). Registration standard for endorsement for scheduled medicines registered nurses (rural and isolated practice). http://www.nursingmidwiferyboard.gov.au/Registration-and-Endorsement/Endorsements-Notations/Registration-standard-for-endorsement.aspx (accessed January 7, 2019).

O'Connell, J. and Gardner, G. (2012). Development of clinical competencies for emergency nurse practitioners: a pilot study. *Australasian Emergency Nursing Journal* 15: 195–201.

Parry, Y., Ullah, S., Raftos, J., and Willis, E. (2015). Deprivation and its impact on non-urgent paediatric emergency department use: are nurse practitioners the answer? *Journal of Advanced Nursing* 72 (1): 99–106. https://doi.org/10.1111/jan.12810.

Queensland Health (2003). *Nurse practitioner project report*. Brisbane: Queensland Government.

Roche, M., Duffield, C., Wise, S. et al. (2013). Domains of practice and Advanced Practice Nursing in Australia. *Nursing and Health Sciences* 15: 497–503.

Rosenfeld, P., McEvoy, M., and Glassman, K. (2003). Measuring practice patterns among acute care nurse practitioners. *Journal of Nursing Administration* 33 (3): 159–165.

Smith, R., Leap, N., and Homer, C. (2010). Advanced midwifery practice or advancing midwifery practice? *Women and Birth* 23: 117–120.

Therapeutic Guidelines (2017). Acute pain: a general approach. eTG complete Nov. https://tgldcdp.tg.org.au/etgcomplete (accessed January 19, 2019).

van Soeren, M. and Micevski, V. (2001). Success indicators and barriers to acute nurse practitioner role implementation in four Ontario hospitals. *AACN Clinical Issues: Advanced Practice in Acute & Critical Care* 12 (3): 424–437.

Walker, D., Lannen, B., and Rossie, D. (2014). Midwifery practice and education: current challenges and opportunities. *Online Journal of Issues in Nursing* 19 (2): Manuscript 4.

Western Australian Department of Health (2003). *Guiding framework for the implementation of nurse practitioners in Western Australia*. Perth: Department of Health Western Australia, Office of the Chief Nursing Officer.

White, L. (2012). Emergency departments need treatment. *Nursing Review* 1326 (472): 20–22.

Willis, E., Reynolds, L., and Keleher, H. (2009). *Understanding the Australian Healthcare System*. Sydney: Elsevier.

CHAPTER 5

Influences on the Development of Advanced Nursing Practice in the UK

Paula McGee

Birmingham City University, Birmingham, UK

Key Issues
- The influence of health policies and reforms of the National Health Service
- The influence of national strategies for nursing
- The regulation of advanced practice
- The influence of nursing organizations
- Educational standards, credentialing and accreditation for advanced nursing practice

LEARNING OUTCOMES
By the end of this chapter you will be able to:
- Critically discuss the importance of policy literacy for advanced nurse practitioners.
- Debate the arguments for and against statutory regulations for advanced nurse practitioners.
- Begin to plan an application for credentialing.

5.1 Introduction

The advent of advanced practice in the UK was announced, in 1994, by the United Kingdom Central Council for Nursing, Midwifery and Health Visiting, in one very short paragraph, as "adjusting the boundaries for the development of future practice, pioneering and developing new roles responsive to changing

Advanced Practice in Healthcare: Dynamic Developments in Nursing and Allied Health Professions,
Fourth Edition. Edited by Paula McGee and Chris Inman.
© 2019 John Wiley & Sons Ltd. Published 2019 by John Wiley & Sons Ltd.

needs and with advancing clinical practice, research, and education, to enrich professional practice as a whole" (United Kingdom Central Council for Nursing, Midwifery and Health Visiting 1994). Unfortunately, there was little further information or guidance to go on and no strategic plan. This left nurses free to explore the idea of advanced practice in whatever way they saw fit, just as they had done in the 1970s in developing specialist roles and educational programs. However, in time, this lack of guidance also created some difficulties, because the Council never quite made clear how this definition of advanced practice would apply to the realities of daily life in practice. It could also not agree, and it spent far too long debating, whether advanced practice was a form or a level of practice. The result was a state of confusion, piecemeal local developments, and a great deal of debate, both useful and acrimonious, as nurses and other health professionals tried to determine the appropriate way forward. There was quite a lot of research, some of which helped illuminate the path. The consensus that emerged was that advanced practice should contain a clinical component, set the pace for changing practice, and be underpinned by formal preparation beyond the level of initial registration. Advanced practice was said to be "firmly grounded in direct care provision or clinical work with patients, families and populations" and "leadership and collaborative practice; improving quality and developing practice; and developing self and others" (Department of Health [DH] 2010a, p. 2). This statement reflected theoretical ideas about advanced practice in which expert and direct patient care formed a core encompassed by other areas of competence. It also helped to differentiate advanced practice roles from others that were more concerned with management.

Against this background, advanced nursing practice continues to develop in the UK. This chapter presents an examination of the main issues and influences that shape it, beginning with a brief overview of the UK's National Health Service (NHS) as the setting in which most nurses are employed. This is followed by a discussion of the continuous cycle of health policies and reforms that began in the late 1990s and the accompanying national strategies for nursing. This discussion is focused on the implications of these changes for advanced nursing practice. Nursing organizations have played important roles in the development of advanced nursing practice. Two factors are addressed in this chapter. The first is the role of the Royal College of Nursing (RCN) in developing standards for the education of advanced nurse practitioners and an accreditation system for universities which provide Master's courses. The College's new credentialing system is explained and illustrated through use of a case study. The second is the quest for statutory regulation by the Nursing and Midwifery Council (NMC); discussion of the reasons why it has not so far succeeded brings the chapter to a close.

5.2 The National Health Service in the UK

The NHS was launched in 1948 by the then Minister of Health, Aneurin Bevan, a former miner, who grew up in deep poverty and became a Labour politician. Until this point, healthcare was available only to those who could pay for it. Bevan regarded this as deeply unjust, because "much sickness and often permanent disability arise from failure to take early action, and this in its turn is due to high costs and the fear of the effects of heavy bills" (Bevan 1952). He used his position to spearhead the establishment of a new, radical approach to healthcare: a state-funded service in which treatment and care were available to everyone, based on clinical need and free at the point of delivery, irrespective of a patient's ability to pay. These founding principles continue to underpin the NHS and are now enshrined in the NHS Constitution, which sets out what the service will provide and what patients and staff have a right to expect (NHS England 2015). The NHS now employs over 1 million staff; the budget for 2017–2018 was £124.7 billion, with an increase of £20.5 billion by 2023–2024 (The Kings Fund 2018). Treatment and care are provided for over 1 million people every day (NHS Confederation 2017). Health policies are intended to address the continued development and adaptation of the NHS in response to changing patient needs and healthcare practice, service design, and delivery, organizational challenges and increasing costs. These factors "act as pressures on policy, sometimes called 'drivers'" for change, but the decisions about how best to address these are ultimately political and reflect the ideology of those in government (Thomson 2016).

5.3 Health Policy

Health policy is a long-term plan of action and targets through which those in government, or aspiring to be in government, hope to achieve the funding, organization, delivery, or any other aspect of services. A new law may be necessary for the implementation of a policy, but it fulfills a different function. Laws set out rules for conduct that are enforced through the police and the courts; failure to comply with rules can result in prosecution. Unlike law, policy and policy formation are a work in progress that can be changed and adapted in the light of events or experience.

Policy and policy formation are subject to multiple influences. The first is the guidance on disease prevention and control issued by international organizations such as the United Nations (www.un.org) and the World Health Organization (www.who.int). The second is from the policy institutes, colloquially known as "think tanks," such as the Joseph Rowntree Foundation (www.jrf.org.uk), which carry out research about specific health-related issues and act as advocates for change. The third is a complex mixture of considerations about the nature of society, demographic trends, regional variations, religious and cultural issues, and what the population will accept as reasonable. Finally, those charged with designing a policy may also exert influence through the approaches that they use (Sangiorgi 2015).

5.4 Influence of Health Policies and Reform of the National Health Service

The Labour government elected in 1997 introduced radical health policies designed to reform the NHS, whilst retaining the core principles of 1948. The policies were aimed at reversing chronic underfunding by previous governments and inequalities generated by a lack of responsiveness to patient need (Ham 2014). The aim was to create a "modern and dependable" service "built around the needs of people, not institutions." It promised more funding, "national standards of excellence," better use of resources, and much more

(DH 1997 pp. 6, 7, and 11). The NHS Plan which followed introduced changes across the whole organization, focusing in particular on "targets and performance management; inspection and regulation; and competition and choice," which were to be overseen by the newly created NHS Modernisation Agency (Ham 2014, p. 8; DH 2000). The roles of front-line staff were to be transformed. Changes for doctors included an increase in the number of general practitioners (GPs) and their involvement in developing local services for local need, new contracts for hospital doctors, more consultants, new specialist registrar posts, and better funding for resources. Changes for nurses included training to take up new roles that would enable them to function more autonomously, for example in managing their own caseloads, leading clinics, and prescribing medication (Table 5.1). The roles of members of allied health professions (AHPs) would also be developed (DH 2003a, b). Clinical leadership would be strengthened by the appointment of experienced senior nurses and AHPs as consultants (DH 2000). Changes for patients included better access to information, more choice over appointments and referrals, and more active participation in healthcare.

Some of these reforms were very successful in making the NHS more responsive to patients' needs. For example, waiting times for hospital appointments and treatment improved. Patient safety gained a higher profile under the auspices of the Patient Safety Agency, which focused greater attention on issues such as hospital cleanliness, food hygiene, and the safety of participants in research. New approaches to care and treatment were developed by nurses and AHPs, who took advantage of opportunities to take on new roles. There were

TABLE 5.1	
The Five year Forward View – models of care.	
Multispecialty community providers (MCPs)	Large GP practices provide a wider range of care by creating multiprofessional teams that can meet the needs of older adults, patients with long-term conditions, and those with multiple health problems
Primary acute care systems	Organizations that provide integrated care by amalgamating GP, hospital, mental health, and community care services
Urgent and emergency care networks	Reducing visits to emergency departments through a number of measures such as evening and weekend access to GPs, enabling pharmacists to take on more responsibilities, and better funding of urgent care for people with mental illness
Specialized care	A drive to concentrate specialist expertise and resources in designated centers
Modern maternity services	A review of maternity care provision as a basis for recommendations regarding future care
Enhanced health in care homes	Plan to work with care homes and the NHS to better address the healthcare needs of residents
Acute care collaborations (originally via smaller hospitals)	Plan to link hospital services as a means of improving efficiency and cutting costs, for example by sharing administration services

Source: Summarized from NHS England (2014), King's Fund (2014).

efforts to improve the working lives of staff; harassment and abuse would no longer be tolerated. Standards and targets were introduced, to good effect, for the care of patients with conditions such as cancer and mental illness; the progress of each healthcare organization toward achieving targets was reviewed regularly via new systems of inspection. However, in this new, tightly controlled NHS, the focus on targets and the consequences of missing them had the potential to encourage creative accounting of progress and less attention to conditions for which there were no published standards. Thus, passing an inspection might not always reflect good performance. Furthermore, the internal market of purchasers and providers introduced by previous Conservative governments was not dismantled, but enhanced by encouraging competition (Ham 2014).

However, policies are not the same as politics, and the incoming Conservative–Liberal Democrat coalition government of 2010 had a different approach. The White Paper issued shortly after the general election set out new health policies. It began with a commitment to the core principles of the NHS and retention of some of the reforms introduced by the previous regime: "putting patients and the public first," "improving health care outcomes," empowering "professionals and providers, giving them more autonomy," and "cutting bureaucracy and improving efficiency" (DH 2010b). These ideas had the potential to increase opportunities for nurses and AHPs, but there was little direct reference to health professionals other than GPs.

Aside from this, what the White Paper actually presented was another radical reform of the NHS, which was formalized in the Health and Social Care Act 2012. These reforms required efficiency savings of £20 billion to be used for reinvestment. Changes to the structure of the health service created an array of new entities to address public health, professional education, monitoring, and regulation. A fourth new entity, NHS England, was to lead the health service for England and became, in turn, responsible for other new bodies such as the NHS Commissioning Board, which now oversees the establishment and work of 195 local Clinical Commissioning Groups (CCGs). These groups are clinically led by elected governing bodies comprising GPs, other doctors, nurses, and lay people; membership consists of GP practices. CCGs assess local needs, promote innovation and research, and purchase services from hospitals, clinics, community services, and other health organizations. They are collectively responsible for spending two-thirds of the NHS budget (NHS Clinical Commissioners 2018, www.nhscc.org). The largest CCG in England serves over 1 million people and controls a budget of £18 billion. Appleby et al. (2015, p. 3) summed up criticisms of these changes in arguing that the impact of the Health and Social Care Act 2012 was "damaging and distracting at a time when the NHS was facing unprecedented financial challenges" and "took time and attention away from the work needed to maintain the improvements in care achieved in the previous decade." Increased workloads, pay freezes, and the use of locum and agency staff as stop-gap measures to ensure patient safety eventually exhausted both efficiency savings and staff. In short, the reforms made a challenging situation worse.

The Five Year Forward View, produced jointly by NHS England, Monitor, and other NHS organizations, introduced more changes that prioritized the integration of services and placed greater emphasis on the prevention of disease: "hard-hitting national action on obesity, smoking, alcohol and other major health risks" (NHS England 2014, p. 4). It called for more engagement with communities "in new ways, involving them directly in decisions about the future of health and care services" (NHS England 2014, p. 13). Seven new care delivery models were put forward as responses to changing healthcare needs, treatments, and technologies, alongside the persistence of health inequalities (Table 5.1). These models provided a basis for the future of the NHS and were deemed necessary because "Monitor, NHS England and independent analysts have previously calculated that a combination of growing demand if met by no further annual efficiencies and flat real terms funding would produce a mismatch between resources and patient needs of nearly £30 billion a year by 2020/21. So to sustain a comprehensive high-quality NHS, action will be needed on all three fronts – demand, efficiency and funding. Less impact on any one of them will require compensating action on the other two" (NHS England 2014, p. 5).

The Forward View was a plan, but putting it into action required major policy changes in commissioning, regulation, quality improvement, and leadership (Ham and Murray 2015). The implications for health professionals and GPs in particular had to be examined. The General Practice Forward View appeared to promise increased funding, better GP support, and technological improvements (NHS Health Education England and Royal College of General Practitioners 2016). However, funding does not seem to have improved. A recent report indicates that between 618 and 777 GP practices will be forced to close by 2022 as a result of underfunding and the current rate of mergers and closures (British Medical Association 2018).

Another set of challenges emerged from proposals to engage with communities "in new ways, involving them directly in decisions about the future of health and care services" (NHS England 2014, p. 13). This is something much talked about, well intentioned, but not always achieved. Lack of commitment at national level, and lack of empowerment of people and professionals to engage meaningfully with one another on an equal basis, are among the many reasons for failure (Foot et al. 2014). Even more contentious was the positioning of this type of engagement alongside volunteering and partnerships with charities. In the UK, millions of people undertake voluntary work every day. Volunteers are unpaid, but they require training, commitment, and the right attitudes, all of which cost money. Charitable organizations that are contracted to provide services have to train their volunteers and ensure that the standard and quality of their work meet the commissioners' requirements. Thus, volunteering has become quasi-professionalized; it is not necessarily a cheap option for those seeking to reduce health service costs.

This reform like the many reforms before it, illustrates the complex issues involved in managing an enormous national organization. Funding and investment present continual challenges as healthcare needs change and costs increase. The seemingly endless reforms and changes of direction devised by politicians rarely seem to solve as much as they promise. The ensuing pressures placed on NHS staff, both front line and in administration, continue to rise, not because these health professionals are intractably inefficient, but because they work with the sick and the dying and those whose illnesses and disabilities just will not go away. What is also noticeable is the pressure heaped on medical staff and the lack of attention to other professions. With the exception of the Labour government's reforms, the potential of nurses and AHPs is not considered in any meaningful way, but only by implication. Advanced nursing practice is not addressed at all.

The latest NHS Plan demonstrates a partial change of direction in recognizing the important contribution of nursing and AHPs to patient care, although there is no reference at all to advanced practice (NHS England 2019). The plan includes improvements to out-of-hospital care so that more patients are cared for at home via GP services, thus reducing pressure on emergency departments. More emphasis is to be placed on preventing major diseases such as cancer and diabetes and tackling health inequalities: "All major national programmes and every local area across England will be required to set out specific measurable goals and mechanisms by which they will contribute to narrowing health inequalities over the next five and ten years" (NHS England 2019, p. 41). Maternity care, services for children, and those for mental health are all to be improved. More will be done to improve the quality of life for people with autism. The importance and acute shortages of nurses, allied health professionals, and doctors to the achievement of these goals are acknowledged alongside plans to increase recruitment. The intentions are laudable, but their effects will not be evident for some time. Even if recruitment does increase, it will take years before new recruits are able to practice; in the meantime, the plan is to rely, as ever, on recruitment from outside the UK.

Nevertheless, advanced nurse practitioners must become *policy literate* by developing a critical understanding about the nature of and complex influences on policy and policy formation; they must also be able to articulate this understanding clearly to others (think about Exercise 5.1 in this regard). Policy literacy informs *policy competence,* the ability to apply understanding to a strategic approach to policy formation. Policy literacy also enables advanced nurse practitioners to engage in *policy advocacy* through organizational and professional channels, to challenge policies that negatively affect patients (Hewison 2009, pp. 23–24).

> **EXERCISE 5.1**
>
> Which health policy has had the most impact on your field of practice in the last two years?
>
> Why is this policy needed?
>
> What are the strengths and weaknesses of this policy?

5.5 Influence of Nursing Strategies

The strategy for nursing that accompanied the Labour government's reforms of the late twentieth century recognized that nurses, who form the largest part of the NHS workforce, were essential to the success of the proposed changes (DH 1999). However, nurses needed to be better equipped to meet the challenges ahead. Changes in initial education followed by life-long learning were introduced to prepare nurses to provide treatment and care for patients in the coming century. Modernized working conditions that took account of the needs of a predominantly female workforce were introduced. The strategy replaced the existing nursing grades with four new ones, as the basis of a revised career structure: healthcare assistants, registered nurse practitioners, senior registered nurse practitioners, and nurse consultants. Senior registered practitioners would be required to have specialist qualifications and Master's degrees. Nurse consultants would be expert, experienced practitioners, clinical leaders with specialist qualifications and Master's or doctoral degrees; they were expected to meet the requirements of higher-level practitioners set out by the United Kingdom Central Council (UKCC) (2002). This new career structure was intended to retain practitioners in clinical practice rather than have them move into education or management. Setting the terminology aside, it is possible to see here some similarities between nurse consultant and advanced nurse practitioner roles. Distinctions between the UKCC's advanced practitioner and the NHS Plan's consultant practitioner were never clarified, and so it would seem that, at this point, the two terms were interchangeable (United Kingdom Central Council for Nursing Midwifery and Health Visiting 1994, 2002; DH 2000).

Unfortunately, as reforms of the NHS continued into the twenty-first century, patient care began to deteriorate. The Mid-Staffordshire Inquiry revealed many disturbing accounts in which patients were neglected, dehumanized, and degraded. Patients were left lying in their own excreta. There were unacceptable delays in providing pain relief and a lack of clear protocols for patient management (Francis 2010). These were not isolated examples of a single institution in which staff had simply lost their way; rather, they were indicative of a much wider malaise, in which patient dignity and compassion for the suffering of others had either been set aside deliberately or completely lost.

That any of this had to be said is a damning indictment of an entire health service overburdened by constant changes of direction, pressures to meet targets, efficiency savings, and a general lack of concern for patients. Nurses were a part but not the whole of this situation. They are the largest part of the workforce, but the work they do is often invisible, incorporating as it does what no one else realizes needs to be done. Nurses are everywhere in the health service: "diagnosing, treating, leading cardiac arrest teams, teaching and assessing" patients, other nurses, doctors, and other professionals. Their clinical and technical skills are vital, but good nursing demands more, because nursing is fundamentally about care. Caring, the heart of nursing, means being truly present with patients and their families. It implies valuing the skilled delivery of those tasks so often referred to as basic care: feeding people, listening to their stories, changing their beds, and making them comfortable. It requires "kindness, empathy, compassion and providing dignity. This is what makes a good nurse," and it is the reason why advanced nurse practitioners are sorely needed (Watson 2018, pp. 198–199). Their clinical and professional leadership is focused on patient care. Nursing is the least valued of the health professions but, as the events at Mid-Staffordshire showed, the absence of the work nurses do has serious consequences for people's lives.

The new nursing strategy which followed the exposure of how badly patient care had deteriorated emphasized patient dignity as a fundamental right. The core values of nursing were restated in terms of compassion for others (see Exercise 5.2); nursing leadership was essential. Nurses needed time and space to perform care activities and support (DH and NHS Commissioning Board 2012; Table 5.2). Commitment to these core values and respect for patient dignity were again emphasized in the most recent strategy, which also reflects the issues raised by the Five Year Forward View (NHS England 2016). It focuses on three themes: "health and well-being, care and quality, funding and efficiency" in order to achieve "better outcomes, better experiences and better use of resources" (NHS England 2016, p. 11). The strategy is intended to demonstrate

TABLE **5.2**

The values and behaviors essential to nursing.

Care	The purpose of nursing
Compassion	The delivery of care based on respect for patient dignity
Competence	Clinical and technical knowledge and skill
Communication	Interpersonal skills; listening to patients and involving them in decisions about their care
Courage	Advocacy on behalf of patients; willingness to try new approaches
Commitment	Taking action to improve care and patient experience

Source: Summarized from Department of Health and NHS Commissioning Board (2012).

the value of nursing through a range of activities that include gathering research-based evidence of the impact of nursing care on achievement of the three themes, more visible leadership, reducing "unwarranted variation" in practice, and ensuring that "improving the population's health is a core component of the practice of all nursing" (NHS England 2016, p. 13). Once again, advanced nursing practice is not an overt feature of this strategy, but it is listed as part of the resources. Advanced nurse practitioners able to steer nursing through the work required by this framework and ensure that high standards of patient care are maintained will be essential to the implementation of this strategy. In doing so, it is essential that they amass and publish systematically collected data on the evidence of the impact of their work on patient care, healthcare organizations, the health of communities, and the nursing profession as a whole.

EXERCISE **5.2**

What is compassion?

As an advanced practitioner, how do you incorporate compassion into patient care?

5.6 Influence of Nursing Organizations

The RCN (2008a, 2010, 2012) has played a particularly important and influential role in addressing standards and education for advanced nurse practitioners. Initial work was based on a combination of the College's own research, the expertise of members, and a wide range of other sources that included the National Organisation of Nurse Practitioner Faculties (www.nonpf.org). This resulted in the identification of domains of advanced nursing practice and the competences required to fulfill them, which facilitated developments in all four UK countries, each of which has published its own definition of and competences required for advanced nursing practice (RCN 2008a). In the College's view, advanced nurses are autonomous practitioners and accountable for their own actions. They are able to assess, diagnose, initiate, and follow through evidence-based treatments for patients without first referring to other health professionals (RCN 2008b). Thus, they can provide complete episodes of care. They can also order investigations, and refer patients to other health professionals within and outside nursing. They provide clinical and professional leadership and act as consultants and teachers for colleagues.

Advanced nurses must be educated at Master's level in order to practice. Courses should include assessment, applied pharmacology and prescribing, research and teaching skills, and ethical practice (RCN 2018c). The requirements of the individual advanced nurse practitioner's post must show parity with similar posts; work activities should focus on direct practice, leadership, teaching, and research. The College's reasoning on these two points is that some employers continue to advertise posts and salaries which do not match the criteria for advanced nursing practice (RCN 2018b).

The College has developed standards for the education of advanced nurse practitioners, and a process whereby universities can apply for accreditation. In considering whether to accredit a university, the College assesses factors such as institutional resources, staffing, research, student support, and assessment processes and standards, especially in regard to practice. Accreditation provides "a strong benchmarking and quality assurance framework" (RCN 2018d, p. 8). It helps to address the variations between Master's courses; each university is still free to develop its own curriculum, as long as it meets the RCN's standards. Graduates of universities whose Master's in advanced practice programs have received accreditation are automatically credentialed free of charge, by the College, as advanced nurse practitioners.

Finally, the College has been instrumental in:

- Addressing some of the common obstacles experienced by advanced practitioners and members of other non-medical professions, particularly in requesting clinical imaging. Guidance for non-medical professionals developed by the RCN was endorsed by the leaders of the professions involved in requesting or responding to requests for imaging (RCN 2008b).
- Providing conferences on issues related to advanced nursing practice.
- Developing resources, for example through the College library.
- Hosting the advanced nursing practice forum, through which nurses can make contact with one another, share experiences, and seek advice about issues in practice.

The NMC has also played an important role in the development of advanced nursing practice. The Council replaced the UKCC in 2002. It received the work of the UKCC's higher-level practice project, but made little progress on the issue of advanced practice for some years. Finally, the Council undertook its own consultation about a post-registration nursing framework, and was able to state that "advanced nurse practitioners are highly experienced, knowledgeable and educated members of the care team who are able to diagnose and treat your health care needs or refer you to an appropriate specialist," and who carried out a specific range of activities (NMC 2005, p. 3; Table 5.3). Furthermore, the Council agreed that advanced practitioners should be registered, and that the role should be defined in a way that was meaningful for patients and the public. The Council also agreed that a policy was needed to accommodate nurses thought to be already working as advanced practitioners.

> **TABLE 5.3**
>
> ## The NMC's first view of advanced nursing practice.
>
> Advanced NPs are highly skilled nurses, with extended skills and knowledge, who can do the following:
>
> Examine patients physically, initiate investigations, and diagnose health problems.
>
> Initiate and make decisions about treatment and care, prescribe medication, or refer patients to other sources of help.
>
> Evaluate and alter treatment and care as appropriate.
>
> Provide leadership and ensure that patients receive high standards of treatment and care.
>
> *Source:* Summarized from Nursing and Midwifery Council (2005).

In 2006, the NMC tried to obtain approval from the Privy Council to open a further sub-part of the nurses' part of the register in order to register advanced nurse practitioners. However, the approval was not granted. The Council for Healthcare Regulatory Excellence (CHRE) (2009), which oversaw the NMC and other professional regulators, argued that "often what is termed advanced practice reflects career development within a profession and is appropriately governed by mechanisms other than additional statutory regulation ... the activities professionals are undertaking do not lie beyond the scope of existing regulation." The Professional Standards Authority (PSA) replaced the CHRE in 2012 and took over its responsibilities. The PSA argued that the whole regulatory system for health professions was no longer fit for purpose and required "a radical overhaul if it is to support rather than stand in the way of the serious changes being proposed for our health and care services. We will not be able to change health and care unless we also change the way it is regulated" (PSA 2015, p. 1).

Advanced nursing practice could be one of the beneficiaries of such an overhaul of professional registration, but there is no guarantee of this. There are a number of considerations to be taken into account when determining the need for statutory regulation. To exemplify these, the PSA proposed a "continuum of risk" when assessing whether new roles and activities require regulation (PSA 2016). The lowest risks can be managed by employers. Next is credentialing, which allows the consistent screening of employees to ensure that they are suitable people with the right qualities and qualifications to work in healthcare. This is followed by voluntary and then, finally, compulsory registration. Decisions about particular occupational groups depend on the level and scale of risk posed by their activities, the environment in which they work, and whether or not they are supervised (Table 5.4). In relating this to advanced nursing practice, there appear to be no accurate figures about the numbers of nurses who have qualified as advanced practitioners, because the title is not protected in law. Consequently, nurses may have job titles including the word "advanced," but may not have undergone formal preparation at Master's level. There is also the issue of what advanced nurse practitioners, properly prepared or not, are expected to do. Advanced nurse practitioners are autonomous but, if they are members of a team, there may be checks and balances in place to reduce risks. Thus, if their work is deemed low risk by their employers, formal regulation may not be needed.

TABLE 5.4

Factors to consider in assessing the risk posed by occupational groups in healthcare.

Questions to ask	Reasons for asking
How many people perform this work?	Small numbers of professionals treating a limited number of patients may not pose a substantial risk; other options may be more appropriate
What safeguards are already in place?	Performance of tasks under supervision or some other monitoring system, such as an employer's policies and procedures, may be enough if the potential for harm is low Greater potential for harm may arise with more autonomous levels of practice and/or specific environments or interventions
What are the potential costs?	The costs of regulation, such as the payment of fees, may mean that people no longer want to do the work, especially if it is not well paid
Do people see this work as posing a risk?	The possible effects on confidence among patients and the public
Could there be any other consequences?	The possibility of unanticipated outcomes

Source: Summarized from Professional Standards Authority (2016).

TABLE 5.5

Credentialing of advanced nurse practitioners: Initial application requirements.

Evidence of registration and qualifications, including prescribing and a transcript of the Master's course (if completed), mapped against the four elements of advanced practice approved by the College: clinical practice, leadership, research, and education. In addition, specialist areas of competence must be included.

A detailed plan of current and regular work activities verified and signed by the employer.

A reference from a clinician verifying that individual is working at an advanced level.

Evidence of professional development: courses, conferences, and other education events.

A statement of good character from the employer verifying that the nurse has not been investigated or found guilty of misconduct.

A fee.

Source: Summarized from Royal College of Nursing (2018d).

There are already some voluntary registers in place. For instance, the Complementary and Natural Healthcare Council (www.cnhc.org.uk) maintains a voluntary register for 16 professions, including cranio-sacral therapists, reiki therapists, massage therapists, and aromatherapists. Voluntary registration can play a part in reassuring the public about an individual's suitability to practice, but there is no legal requirement to join. In addition, there appear to be several other organizations that also maintain registers of complementary therapists, so it may be difficult to trace which one an individual is registered with. Statutory regulation means that, in order to practice, individuals must meet the standards and educational requirements for registration with an approved regulatory body. In healthcare there are nine such bodies. In addition to maintaining registers, they are also responsible for professional discipline and can, if needed, remove an individual's right to practice. The statutory regulation of health professions covers activities that are deemed very high risk. If there are sufficient numbers of advanced nurse practitioners engaged in practice that is truly high risk, then there may in future be a case for extending statutory regulation to include them. This could be as a special category of nurse, under the auspices of the NMC, or as a new professional group.

The quest for some sort of professional regulation, or at the least formal recognition of advanced nursing practice, is also hampered by the fact that there is no "legal or statutory limitation on the scope of practice of a nurse in the UK which means that nursing has developed over time to include many advanced nursing and specialist healthcare roles which meet the changing healthcare needs of the public" (NMC 2017, p. 2). As long as these practitioners have to maintain and revalidate their nursing registration, then their advanced practice can be considered as being within the current scope of nursing. This is the argument put forward by the NMC in response to a consultation about whether advanced critical care practitioners and surgical care practitioners should be regulated through a new, separate register (Department of Health and Social Care [DHSC] 2017). The Council also raised the issue of how dual registration could be managed; whether or not practitioners might choose between the two; and what might happen if they relinquished their nursing registration but continued to undertake some nursing work (NMC 2017). At the time of writing, no decisions have been made and the DHSC has not yet reported on the outcome of the consultation. However, there is often more than one way of addressing a problem.

CASE STUDY

In 2018, the RCN began offering credentialing to advanced nurse practitioners. This is intended to "provide formal recognition for each nurse, their colleagues, employers and most importantly, patients and the public, of the advanced level of expertise and skill that nurses awarded the credential have achieved" (RCN 2018a, p. 4). Credentialing (Table 5.5) involves making an application and undergoing an assessment by a team at the College. Successful applicants will receive a certificate and a badge; they will also be included in a database accessible by the public. Credentialing is valid for three years, at the end of which the advanced nurse practitioner may reapply. It must be emphasized that a credential is not a register but, in the current absence of any statutory regulation, it provides assurance that individual nurses are safe and competent to practice at an advanced level.

Ashley has completed a postgraduate diploma in diabetes care and a Master's degree in advanced practice. Her dissertation focused on the care of young people with Type 2 diabetes. She has been employed as an advanced nurse practitioner in diabetes care in a large NHS hospital. When she was appointed three years ago, she was required to work as part of the multidisciplinary team providing care for people with diabetes. Her responsibilities focused mainly on the management of foot ulcers and the care of individual patients frequently admitted to hospital because of poorly controlled diabetes. She also worked in the diabetes clinic in the outpatient department, where she provided education for patients and monitored those whose diabetes was well controlled.

Ashley now leads a team that covers a range of activities. These include a support group for people who are newly diagnosed with diabetes; a service for young people with Type 2 diabetes; liaison with the children's hospital for patients transferring to adult services; and a joint clinic with midwives to improve care for young women who are pregnant. She teaches students undertaking courses in diabetes care at the local university, junior doctors, and other colleagues.

There are four types of application for credentialing:

- Model A is for applicants whose Master's course is accredited by the College.

- Model B is for nurses whose Master's course was not accredited.

- Model C applies to nurses whose Master's course had a clinical focus.

- Model D is for applicants who do not have a Master's degree. This route is open only until 2020 (RCN 2018a, 2018e).

Before reading on, consider Exercise 5.3.

EXERCISE 5.3

Which model should Ashley use to apply for credentialing?

If Ashley's Master's degree was accredited by the College, then she can apply using Model A. If it was not, then she should use Model B.

Ashley will need to submit a substantial set of documents based on four elements: qualifications, experience, competence, and the evidence to support these. The College's handbook provides guidance on these issues (RCN 2018e). In some ways this is not unlike the process required for revalidation, but credentialing goes beyond that, because it requires verification of competence at such a high level of clinical practice. Ashley's job has clearly changed considerably in three years. This is not unusual, but she will now have to map her regular activities against the four elements of advanced practice and agree the result with her manager. The emphasis here is on making explicit the nature of her normal working week or month by specifying her activities during each part of every day. In this context, it is not clear whether this includes all her activities, because some, such as liaison with the children's hospital, may take place only occasionally. The reference from a clinician is another important document. Ashley's referee must be able to comment knowledgeably about her advanced nursing practice role and verify her competence. The clinician cannot be the same person as her employer.

Now do Exercises 5.4 and 5.5.

EXERCISE 5.4

Create a table as shown here. In each box enter what you do, each day, in a normal working week, and roughly how much time it takes. Some examples are given to help you begin.

	Mon	Tues	Wed	Thurs	Fri	Sat	Sun
Morning	Your advanced nurse-led clinic 3 hours						
Afternoon			Ward round 2 hours				
Evening							
Night duty							

EXERCISE 5.5

Take each item from the table in Exercise 5.4 in turn and identify how it links with the four pillars of advanced practice. It is not necessary to link all four to each item, but they should all feature in your working week. More than one pillar may apply. If this happens, you will need to decide which pillar is most important. Try to be precise and give details. The questions set out in the following example will help you to begin.

The four pillars are direct clinical practice, leadership and collaborative practice, improving quality and developing practice, and developing the self and others. In addition, specialist areas of competence must be included.

Example: Your advanced nurse-led clinic

What does this clinic involve?	Relevant pillar
What is the purpose of the clinic?	Clinical practice
What do you do in clinic that is different to the role of other nurses? For example, do you examine and diagnose patients and initiate treatment?	Research and specialist competences
Do you refer patients for investigations such as blood tests or clinical imaging?	
Is your practice evidence based?	
What specialist competences do you have? How do you apply these in the clinic?	
How would you describe your advanced nurse practitioner role in relation to other health professionals in the clinic?	Leadership
Did you initiate the clinic and if so why? What research evidence did you access to help you?	Research
Did you have to negotiate with colleagues to set up the clinic?	
Do you lead the clinic? What does this involve?	
How you changed practice in this clinic? How have you done so?	Research skills and leadership
Have you kept a record of what you changed and why?	
What evidence have you collected about the impact of improvements that you have initiated?	
Have you presented this evidence at a conference or published it in a professional journal?	
Do you teach patients about their condition and/or ways to improve their health?	Education
Do you share your expertise with other nurses and other colleagues?	Specialist competences
Do you share your expertise through conference presentations, posters, or special interest groups?	

5.7 Conclusion

The importance of advanced practice in the provision of healthcare does not feature strongly in recent healthcare reforms. Despite this, advanced nurse practitioners have clarified the competences required at this level and the key components of the preparation they require. They still need to develop a stronger voice that articulates to commissioners and politicians the contribution that advanced nurses make to healthcare.

Key Questions

1. As an advanced nurse practitioner, what evidence is needed to demonstrate the effectiveness of your role? Who should collect this and how should they do so?
2. How might you, as an advanced nurse practitioner, improve your knowledge and understanding of the role and priorities of the CCG in relation to the service in which you work?
3. To what extent would statutory regulation contribute to your advanced nurse practitioner role?

Glossary

British Medical Association (BMA; www.bma.org.uk): the trade union and professional body for doctors in the UK.

NHS Constitution (www.gov.uk): sets out the guiding principles of the NHS, including patients' rights and responsibilities.

NHS England (www.england.nhs.uk): leads the National Health Service for England. Following devolution, Scotland, Wales, and Northern Ireland have their own organizations.

Nursing and Midwifery Council (NMC; www.nmc.org.uk): the professional regulator for nurses and midwives in the UK.

Patient Safety Agency: a body with a wide range of responsibilities that is now part of NHS Improvement (www.improvement.nhs.uk), which oversees healthcare providers.

Privy Council (https://privycouncil.independent.gov.uk): the body of advisors to the Queen in the UK.

Professional Standards Authority (www.professionalstandards.org.uk): an independent body that oversees the regulatory bodies of nine health professions, including the Health and Care Professions Council, Nursing and Midwifery Council, General Medical Council, General Pharmaceutical Council, and General Osteopathic Council. It also oversees other organizations such as the Complementary and Natural Healthcare Council, which maintains voluntary registers and has a regulatory function.

Royal College of Nursing (www.rcn.org.uk): a trade union and professional body for nurses, midwives, and healthcare assistants in the UK.

References

Appleby, J., Baird, B., Thompson, J., and Jabbal (2015). *The NHS under the Coalition Government Part Two: NHS Performance*. London: King's Fund.

Bevan, A. (1952). *In Place of Fear*. London: Heinemann.

British Medical Association (2018). GP closures expected as Forward View falls short. https://www.bma.org.uk/news/2018/june/gp-closures-expected-as-forward-view-falls-short (accessed January 8, 2019).

Council for Healthcare Regulatory Excellence (2009) Advanced Practice: Report to the four UK Health Departments. Unique ID 17/2008. https://www.professionalstandards.org.uk/docs/default-source/publications/advice-to-ministers/advanced-practice-2009.pdf?sfvrsn=6 (accessed January 8, 2019).

Department of Health (1997). *The New NHS. Modern. Dependable. Cm 3807*. London: Stationery Office.

Department of Health (1999). *Making a Difference: Strengthening the Nursing, Midwifery and Health Visiting Contribution to Health and Healthcare*. London: DH.

Department of Health (2000). *The NHS Plan: A Plan for Investment. A Plan for Reform*. Wetherby: DH.

Department of Health (2003a). *Implementing a Scheme for Allied Health Professionals with Special Interests*. London: DH.

Department of Health (2003b). *Ten Key Roles for Allied Health Professionals*. London: DH.

Department of Health (2010a). *Advanced Level Nursing: A Position Statement*. London: DH.

Department of Health (2010b). *Equity and Excellence: Liberating the NHS. Cm 7881*. London: Stationery Office.

Department of Health and NHS Commissioning Board (2012). *Compassion in Practice. Nursing, Midwifery and Care Staff, Our Vision and Strategy*. Leeds: DH.

Department of Health and Social Care (2017). *The Regulation of Medical Associate Professions in the UK*. London: Department of Health and Social Care.

Foot, C., Gilburt, H., Dunn, P. et al. (2014). *People in Control of their Own Health. The State of Involvement.* London: King's Fund.

Francis, R. (2010). *Independent Inquiry into Care Provided by Mid Staffordshire NHS Foundation Trust January 2005–March 2009. Chaired by Robert Francis QC.* London: Stationery Office.

Ham, C. (2014). *Reforming the NHS from Within. Beyond Hierarchy, Inspection and Markets.* London: King's Fund.

Ham, C. and Murray, R. (2015). *Implementing the NHS Five Year Forward View: Aligning Policies with the Plan.* London: King's Fund.

Hewison, A. (2009). UK health policy and health service reform. In: *Advanced Practice in Nursing and the Allied Health Professions*, 3e (ed. P. McGee), 15–28. Oxford: Wiley-Blackwell.

King's Fund (2014). The Five Year Forward View new models of care. https://www.kingsfund.org.uk/projects/nhs-five-year-forward-view (accessed January 19, 2019).

King's Fund (2018). NHS funding: what we know, what we don't know and what comes next. https://www.kingsfund.org.uk/blog/2018/06/nhs-funding-what-we-know (accessed January 8, 2019).

NHS Clinical Commissioners (2018). About CCGs. https://www.nhscc.org/ccgs (accessed January 8, 2019).

NHS Confederation 2017 NHS statistics, facts and figures. https://www.nhsconfed.org/resources/key-statistics-on-the-nhs (accessed January 8, 2019).

NHS England (2014). The Five Year Forward View. https://www.england.nhs.uk/wp-content/uploads/2014/10/5yfv-web.pdf (accessed January 8, 2019).

NHS England (2015). The NHS Constitution. https://assets.publishing.service.gov.uk/government/uploads/system/uploads/attachment_data/file/480482/NHS_Constitution_WEB.pdf (accessed January 8, 2019).

NHS England (2016). Leading change. Adding value. A framework for nursing, midwifery and care staff. https://www.england.nhs.uk/wp-content/uploads/2016/05/nursing-framework.pdf (accessed January 8, 2019).

NHS England (2019). The NHS long-term plan. https://www.england.nhs.uk/long-term-plan (accessed January 19, 2019).

NHS Health Education England and Royal College of General Practitioners (2016). General Practice Forward View. https://www.england.nhs.uk/wp-content/uploads/2016/04/gpfv.pdf (accessed January 8, 2019).

Nursing and Midwifery Council (2005). Implementation of a framework for the standard of post registration nursing. Agendum 27.1 C/05/160. http://aape.org.uk/wp-content/uploads/2015/02/NMC-ANP-Dec051.doc (accessed January 8, 2019).

Nursing and Midwifery Council (2017). NMC response to the Department of Health consultation 'The regulation of medical associate professions in the UK'. https://www.nmc.org.uk/globalassets/sitedocuments/consultations/nmc-responses/2017/nmc-response-map-consultation.pdf (accessed January 8, 2019).

Professional Standards Authority (2015). *Rethinking Regulation.* London: PSA.

Professional Standards Authority (2016). *Right-Touch Assurance: A Methodology for Assessing and Assuring Occupational Risk of Harm.* London: PSA.

Royal College of Nursing (2008a). *Advanced Nurse Practitioners. An RCN Guide to the Advanced Nurse Practitioner Role, Competencies and Programme Accreditation.* London: RCN.

Royal College of Nursing (2008b). *Clinical Imaging Requests from Non-medically Qualified Professionals.* London: RCN.

Royal College of Nursing (2010). *Advanced Nurse Practitioners. An RCN Guide to the Advanced Nurse Practitioner Role, Competences and Programme Accreditation.* London: RCN.

Royal College of Nursing (2012). *Advanced Nurse Practitioners. An RCN Guide to Advanced Nursing Practice, Advanced Nurse Practitioners and Programme Accreditation.* London: RCN.

Royal College of Nursing (2018a). *Advanced Level Nursing Practice. Section 2: Advanced Level Nursing Practice Competencies.* London: RCN.

Royal College of Nursing (2018b). *Advanced Level Nursing Practice. Section 1: The Registered Nurse Working at an Advanced Level of Practice.* London: RCN.

Royal College of Nursing (2018c). *Advanced Level Nursing Practice. Royal College of Nursing Standards for Advanced Level Nursing Practice.* London: RCN.

Royal College of Nursing (2018d). *Advanced Level Nursing Practice Section 3: RCN Accreditation and Credentialing.* London: RCN.

Royal College of Nursing (2018e). *RCN Credentialing for Advanced Level Nursing Practice. Handbook for Applicants.* London: RCN.

Sangiorgi, D. (2015). Designing for public sector. *Foresight* 17 (4): 442–448.

Thomson, K. (2016). Policy in health. In: *Sociology for Nurses*, 3e (ed. E. Denny, S. Earle and A. Hewison), 275–296. Cambridge: Polity Press.

United Kingdom Central Council for Nursing Midwifery and Health Visiting (1994). *The Future of Professional Practice – The Council's Standards for Education and Practice Following Registration*. London: UKCC.

United Kingdom Central Council for Nursing, Midwifery and Health Visiting (2002). *Report of the Higher Level of Practice Pilot and Project*. London: UKCC.

Watson, C. (2018). *The Language of Kindness. A Nurse's Story*. London: Chatto and Windus.

PART 2

Advanced Practice in Allied Health Professions

The Development of Advanced Practice in the Allied Health Professions in the UK

Paula McGee

Birmingham City University, Birmingham, UK

Key Issues
- The range of allied health professions
- Factors influencing the development of advanced practice in allied health professions
- Current issues in advanced practice in allied health professions

LEARNING OBJECTIVES

By the end of this chapter you will be able to:
- Discuss the development of advanced practice in two allied health professions
- Critically examine current issues in advanced practice in allied health professions
- Discuss the questions to be asked in assessing the impact of an advanced practice post

6.1 Introduction

In the UK, 14 professions are formally listed as allied health professions. Their members form the third largest professional workforce in the National Health Service (NHS); a significant number can also be found in social care and in the

Advanced Practice in Healthcare: Dynamic Developments in Nursing and Allied Health Professions, Fourth Edition. Edited by Paula McGee and Chris Inman.
© 2019 John Wiley & Sons Ltd. Published 2019 by John Wiley & Sons Ltd.

voluntary, higher education, and independent sectors. Each profession brings specific knowledge, skill, and expertise to the care and treatment of patients in diverse settings, ranging from initial emergency care to rehabilitation (Table 6.1). Most require degree-level preparation; 13 are regulated by the Health and Care Professions Council (HCPC; www.hcpc-uk.co.uk) and osteopaths by the General Osteopathic Council (www.osteopathy.org.uk/home). There is also a range of other professions which are not normally classed as allied health professions, although they fulfill important roles in healthcare. These include pharmacists, psychologists, and chaplains who work with patients in the NHS and other settings; some, but not all, are regulated by the HCPC.

Each of the allied health professions has developed an approach to advanced practice in response to multiple factors that necessitated or encouraged change. Initially each profession pursued its own pathway, but over time it has become clear that the core competences of advanced practice are common to all professions, as well as the additional competences required in each specific field. This chapter is the first of three that examine advanced practice in allied health professions. Here, the focus is on the factors that have contributed to the development of this level of practice with particular reference to two professions: physiotherapy and paramedic practice. The chapter then moves on to examine some of the factors that still need to be addressed as advanced practitioners in allied health professions continue to expand their contributions to patient care and the importance of determining the effectiveness of advanced roles.

This chapter is followed by a more detailed account of current advanced practice in speech and language therapy. This is based around a case study which demonstrates how an advanced therapist contributes to patient care by coaching and guiding a less experienced colleague. The situation outlined shows the advanced therapist "working at the edge of the evidence base," applying her enhanced competences to manage the risks inherent in performing a videofluoroscopic swallow study on a child with special needs. This is a highly specialized procedure. Enhanced assessment skills informed by a thorough, critical knowledge of the evidence surrounding both the clinical problem and the videofluoroscopic procedure are required to determine whether it should be performed; the advanced therapist must also have achieved the required level of competence to carry it out. Clinical and sensitive interpersonal expertise come together in this situation in working across traditional

TABLE 6.1	
Allied health professions.	
Art therapists	**Operating departmental practitioners**
Chiropodists/podiatrists	Osteopaths
Dietitians	Paramedics
Diagnostic radiographers	Physiotherapists
Drama therapists	Prosthetists and orthotists
Music therapists	Speech and language therapists
Occupational therapists	Therapeutic radiographers
Orthoptists	

Source: Summarized from National Health Service England (2017).

boundaries of practice to find an innovative solution to the child's needs. The chapter also shows the importance of continuity of care and treatment. Both the advanced and the less experienced therapists had known the child and the family for some years. Continuity of care is important in sustaining trust between professionals, patients, and families, but is often overlooked in an increasingly busy health service.

The third chapter in this set focuses on advanced practice in the radiography professions. New imaging technologies have required radiography professionals to develop new skills and ways of working; increased demand for radiography services provided additional impetus for change. This chapter presents a cogent account of the changes introduced so far, followed by a critical discussion of current issues surrounding advanced practice in the radiography professions. Of particular note here is the rate of technological development; what is deemed "advanced" at this moment, because it is new, rapidly becomes routine practice. Thus, advanced radiography practice is in a constant state of flux in which practitioners have to reposition themselves in response to change.

6.2 Background to the Development of Advanced Practice in Allied Health Professions

The healthcare reforms begun following the election of the Labour government in 1997 aimed to provide better patient-focused care and treatment, ensure quicker and more efficient access to services, reduce health inequalities, and promote health (National Health Service Modernisation Agency 2004). The achievement of these reforms required changes in working practices, realigning the workforce with the realities of the work to be done. Inherent in this was the redistribution of workloads and the exploitation of underutilized resources. Allied health professionals were regarded as one such resource, with the potential to act as the first point of contact with the health service, diagnose and treat patients, and refer them on to other professionals as necessary. They were seen as having the potential to promote health, request diagnostic tests, treat, and even prescribe within stated protocols. Allied health professionals could also manage and lead teams and play a central role in the planning and delivery of healthcare (Table 6.2). Thus, members of allied health professions were actively encouraged to use their knowledge and skills in new ways and pioneer new practice. Providing opportunities to do so, coupled with plans for developments in both education and career pathways, offered an attractive package with the anticipated benefit of increasing the retention of highly skilled, experienced practitioners in direct patient care settings (Department of Health [DH] 2003a, b). Each profession approached these opportunities separately, as there was no overarching national strategy to facilitate development.

In the twenty-first century, health reforms and policies must also take account of demographic changes. In 2016, the total population of the UK was 65.6 million, of which 18% were aged 65 years or more. Over half a million people, including a growing number of men, were estimated to be aged 90 or over, the highest number ever recorded. Approximately 15 000 of this half a million were aged over 100. Whilst they represent only a fraction of the total population, the number of very old people has risen year on year from 1986 and continues

---

TABLE 6.2

Ten key roles for allied health professionals.

To provide a first, and in some cases only, point of contact with health services

To provide complete episodes of care by assessing, initiating investigations, diagnosing, and treating patients within established protocols

To discharge and/or refer patients to other services, working with protocols

To educate and guide colleagues and other professionals, patients, and carers

To develop new ways of working that transcend the traditional boundaries of practice in their field

To provide clinical and professional leadership

To ensure that practice is based on the best available research evidence

To promote health

To participate in planning and policy development at organizational level

To work collaboratively with other professions and services

Source: Summarized from Department of Health (2003a, b).

---

to grow more quickly than other age groups (Office of National Statistics [ONS] 2017). Older adults, and especially the very elderly, are more likely to experience multiple health problems as a result of aging processes, such as cognitive decline, reduced mobility due to arthritic change or stroke, Type 2 diabetes, cataracts, or heart disease. Therefore, treatment and care require the application of a mixed economy of knowledge and skills, not only to manage a complex range of symptoms, but also to maintain dignity and independence for as long as possible. Allied health professionals are a vital part of this mixed economy because of their expertise in enabling people to cope with the demands of daily living through interventions provided by, for instance, occupational therapists and physiotherapists, or the application of creative arts, drama, or music therapy to preserve a sense of self among people with Alzheimer's disease.

In addition, the impact of new knowledge of the causes of disease, new medicines, improvements in surgical techniques and procedures, and an emphasis on evidence-based practice means that many people with long-term conditions, who would previously have died, are now living for much longer. Cystic fibrosis provides a useful example of this trend. This is a genetic disease in which the lungs and digestive system become clogged with mucus. In the 1950s, children born with this condition had a life expectancy of about five years. The development of new drugs to clear mucus and treat infections, new interventions such as lung transplant and gene therapy, improved approaches to the management of patients' nutritional needs, and physiotherapy have all contributed to a current predicted life expectancy of about 47 years (Jones 2015; Elbron 2016; Cystic Fibrosis Trust 2018). This example also helps to illustrate the importance of a multidisciplinary approach that includes the expertise of doctors, respiratory nurses, physiotherapists, dietitians, pharmacists, and others such as psychologists and counselors, who may also be needed because, although there is evidence of a declining death rate, people with cystic fibrosis have a reduced chance of reaching old age.

Before reading on, consider Exercise 6.1.

EXERCISE 6.1

Thinking of your own caseload, is there one or more patient group(s), with a specific condition, now living longer than previously expected? How has life expectancy changed and what factors have contributed to this?

Changes in patient need also reflect an increased emphasis on enabling people to remain healthy. Changes in behavior are the most important factors in tackling an estimated 40% of the burden of disease; smoking, high alcohol intake, and an unhealthy diet are currently considered to be the major contributors to the onset of ill health and to increase the chances of early death (Public Health England 2016). In this context, allied health professionals have important roles to play in health education. For example, dietitians have the knowledge and skills required to teach patients and the general public about behavior change and in supporting people in adapting their lifestyles. Similarly, paramedics and physiotherapists have opportunities through their contacts with patients to encourage smoking cessation and direct them to appropriate sources of help.

These examples of changing patient need reveal a complex web in which diverse professions must work together to manage or resolve health problems. No one discipline or health practitioner can provide all the care and treatment for an increasing number of patients. What is currently needed most is multidisciplinary teams located in primary care. Health policies aimed at reducing hospital stays and the transfer of previously hospital-based services to GPs' surgeries mean that the majority of patients, including those with multiple and complex needs, are in community settings. The home and community facilities are now places of high patient need, in which members of all health professions, including those in allied health, must work collaboratively and communicate effectively to provide a coherent, holistic approach to care and treatment. Moreover, members of these teams must be versatile, able to work with patients who have multiple, and sometimes competing, health needs. This type of working requires a large repertoire of knowledge and skill, a mixture of generalist and specialist expertise far greater than that of any one individual. Achieving effective multidisciplinary working presents numerous challenges to established practices based on treating and managing a single disease or event. Reconfiguration of the workforce and professional education that actively prepares professionals to work in multidisciplinary teams are essential to bringing about change; they offer opportunities to allied health professionals to develop and expand their practice (Imison and Bohmer 2013).

The Five Year Forward View (NHS 2014) provided a plan for change in health services in England. This featured factors such as new models of care that suited local need, robust approaches to improving public health, and facilitating research and innovation by "streamlining approval processes" and thus containing costs. Additional features included reductions in the costs of randomized controlled trials (NHS 2014, p. 33), more investment in new technologies, and plans to address the separatism between mental and physical health services, primary and secondary care, health and social care provision. In response to this review, the Chief Allied Health Professions Officer led the development of a framework for allied health professionals using an innovative survey based on crowdsourcing. This is an internet-based strategy based on broadcasting a particular issue or problem to members of the public to gather their ideas or solutions. In this instance, crowdsourcing netted over 16 000 responses from allied health professionals, patients, carers, other health and care staff, and members of the public. These were complemented by face-to-face meetings in different parts of the UK and a review of health policies (NHS England 2017). The framework is intended for managers and leaders and focuses on three factors: impact, commitment, and priorities. *Impact* refers to delivering cost-effective outcomes for individual patients and for populations. This is to be achieved through improving health, service integration, and finding solutions to issues in specific services. *Commitment* refers to the location and the way in which services are delivered to individuals and groups. Informing both are four *priorities*: leading change, developing new skills, using technology, and providing evidence of the contribution of allied health professionals to the outcomes achieved. The framework sets out the responsibilities of the Chief Allied Health Professions Officer, leaders, and allied health professionals themselves. It includes a range of questions for staff in leadership positions to enable them to identify how to make the best use of their allied health professional workforce and demonstrate value for money (NHS England 2017). This framework represents a creative approach to articulating the expertise and potential of allied health professions, but, at the time of writing, its effectiveness is unclear.

6.3 Advanced Practice in Allied Health Professions

The development of advanced practice has progressed steadily since the beginning of the twenty-first century and is now an established part of modern professional thinking. Despite the lack of a national strategy, similarities seem to be emerging in terms of how advanced practice is located in professional practice. The two professions discussed in this section place it between qualified and consultant levels; thus, advanced practice is not the apex of a career, but a step toward it. Physiotherapy provides an example of a long-established profession, founded in 1894; the development of advanced practice was discussed in the previous edition of this book as it was already well underway, and this chapter presents the changes that have taken place since. In contrast, paramedic practice is a relatively new allied health profession, but one in which there has been considerable development in recent years. Discussion of these developments reveals agreement about the core elements of advanced practice and the competences required.

6.4 Advanced Practice in Physiotherapy

The Chartered Society of Physiotherapy (CSP; McGee and Cole 2009) initially drew on the work of Benner (1984) and other sources in nursing and identified three roles beyond graduation: *clinical specialist* roles in specific fields, *extended scope practitioners* working outside the normal range of practice, and *consultant* roles focused on direct practice with patients. However, the profession has now moved well beyond this, generating its own professional literature, abandoning the term *extended scope practitioner*, and clarifying the advanced practitioner role. The Physiotherapy Framework (CSP 2013) set out four levels of practice in which the core elements of the profession's work remain constant, but are applied in different ways in response to three factors: the level of complex need, the predictability of the context or outcomes, and the practitioner's sphere of influence. Whilst the framework provided a useful guide to the similarities and differences between the four levels, it did not offer a definition of advanced practice, although it did state that the advanced practitioner worked beyond the level of an experienced graduate. The advanced practitioner's caseload was focused on patients who had complex needs and situations in which the outcomes were not predictable. The sphere of influence included colleagues in the multidisciplinary team, in hospital and community settings, and outside the workplace.

More recently, the CSP (2016) has sought to clarify advanced practice as one of the four levels of qualified practice. The term "advanced practice" replaces and moves beyond the scope of the extended role practitioner and extended scope of practice. Advanced practice is a level of practice "that enables physiotherapists to incorporate advanced level skills and knowledge … Advanced Practice Physiotherapists have the skills to address complex decision-making processes and manage risks in unpredictable contexts. Physiotherapists incorporating advanced practice will have completed an advanced programme of studies and/or are able to demonstrate the ability to work at an advanced/Master's level of practice" (CSP 2016, p. 4). Thus, an advanced practice physiotherapist may or may not have completed Master's-level preparation, but must be deemed competent to perform at an advanced level.

The advanced practitioner can progress to yet another level and become a consultant practitioner, who "works within complex, unpredictable and normally specialised contexts that demand innovative work that may involve extending the current limits of knowledge. Practice at this level provides opportunities to have a broader sphere of influence" (CSP 2013, p. 11). Both may have local and national reputations, but the consultant's is also international. Both engage in direct practice, but the consultant is an expert. The advanced practitioner may be a leader, or be involved in research, service development, or education. The consultant engages in all of these activities (CSP 2016). There are currently about 50 consultant physiotherapists in the UK, but the number of advanced practitioners is not known.

The strengths of the CSP's approach lie in attempting to differentiate between levels of practice as a basis for explaining what advanced physiotherapy practice is and where it fits into the profession. This is important in promoting an understanding of the unique characteristics of this level of practice among both other members of the physiotherapy profession and the wider healthcare workforce. Patients too need to understand what an advanced physiotherapist can do to help them. Finally, the CSP's approach can be seen as helpful in establishing job profiles and pay. In addition, the CSP offers evidence of the effectiveness of advanced practitioners, for example in fall prevention among the elderly, arguing that this level of practice is clinically and cost effective and, therefore, represents an appropriate use of physiotherapists as a resource (CSP 2016).

6.5 Advanced Practice Paramedics

The paramedic role is to act as a first point of contact for people with a wide variety of health problems, resulting, for example, from trauma, acute or long-term physical or mental health conditions, and other emergencies. Paramedics assess, diagnose, and treat patients, referring them on to other services if appropriate. The development of paramedic practice is fairly recent in comparison to other health professions. Entry to the professions can be achieved via a course in paramedic science, which may be at diploma, foundation degree, or Bachelor's degree level. A degree apprenticeship route has also been introduced (https://www.healthcareers.nhs.uk).

The College of Paramedics has identified four fields of paramedic practice: clinical, education, management, and research. In this context advanced practice is a level, within the clinical field, between specialist and consultant (you may want to consider how this relates to your own field in Exercise 6.2). Advanced paramedics are defined as "experienced, autonomous allied health professionals who have undertaken further study and skill acquisition to enable them to be able to deliver a more appropriate level of assessment and indeed care to patients in the community and access many more referral pathways." Master's-level preparation is required for this level of practice, plus at least three to five years of experience post initial qualification (College of Paramedics 2015, p. 41). As in physiotherapy, advanced practice is a level below that of consultant. Consultant paramedics are expected to work strategically, developing new practice and care pathways as well as taking an active role in research and audit. PhD-level preparation is expected for this level of practice (College of Paramedics 2015).

EXERCISE 6.2

In your professional field, what is the difference between qualified, advanced, and consultant practice?

Advanced paramedic practitioners are regarded as essential in being "innovators and role models to take the profession forward" (College of Paramedics 2017, p. 7). A review of current evidence by the National Institute for Health and Care Excellence (NICE; 2017) led to a recommendation that increasing the number of advanced paramedic practitioners able to assess and treat a range of medical emergencies could help to reduce pressures on emergency departments, reduce hospital admissions, and improve patient satisfaction. In line with this recommendation, advanced paramedics were allowed to become independent prescribers from April 1, 2018. Whilst it might be more expensive to employ advanced practitioners than less experienced paramedics, the costs would be offset by the benefits of the posts. It was not deemed appropriate to train all paramedics to advanced level, as less experienced practitioners needed time to develop the skills and expertise required as a foundation for progress to more advanced roles.

6.6 Current Issues in Advanced Practice in Allied Health Professions

Physiotherapy and paramedic practice have clearly made considerable progress in defining advanced practice in their respective fields, identifying their own levels of practice, and developing their own career frameworks and scope of practice. Radiography, speech and language therapy, occupational therapy, and other professions have done the same. It is now accepted that there are levels of practice beyond initial qualification, and that the advanced level takes years to achieve through a combination of a range of experience with patients/clients and formal education at Master's level. This acceptance reflects a growing mastery of autonomous practice in which knowledge, clinical skills, and critical reasoning skills are applied to the care of patients who may have single or multiple needs. Advanced allied health practitioners are now able to meet many of the roles envisaged in early twentieth-century healthcare reforms (Table 6.2), for example by providing complete episodes of evidence-based care, educating others, developing new ways of working, and promoting health. Current evidence indicates that they are effective. For example, an advanced practitioner physiotherapist serving four GP practices in North Wales saved 1983 appointments with doctors over a period of nine months and had high levels of patient satisfaction (Caine and Wynne 2016). Reports collated by NICE (2017) also point to the important contributions of advanced paramedics to emergency care. There is, therefore, no question that advanced allied health professionals are fulfilling much-needed roles in healthcare.

However, there are still some issues to be addressed. First, allied health professions have not, historically, enjoyed quite the same profiles and status as medicine and nursing, and still do not seem to have the same degree of influence. This may, in part, be due to lack of public understanding about the work they do, but allied professionals themselves are not always very good at explaining this. They are "often better at describing individual patient level improvements but often find it hard to concisely articulate population level impact which is needed to establish value" (NHS England 2017, p. 12). In other words, allied health professionals do not always do themselves justice in explaining what they do to those with commissioning, budgetary, and managerial responsibilities. Failure to communicate effectively leads inevitably to a muted voice in healthcare systems. This is evident in the lack of clear representation of allied health professions at senior levels of decision making in the NHS. For example, in each of the four countries, the Chief Medical Officer and Chief Nursing Officer are the chief advisors to the government on matters relating to their professions, and play a leading role in the development of health policies. Similarly, at NHS Trust level, the medical and nursing directors are normally members of Trust boards. In contrast, the Chief Allied Health Professions Officer represents all allied health professions at governmental level; representation on Trust boards is variable. Lack of representation may in turn have an impact on organizational knowledge of the potential of allied health professions to meet the changing healthcare needs of patients in the twenty-first century. It is, therefore, essential that allied health professionals develop a stronger voice generally, but especially with regard to advanced practice. Allied health professionals need to be more assertive; they are the experts in their respective fields but, if they cannot articulate what it is they do and how they contribute to both individual patient care and overall service provision, the contribution of their advanced practice roles to patients and services will not be fully appreciated. Consider Exercise 6.3 in relation to the organization where you work.

Second, advanced practice is regarded as a combination of breadth of experience, Master's-level preparation, and four core components: direct expert practice; leadership; education and research; and advanced, profession-specific expertise. These elements are now seen as generic, shared by nursing and all allied health professions. Unfortunately, having arrived at this point, each country in the UK is now pursuing its own way forward. NHS Health Education England (2017) has issued the following definition of advanced practice:

> Advanced Clinical Practice is delivered by experienced registered healthcare practitioners. It is a level of practice characterised by a high level of autonomy and complex decision-making. This is underpinned by a masters level award or equivalent that encompasses the four pillars of clinical practice, management and leadership, education and research, with demonstration of core and area specific clinical competence.
>
> Advanced Clinical Practice embodies the ability to manage complete clinical care in partnership with patients/carers. It includes the analysis and synthesis of complex problems across a range of settings, enabling innovative solutions to enhance patient experience and improve outcomes. (NHS Health Education England 2017, p. 8)

EXERCISE 6.3

How could advanced practitioners from different professions collaborate in your employing organization?

This definition applies only to England. It also heralds yet another framework, which sets out what advanced practitioners should be able to do with regard to clinical practice based around the principles of workforce governance, accountability, education, and development. Northern Ireland has issued separate strategies for nursing and allied health professions (Department of Health and Social Services and Public Safety 2012, 2016). Scotland is also pursuing its own agenda. There are, of course, many similarities between the various documents produced by each country. They may yet all prove to be useful steps in the development of advanced practice, but the overall impression is that each country is pursuing its own path, which raises concerns that all these documents will simply add to the plethora of definitions of advanced practice already available and the multitude of frameworks already produced by both individual professions and government departments.

Compiling yet more definitions and frameworks gives the impression of progress, but it skirts neatly around other issues, for example public protection. The title "advanced practitioner" and registration seem to feature little in the discourse at present. This is cause for concern, given the results of a recent survey of job titles in nursing, which found 323 advanced nurse practitioner postholders who were not on the UK nursing register (Leary et al. 2017). Anyone can call themselves an advanced practitioner, or even be named as such by their employers. A similar survey is needed to determine whether there are any unqualified advanced allied health practitioners, and the professions also need to consider how best to ensure that patients are protected. The consequences of diagnosis and treatment by unqualified individuals places patients at risk and does little to reassure the public that genuine health professionals are able to perform advanced levels of practice.

The third issue is that expanding and developing practice in allied health professions as envisaged in health policies and reforms did not and has not reduced other aspects of the workload. Prior to the advent of advanced practice, physiotherapists, occupational therapists, prosthetists, and others were not waiting for patients to fill their caseloads, nor have patients since ceased to need foot care, X-rays of their fractures, or rehabilitation. These patients still require care and treatment, all of which limits the time available for more advanced work. The introduction of the new workforce of assistant practitioners was helpful, in that it provided a staff group to whom qualified practitioners could delegate a range of routine, day-to-day tasks, thus freeing up qualified professionals to spend more time with patients who are perceived to have greater needs.

Assistant practitioners are now an established group within the NHS. They are generic workers who have been educated to perform some of the work previously undertaken only by qualified health professionals. The core competences include the assessment of patients without complex needs, ensuring that patients have adequate nutrition and fluids, working in a team, applying health and safety and infection-control measures as appropriate, and communicating effectively (Skills for Care and Skills for Health 2013). Role- or job-specific competences may include the provision of personal care, assessing patients' needs for aids at home, and working with people who have mental health problems. Assistant practitioners work in a variety of care settings, both in hospitals and in the community, and may work across traditional professional boundaries, although there is variation between employing organizations (Miller et al. 2014). There are multiple training routes for assistant practitioners – foundation degrees, National Vocational Qualifications, and apprenticeships – and employers are free to choose the route which best services their organizational needs. Consequently, there is variation in the content of training courses, which is a cause for concern. Additional concerns focus on the lack of opportunities for career progression, despite the fact that assistant practitioners can join allied health professional organizations. Overall, there is a certain irony in encouraging the development of advanced practice whilst at the same time introducing support staff to enable that development to take place. This may serve to separate advanced practitioners from the realities of performing the day-to-day tasks undertaken by assistants and qualified practitioners, as opposed to delegating and supervising them, and thus lead to some deskilling.

Fourth, the rhetoric about the need for new ways of working is not always easy to achieve. Organizational culture, the "way we do things round here," and traditional interprofessional relations are not easy to change. Despite the progress made, allied health practitioners may still experience obstacles to their work. For example, requests for clinical imaging have traditionally been made via a doctor; radiographers could accept referrals from other, designated professionals provided they were deemed competent to act in this way. However, local variations in practice meant that advanced practitioners could experience difficulties in getting their referrals accepted. This situation was resolved through multiprofessional collaboration between the Royal College of Nursing, Society and College of Radiographers, Chartered Society of Physiotherapists, General Osteopathic Council, General Chiropractic Council, NHS Alliance, and Royal College of Radiologists. The collaboration produced guidance on referrals; this included a requirement for employers to maintain a list of competent referrers, their individual profession, what images they could request, and the need for clear referral pathways (Royal College of Nursing 2008). This represents one approach to resolving barriers to advanced practice, but it requires considerable effort, commitment, and time. Addressing barriers to advanced practice remains an issue both for individual practitioners and for professions as a whole.

Finally, there is the issue of determining the impact of advanced allied health practices, an issue emphasized by NHS Health Education England (2017). At present, there does not appear to be agreement on how this should be done, and the subject does not seem to have been widely addressed by the allied health professions themselves. Examination of the impact of advanced and consultant nurses suggests that these levels of practice do seem to have some positive effects. For example, Klassen et al. (2009) evaluated the impact of a newly created advanced nurse practitioner post in a nursing home in Winnipeg. The use of multiple methods revealed a reduction in the use of medication, polypharmacy, and hospital admissions, and an increase in family, but not patient, satisfaction. The impact of a single post shows what one individual can achieve, but it does not provide robust evidence for the profession or service commissioners. Similar criticisms have been made of studies in allied health. A systematic review of the effects of extended roles in physiotherapy, occupational therapy, and speech and language therapy on patient care, colleagues, and health services revealed a lack of randomized controlled trials, a tendency to focus on description, and a lack of precise data (Saxon et al. 2014). For example, "outcomes in terms of reduced waiting times do not consistently specify to which point in the patient's journey" (Saxon et al. 2014).

CASE STUDY

One year ago, a healthcare organization appointed an advanced practitioner in the physiotherapy department. The aim of the post was to provide treatment and care for patients with musculoskeletal problems, for example chronic pain and other long-term conditions affecting patients' ability to work, and short-term problems such as back pain. The postholder would spend half of each week based in hospital clinics and the other half in community services to which patients can self-refer. After one year, the impact of the post is to be assessed.

What factors should be considered in determining the impact of this post?

Advanced practitioners undergo lengthy and expensive preparation. They can be costly to employ and much is often expected of them. Employers need to know how and where to make the best use of them. Moreover, advanced practitioners themselves need to know, as part of job satisfaction, whether they are really making a difference. The problem is that determining impact is not always easy; advanced practitioner posts differ, often within the same organization, so setting rigid criteria is not helpful. This may explain why so many studies seem to rely on asking patients or colleagues for their views and experiences. Factors such as patient satisfaction are very important, but impact involves more than this. Impact is effect, so determining impact begins with the question: "What is the effect of this post on (i) patient care; and (ii) this organization?" It is the effect of the post rather than the individual that matters. The competence and capability of the postholder are a complementary issue, but one that can be assessed in other ways. Focusing attention on the effect of the post takes away issues of personality, individual likes and dislikes, and other personalized factors. Asking "What is the effect of this post on (i) patient care; and (ii) this organization?" leads to a further series of questions that act as a guide to gathering evidence of impact (Table 6.3). This can be used to inform decision making about the post and further action. Thus, assessment of impact is really a continuous cycle that runs concurrently, rather than separately from, the advanced practice post (Figure 6.1).

TABLE **6.3**	
Questions for determining the impact of an advanced practice post.	
1. What is the aim(s) of the post?	An advanced practitioner post is usually set up in response to some perceived need and the actions required to address it. Allied to this are issues concerning patient safety, lines of accountability and responsibility, arrangements for supervision and training, the location of the post, and the support systems required to facilitate achievement of the aims. This preparatory material is useful, because impact may both affect and be affected by these issues. For example, this case study omits lines of responsibility; where these are unclear, managerial oversight and support may be weak, which may in turn affect the extent to which the aim(s) are achieved.
2. What evidence is needed?	The impact on patient care and on the organization will require different forms of evidence. Consequently, evidence may be gathered from multiple sources and include quantitative and qualitative data; financial data should also be included where appropriate, for instance in demonstrating efficiency savings. Regardless of the approach used, it is the quality of the data that matters most; good data will show clear evidence of changes.
	In this case study, quantitative data might include reductions in requests for doctors' appointments, improvements in self-management among patients with short-term problems such as backache, and increased patient satisfaction scores. Qualitative data might include interviews with patients or relatives.
3. How, when, and where should this evidence be collected?	Methods used should fit within and not obstruct the work of the postholder or others. Decisions will be required about when and where data will be recorded, whether a sample is sufficient, or whether every item of information is required. For example, reductions in hospital stays may require quantitative data collected daily over a specific period of time, whereas information about particular aspects of care may be episodic.
4. Who is responsible for collecting the evidence?	Responsibility for collecting evidence should not be left solely to the postholder. Managers too must collect evidence as part of their roles in overseeing advanced practitioners.
5. Which stakeholders should be consulted/involved?	These may be patients, relatives, carers, senior staff, commissioners, or anyone with a significant association with the post. Evidence may be qualitative or quantitative in nature.
6. Who will collate the evidence into a report?	This is a managerial responsibility, although the advanced practitioner postholder may collaborate in compiling this.
	The report should specify, as appropriate, the impact of the post on (i) patient care; and (ii) this organization. Good evidence of impact is that which can be shared with others and used as a basis for developing practice, services, or both.
7. In which committee(s) should the report be presented?	This depends on the organization, but an additional consideration is where the item is placed on the committee's agenda. Items toward the end of the agenda may be overlooked because those attending are anxious to leave.

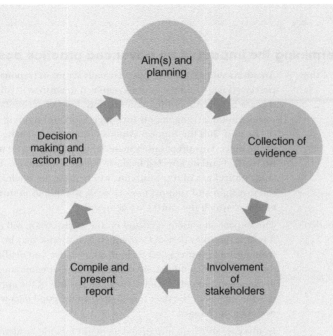

FIGURE 6.1 Assessment of impact as a continuous process.

6.7 Conclusion

Allied health professions have seized the opportunities offered, by health policy and service reforms, to expand their fields of practice and develop their potential. Advanced practitioners work in diverse settings, either as members of multidisciplinary teams caring for individuals with long-term and complex needs, or as front-line staff providing complete episodes of care. Nevertheless, there are still challenges to be addressed, particularly in terms of articulating the contribution of advanced allied health professionals to patient care and senior managers. The full impact of these advanced posts is not yet realized and more research is needed to ensure that this impact is appreciated.

Key Questions

1. Advanced practice is regarded as a combination of breadth of experience, Master's-level preparation, and four core components: direct expert practice, leadership, education and research, and advanced, profession-specific expertise. Could advanced practitioners become a separate profession?

2. As an advanced allied health practitioner, how would you explain your role to a senior manager?

3. How is the use of modern technology contributing to your work as an advanced allied health practitioner?

Glossary

Chartered Society of Physiotherapy (www.csp.org.uk): the professional organization for physiotherapists.

College of Paramedics (www.collegeofparamedics. co.uk): the professional organization for paramedics.

General Osteopathic Council (www.osteopathy. org.uk/home): regulates osteopaths in the UK, maintains a register of qualified individuals, sets standards, and approves training programs.

General Pharmaceutical Council (www.pharmacy regulation.org): regulates pharmacists, pharmacy technicians, and pharmacy premises. The Council maintains a register of qualified individuals, sets standards, and approves training programs.

Health and Care Professions Council (**HCPC**; (http://www.hcpc-uk.co.uk): regulates 16 health and care professions in the UK, maintains a register of qualified individuals, sets standards, and approves training programs for those professions.

Health Education England (https://hee.nhs.uk): responsible for education and training courses for health professionals.

National Health Service (NHS) England (https://www.england.nhs.uk): responsible for the health service in England, including strategic planning and commissioning services. Scotland, Wales, and Northern Ireland have their own, equivalent organizations.

National Institute for Health and Clinical Excellence (**NICE**; www.nice.org.uk): provides evidence-based guidance, advice, resources, and information for health and social care professionals.

Paramedics: provide emergency and life-saving treatment and care for individuals suffering from trauma or from illness requiring immediate intervention. Paramedics provide services in homes, places of work, at road traffic accidents, and in other community settings. They also work in hazardous areas such as offshore oil rigs, and remote areas and alongside other emergency and law enforcement agencies, offshore oil rigs, and remote areas.

Physiotherapy: the UK's term for the holistic application of physical exercises, education, massage, and other interventions to facilitate recovery from illness or trauma, or manage disability. The practice of physiotherapy varies from country to country, as does the term itself.

Public Health England (**PHE**; https://www.gov.uk/government/organisations/public-health-england): part of the NHS, responsible for improving health and reducing health inequalities through evidence-based campaigns that promote understanding of disease and healthier lifestyles, preparing for and responding to emergency situations.

Skills for Care (www.skillsforcare.org.uk): an organization that supports employers in developing the workforce skills and procedures required for the provision of efficient, cost-effective, and flexible social care services.

Skills for Health (www.skillsforhealth.org.uk): an organization that supports employers in developing the workforce skills and procedures required for the provision of efficient, cost-effective, and flexible health services.

References

Benner, P. (1984). *From Novice to Expert: Excellence and Power in Clinical Nursing Practice*. Menlo Park, California: Addison Wesley.

Caine, R. and Wynne, C. (2016). Advanced practitioner physiotherapists in primary care. *Physiotherapy* 102 (Supplement 1): eS142.

Chartered Society of Physiotherapy (2013) The physiotherapy framework. https://www.csp.org.uk/professional-clinical/cpd-and-education/professional-development/professional-frameworks (accessed January 8, 2019).

Chartered Society of Physiotherapy (2016) Advanced practice in physiotherapy. Understanding the contribution of advanced practice in physiotherapy to transforming lives, maximising independence and empowering populations. https://www.csp.org.uk/publications/advanced-practice-physiotherapy (accessed January 8, 2019).

College of Paramedics (2015). *Paramedic Career Framework*, 3e. Bridgwater: College of Paramedics.

College of Paramedics (2017). *Paramedic Scope of Practice Policy*. Bridgwater: College of Paramedics.

Cystic Fibrosis Trust (2018) Survival statistics – what if I'm already 30? https://www.cysticfibrosis.org.uk/news/survival-statistics-what-if-im-already-30 (accessed January 8, 2019).

Department of Health (2003a). *Implementing a Scheme for Allied Health Professionals with Special Interests.* London: DH.

Department of Health (2003b). *Ten Key Roles for Allied Health Professionals.* London: DH.

Department of Health and Social Services and Public Safety (2012). *Improving Health and Well-Being through Positive Partnerships. A Strategy for the Allied Health Professions in Northern Ireland 2012–17.* Belfast: DHSSP.

Department of Health and Social Services and Public Safety (2016). *Advanced Nursing Practice Framework. Supporting Advanced Nursing Practice in Health and Social Care Trusts.* Belfast: Northern Ireland Practice and Education Council for Nursing.

Elbron, J.S. (2016). Cystic fibrosis. *The Lancet* 388: 2519–2531.

Imison, C. and Bohmer, R. (2013). *NHS and Social Care Workforce: Meeting Our Needs Now and in the Future? About Time to Think Differently* series. London: King's Fund.

Jones, A. (2015). *Life Expectancy of People with Cystic Fibrosis. Expert Commentary on Important New Evidence.* London: National Institute for Health and Care Excellence. http://www.nice.org.uk (accessed January 8, 2019).

Klassen, K., Lamont, L., and Krishnan, P. (2009). Setting a new standard of care in nursing homes. *Canadian Nurse* 105: 24–30.

Leary, A., Maclaine, K., Trevatt, P. et al. (2017). Variation in job titles within the nursing workforce. *Journal of Clinical Nursing* 26: 4945–4950.

McGee, P. and Cole, D. (2009). Advanced practice in allied health professions. In: *Advanced Practice in Nursing and the Allied Health Professions*, 3e (ed. P. McGee), 29–42. Oxford, UK: Wiley-Blackwell.

Miller, L., Williams, J., Marvell, R., and Tassinari, A. (2014). *Assistant Practitioners in the NHS in England.* Bristol: Skills for Health.

National Health Service (2014) The Five Year Forward View. https://www.england.nhs.uk/wp-content/uploads/2014/10/5yfv-web.pdf (accessed January 8, 2019).

National Health Service England (2017). *Allied Health Professions into Action. Using Allied Health Professionals to Transform Health, Care and Wellbeing.* London: NHS England.

National Health Service Health Education England (2017) Multi-professional framework for advanced clinical practice in England. https://www.hee.nhs.uk/our-work/advanced-clinical-practice/multi-professional-framework (accessed January 8, 2019).

National Health Service Modernisation Agency (2004) 10 high impact changes for service improvement and delivery. https://www.england.nhs.uk/improvement-hub/publication/10-high-impact-changes-for-service-improvement-and-delivery (accessed January 8, 2019).

National Institute for Health and Care Excellence (2017) Emergency and acute medical care in the over-16s: service delivery and organisation. Draft for consultation. https://www.nice.org.uk/guidance/ng94 (accessed January 8, 2019).

Office of National Statistics (2017) Estimates of the very old (including centenarians): 2002 to 2016. https://www.ons.gov.uk/peoplepopulationandcommunity/birthsdeathsandmarriages/ageing/bulletins/estimatesoftheveryoldincludingcentenarians/previousReleases (accessed January 8, 2019).

Public Health England (2016). *Strategic Plan for the Next Four Years: Better Outcomes by 2020.* London: Public Health England.

Royal College of Nursing (2008). *Clinical Imaging Requests from Non-medically Qualified Professionals.* London: RCN.

Saxon, R., Fray, M., and Oprescu, F. (2014). Extended roles for allied health professionals: systematic review of the evidence. *Journal of Multidisciplinary Healthcare* 4 (7): 479–488.

Skills for Care and Skills for Health (2013). *National Minimum Training Standards for Healthcare Support Workers and Adult Social Care Workers in England.* Leeds: Skills for Care and Skills for Health.

CHAPTER 7

Advanced Practice in the Radiography Professions

Nick White and Helen White

Birmingham City University, Birmingham, UK

Key Issues
- To reflect the current status of advanced practice roles and the development of advanced practitioners within the radiography professions, primarily considering diagnostic radiographers, therapeutic radiographers, and sonographers
- Using examples from radiotherapy and imaging services, it will provide a synopsis of the contextual detail of advanced practice role development in the UK
- To discuss how the developments and evolution of the role of the radiographer have resulted in the current status and practice of the advanced practitioner radiographer.

LEARNING OUTCOMES

By the end of this chapter you will be able to:

- Evaluate the concept of advanced practice within the context of imaging and cancer service delivery.
- Appraise the role of an advanced practitioner within therapeutic radiography, diagnostic radiography, and medical ultrasound.
- Debate contemporary issues associated with advanced practice in the radiography professions.

7.1 Introduction

In the UK, non-medical allied health professionals administering radiation to patients for therapeutic purposes and imaging constitute the radiography work-force. It would, however, be useful to be clear that when we talk about

Advanced Practice in Healthcare: Dynamic Developments in Nursing and Allied Health Professions,
Fourth Edition. Edited by Paula McGee and Chris Inman.
© 2019 John Wiley & Sons Ltd. Published 2019 by John Wiley & Sons Ltd.

radiography, we are not talking about one profession. There are at least two professions that fall under the umbrella term "radiography": *therapeutic radiographers* as cancer specialists working in radiotherapy and cancer services; and *diagnostic radiographers* working in imaging services. Therapeutic radiographers are professionally responsible for the planning and delivery of accurate radiotherapy treatments. The diagnostic radiographer's scope of practice is centered in medical imaging, examinations for which are usually undertaken following referral from a suitably qualified medical staff member on the basis of clinical need. Diagnostic radiographers have traditionally undertaken postgraduate study, for example specializing in ultrasound imaging to become sonographers, or specializing in breast X-ray imaging to become mammographers.

Technological developments have led to the development of advanced practice in imaging modalities such as computed tomography (CT), magnetic resonance imaging (MRI), or nuclear medicine, including molecular imaging, as well as the development of expert skills in reporting on images. Within radiotherapy, advanced practice roles can be found in the pre-treatment and planning of radiotherapy treatment, in treatment of both external-beam radiotherapy and brachytherapy, or in post-treatment and ongoing patient support roles, including palliative care.

7.2 Worldwide Variation in the Adoption of Advanced Practice in Radiography

The UK recognizably leads the world in its development of advanced practice in radiography. Global differences in the adoption and approach to role advancement have been sought to be classified, with the UK and USA having well-established systems. However, there is sporadic development in Europe, despite the need for more clearly defined role advancement (Nightingale and McNulty, 2016). For example, in Denmark, image reporting roles for diagnostic radiographers have only recently been introduced (Buskov et al., 2013). Global adoption of such advanced practice roles appears to be inextricably linked to the many differing healthcare systems and structures that exist worldwide, and the financial and political frameworks associated therewith. In many countries the professions of diagnostic and therapeutic radiography remain unrecognized and lack any rigid program of education or professional organization. For these, advanced radiographic practice remains conceptual and some way off (Cowling, 2008).

Before reading on, consider Exercise 7.1.

EXERCISE 7.1

How does the role of the radiographer, advanced practitioner, and consultant practitioner radiographer differ across Europe and the rest of the world?

7.3 Four-tier Service and Advanced Practice in Radiography

The College of Radiographers has been working to define the four-tier radiography service for many years. Due to the prioritized aims of the National Health Service (NHS) Cancer Plan (Department of Health, 2000), this was initiated in breast imaging, radiotherapy, and then imaging, including ultrasound. The aim was to develop a workforce that could expand cancer services, against a backdrop of critical radiographer, radiologist, and oncologist shortages. The Radiography Skills Mix Project (Department of Health, 2000), was initiated to benefit patients through the design of a clinical team focused on patient care needs rather than professional boundaries. It was also intended to benefit radiographers of both professions through a defined career progression structure and professional leadership. The four tiers were identified as *assistant practitioner, registered practitioner, advanced practitioner*, and *consultant practitioner*.

In their working lives, diagnostic and therapeutic radiographers have been specializing in existing roles and developing new ones, creating their advanced practice roles. Arguably, the initial emphasis for advanced practice was solely on the development of clinical expertise and skill, though this was developed to include wider role expectations. For example, the Department of Health (2013) mandated Health Education England (HEE) to ensure that the NHS workforce was research and innovation aware as a basis for service improvement and benefits to patient care. Cancer Research UK (2014), in its joint paper with NHS England, emphasized the enablement of therapeutic radiographers in advanced and consultant practitioner roles to further develop skills in, for example, radiotherapy treatment planning, to have positive impacts on service development.

While the emphasis of *Team Working in Clinical Imaging* (RCR and SCoR, 2012, p. 13) was important for team relationships between radiologists and diagnostic radiographers, it also highlighted the significant role of the advanced practitioner with "expert skills and knowledge in a defined field or fields of reporting" in contributing to patient management through the writing of clinical reports. The expectation, therefore, remains that clinical expertise is the basis of all advanced and consultant practice in both depth (specialist) and breadth (generalist).

Increasing service demands and an aging population have proved to be powerful drivers in the development and adoption of advanced practice roles, as has the rapid evolution of patient treatment technologies and changing patterns of patient care delivery, including seven-day working within the NHS. Changes to the skills mix have also provided opportunities for the adoption of advanced radiographic practice, although local demands and variation in service design have tended to lead to patchy implementation in certain areas (Henderson et al. 2016). The wider impact of advanced practice roles themselves also warrants further scrutiny with respect to measurable data such as potential improvements to patient outcomes. The College of Radiographers (2010) has sought to outline the advanced practice role within a defined scope of practice, and it is important to emphasize here that this scope is philosophically based on radiographers operating as autonomous and highly educated practitioners capable of enhancing service delivery and improving patient care. It is important also to distinguish radiographic advanced practice as being a matter of skills development rather than merely skills substitution. Advanced practice roles in radiography are therefore not simply a short-term solution to staffing shortages among the medical workforce via backfilling of duties traditionally discharged by medical personnel, but offer much more to the benefit of the patient.

The phrase "advanced practice" is well worn, suggesting that it should be easy to define and that all would be clear on what this means. Yet, there has been much discussion around this subject, particularly in how the title is used across professions and across healthcare providers. In an attempt to create a common language for the description of roles across all allied health professions (AHPs), *Modernizing AHP Careers* (Department of Health, 2007a) initially described a competence framework to highlight the common elements for competence-based workforce planning, linking this to educational requirements and career progression across all AHPs. Discussion over 10 years has, however, now importantly culminated in the design of the Multi-professional Framework for Advanced Clinical Practice (ACP) in England (HEE 2017b). This presents a definition of ACP that works across professional boundaries and defines a level of practice rather than a specified job role. Alongside the requirements for registration, competence, and capabilities, the individual is expected to have experience and to hold a Master's-level award, or equivalent, that encompasses "the four pillars of clinical practice, leadership and management, education and research, with demonstration of core capabilities and area specific clinical competence." ACP should embody "the ability to manage clinical care in partnership with individuals, families and carers. It includes the analysis and synthesis of complex problems across a range of settings, enabling innovative solutions to enhance people's experience and improve outcomes" (HEE 2017b, p. 8). Demonstrating capability and competence across the four pillars may present some interesting challenges to employers, particularly where individuals may be titled "advanced practitioner" but demonstrate a range of differing interpretations of this title. Some rationalization may be required as individuals and employers review roles in light of this definition, with it being likely for some individuals to need support as capabilities are developed across all four pillars to complement clinical expertise.

Before reading on, think about your answers to Exercises 7.2 and 7.3.

EXERCISE 7.2

Discuss the impact that the adoption of advanced practice roles for radiographers has had on service provision within the UK and in the rest of the world.

EXERCISE 7.3

Identify the core characteristics and domains of practice expected of an advanced practice radiographer working within the UK.

7.4 Educational Preparation for Advanced Practice Roles in Radiography

The College of Radiographers has established that those discharging advanced practice roles and responsibilities must be suitably trained and educated in order to provide effective service delivery and quality, and in turn to provide education and training to their peers as part of their recognized core responsibilities. This usually requires the radiographer to undertake a postgraduate qualification, given that the minimum threshold for registration in the UK as a radiographer, therapeutic or diagnostic, is a Bachelor's degree with honors.

The College of Radiographers has adopted a robust educational and career framework (CoR 2013) that determines the expected professional attributes of the advanced practitioner and currently supports the study of education programs at postgraduate (i.e. Master's) level. The association with education at this level places diagnostic radiographers, therapeutic radiographers, and sonographers on an equitable footing with other AHPs, and, as a consequence, there are opportunities for shared interprofessional learning, both in practice and within defined programs of study. In addition, such programs ordinarily embed some degree of research training and theory into their structure, which aligns the professional development of radiographers in research as an espoused core domain supporting development toward advanced standing.

There is, however, considerable debate surrounding the *amount* of Master's-level study that should be expected. For example, many programs of study leading to an award in radiographer image reporting require students to complete their training without completion of a full Master's degree; students exit with a postgraduate diploma or certificate. Similarly, within ultrasound, most UK students currently complete their training without undertaking a full Master's award. Mammography is a postgraduate qualification too, usually undertaken by diagnostic radiographers and, on occasion, therapeutic radiographers, but mammographers similarly do not always hold a named postgraduate award, and if they do, this is usually the result of an individual's decision rather than an employer's requirement. While most employers continue to recognize the postgraduate diploma or postgraduate certificate as the threshold for advanced standing, there seems little financial or professional impetus for completion of the full award. This may change with the expectation held within the ACP Framework (HEE, 2017a).

Consultant practice is the next level beyond advanced practice. Recent guidance about the expectations of the consultant practitioner radiographer (CoR, 2017) will no doubt help with establishing the clarity of boundaries between the two levels. Consultant practice requires doctoral-level study and a highly developed clinical role, ordinarily incorporating research and service design, enhancement, and evaluation. Consultant radiographers themselves have been well received into clinical practice and recently there have been new opportunities for the development of clinical-academic roles, whereby the consultant radiographer divides their time between practice and academia.

7.5 Defining Advanced Practice – Do Role Specialism and Role Extension in Radiography Truly Lead to "Advanced Practice"?

The professional aims of the advanced practitioner in diagnostic imaging, radiotherapy, and ultrasound are contributions toward evidence-based practice, leadership, knowledge transfer, and clinical expertise. Skill mix policy and practice developments have witnessed a move away from task orientation, such that today the radiographer's role is defined more by the patient's individual pathway and the provision of high-quality care, with an attendant widening scope of practice that may cross professional boundaries. The advanced practitioner therapeutic radiographer, for example, may have responsibility for patient management and support throughout their radiotherapy treatment pathway, from referral, to pre-treatment planning, treatment coordination, and follow-up, while acting as an important lynchpin within the multidisciplinary oncology team. Being able to demonstrate cost effectiveness and meet national cancer targets is, however, emphasized as these staffing models and advanced practice therapeutic radiographers are implemented within the radiotherapy workforce, as discussed within the College of Radiographers' (2009) guidance in response to the Cancer Reform Strategy (DH, 2007b). Although both documents have since been superseded, this remains a pertinent position.

There is still a lack of evidence based on a thorough analysis of the wider role that advanced practice diagnostic radiographers play with respect to achieving improved patient outcomes (Hardy et al. 2016). However, despite this, there is clear evidence from practice that both diagnostic and therapeutic radiographers have developed their skills and roles, which has, in turn, realized greater service capacity and reduced pressure on radiologists and oncologists. Image-reporting radiographers, for example, undoubtedly provide some alleviation in service pressures, and evidence shows their image-reporting skills to be as good as those of their radiologist colleagues (England et al. 2010).

Ideally, an advanced practice radiographer's role should evidence clear alignment with the four core pillars of advanced practice espoused by the Society and College of Radiographers, but closer scrutiny of the radiography workforce suggests this alignment is often indistinct and not universally adopted. For example, Milner and Snaith (2017) have reported examples of advanced practice radiographers, stating that they consider leadership responsibilities to be unnecessary within their scope of practice. Similarly in this work, there is evidence that the adoption of research as a core responsibility is patchy. It is possible that those currently discharging roles nominally as advanced practitioners are in fact *specialist* rather than *advanced* according to the core domains of practice. Certainly, much of the published work addressing advanced practice in radiography focuses on advanced clinical skills and competence, which leads Milner and Snaith (2017) to suggest that there is a disproportionate focus on ability rather than influence. This may, in part, stem from a lack of a standardized and recognized minimum qualification for advanced practitioners, particularly where a research or leadership component may not have been included within an individual's Master's-level study. This may also be compounded by a lack of clarity surrounding job titles and associated terminology, some of which may now be considered further with the recent release of the ACP framework (HEE, 2017b).

In truth, it is likely that there are individual radiographers whose extended role means that their high-level clinical skills, such as image reporting, might be commensurate with those traditionally undertaken by clinicians; however, these practitioners may not wish to undertake additional research or leadership responsibilities, and desire to remain embedded closely in clinical practice and patient care. Similarly in nursing practice, advanced practice responsibilities may be perceived to reduce the traditional sense of professional identity. This may, for example, arise from a purely competence-based approach rather than via adoption of a more holistic view of the provision of patient care (Rolfe 2014). This position too may potentially change as the new HEE (2017b) definition becomes embedded in clinical practice and terminology.

Whilst the inherent advantages of the adoption of advanced practice opportunities have been suggested here, it should also be borne in mind that, at the individual level, there are likely to be many practicing radiographers for whom the adoption of advanced practice roles exceeds their professional goals or individual career aspirations, and for whom it would seem unfair to view advanced practice as the natural progression or professional norm. Griffiths (2013) has warned of the unintended consequences of the rapid adoption of advanced practice roles leading to the rock star radiographer effect, in which newly qualified radiographers naively identify advanced practice responsibilities as usual, without recognition of the importance of providing accurate and useful, albeit routine, imaging and high-quality care for the patient.

McGee and Cole (2009) have previously sought to assess whether the adoption of new radiography and sonography roles may legitimately be considered as advanced practice. Their framework espouses professional maturity, challenging the status quo, and the ability to innovate as the foundations of advanced practice. Using the advanced practice therapeutic radiographer to illustrate, it is clear that a typical advanced practitioner is able to advise on the adoption of new treatment protocols and adopt new practices which embed rapidly developing radiotherapy technologies to positively affect patient care. Arguably, none of these features is achievable without the presence of advanced practitioners; they champion professional practice development and service delivery rather than merely support it.

Before reading on, consider Exercise 7.4.

EXERCISE 7.4

Summarize the debates that surround attempts to distinguish the differences between extended role and advanced practice within radiography:

- For diagnostic radiographers
- For therapeutic radiographers

7.6 Taking Stock: The Deployment of Advanced Practitioners within the Diagnostic Imaging, Radiotherapy, and Ultrasound Communities of Practice

Advanced radiographer and sonographer practitioners are now to be found in a wide variety of roles throughout the NHS in the UK and in many parts of the rest of the world. These advanced practitioners influence patient pathways and patient management, and are usually able to demonstrate an enhanced level of clinical skill. In diagnostic radiography, a catalyst for the adoption of advanced practice roles has undoubtedly been the dual pressure of advancing technologies and staff shortages. A product of this has been the implementation of new ways of working and the reassessment of the skills mix, so that advanced practice has been cemented within the career structure for the diagnostic radiographer. In particular, the rapid expansion of the provision of cross-sectional imaging, primarily CT and MRI, has afforded new opportunities for skills development. In these areas of diagnostic radiography practice, advanced practitioners operate autonomously and will undertake all aspects of the imaging process, from referral to imaging the patient, assessing, and reporting on the clinical findings of scans. Advanced practitioner diagnostic radiographers will also assess patients prior to the use of intravenous contrast media, and undertake risk assessment and advanced clinical decision making, including drug administration and image reporting. Such advanced roles in cross-sectional imaging have become so widely adopted that we now see a blossoming of new and innovative roles for advanced practitioners which indicate further subspecialisms, such as CT head reporting, CT coronary angiography, and MRI practice.

Elsewhere, advanced practitioner diagnostic radiographers routinely provide expert formal (written) reports of medical images and influence patient care thereafter. In many hospitals, patients with routine or minor trauma injury, for example, undergo assessment, diagnosis, and decision making that is radiographer led. Such roles are widely established in the assessment of imaging of the appendicular and axial skeleton, and with respect to regional anatomy such as chest and abdomen image reporting. These roles are supported by a number of accredited postgraduate education programs across the UK which aim to prepare radiographers for such roles. Woznitza (2014) evidences the deployment of diagnostic radiographers in providing definitive reports in chest radiography and mammography and, in the case of reporting of skeletal images, advanced practice diagnostic radiographers' performance is demonstrably as good as their radiology colleagues, with high levels of sensitivity and specificity reported. It is also not uncommon to witness advance practice radiographers managing their own caseloads and taking ownership of discrete work area responsibilities, as illustrated in the following case study of an advanced practitioner diagnostic radiographer.

CASE STUDY | The Role of the Advanced Practitioner Reporting Radiographer within Cancer Referral Pathways

Mr. Jones is a 69-year-old retired school teacher who visits his general practitioner following repeated bouts of shortness of breath, unexpected weight loss, and a persistent unproductive cough. The doctor, suspecting a sinister underlying diagnosis, arranges a chest X-ray at the patient's local hospital and the patient attends as a priority, as a "walk-in" referral. The patient's chest is X-ray imaged by a practitioner diagnostic radiographer, and the images are passed to an advanced practitioner diagnostic radiographer for immediate (or "hot") image reporting. The advanced practitioner is an expert in image interpretation, and is appropriately trained and experienced, often being referred to as the "reporting radiographer." In reviewing the image, the advanced practitioner identifies a lesion in the patient's left lung and writes a diagnostic report indicating the clinical findings of the chest X-ray. Lung cancer is suspected. The advanced practice diagnostic radiographer concludes that a referral onward for further imaging such as CT imaging is necessary, and within the image report documents

a recommendation that the patient be fast-track referred on to an oncology patient management pathway.

More widely, this advanced practitioner discharges an extended scope of practice that articulates with the underlying pillars of advanced practice. The clinical role indicated in this case study reflects a system of work defined by the advanced practitioner, and the diagnostic radiographer also undertakes a role at the local university in the education and assessment of postgraduate image-reporting radiographers, as well as in the education of trainee radiologists at both university and in practice. The postholder also participates in research and development activities within the clinical department, and attends national conferences and working groups presenting project work and sharing best practices – this being supported by the split role of clinical expert and educator within higher education.

1. Describe the duties and responsibilities undertaken by this diagnostic radiographer that

distinguishes them as an expert within their scope of practice as an advanced practitioner.

2. Summarize the impact that the advanced practitioner has within the context of improved patient management and potential clinical outcomes.

3. Describe the distinguishing features of this diagnostic radiographer's role which support their position within the scope of advanced practice. What supporting resources are required to enable the development of such roles?

Within therapeutic radiography, advanced practice roles are similarly established and, given the complexities of a typical radiotherapy treatment pathway, an arguably more varied range of advanced practice roles have evolved than is seen within diagnostic radiography. Advanced practitioners are now embedded throughout the radiotherapy treatment pathway and provide focused specialist skills within areas such as pre-treatment planning, dosimetry, treatment site specialism, and technical innovation. Advanced practitioners may also lead in areas such as brachytherapy treatment administration, on-treatment clinical review, quality assurance, and research. Such roles are now supported by education programs at a suitable level commensurate with advanced practice. However, the earlier work of Eddy (2008) has been vindicated in the warning that the chicken-and-egg situation of the pace of change has led some higher education institutions to wait and see which advanced practice roles become established before subsequently designing programs to support these.

The education of sonographers in the UK is predominantly at postgraduate level, and many sonographers will have established responsibilities, within which are embedded the core attributes of an advanced practitioner. Autonomous practice involving detailed analysis of dynamic images is accompanied by the need to diagnose pathologies from ultrasound images in real time and adapt techniques to suit individual clinical cases. Provision of a written report which may require recommendations for ongoing patient management to the referring clinician, is also required. In certain circumstances the sonographer will be required to break bad news as part of their responsibilities. In addition, sonographers will often manage the imaging throughput within their department and need to undertake leadership and service management more generally. Likewise, many sonographers' postgraduate education has equipped them with some theoretical knowledge of research, as this is a core requirement within the majority of postgraduate diploma qualifications, and also service design, which should enable them to undertake service evaluation and research. This should enable sonography practice to be firmly anchored to a sound evidence base. In line with the previous discussion, however, there are also sonographers where this is not the case. The wide scope of ultrasound practice has also allowed for the development of subspecialisms, as witnessed in diagnostic radiography and therapeutic radiography, such as ultrasound-based musculoskeletal or vascular imaging, which some view as further advanced practice within sonography.

At the time of writing, ultrasound practices are undergoing a review driven by significant workforce shortages, which has raised questions about whether all aspects of ultrasound practice are truly advanced in nature, and whether there is scope to develop education for sonographers to discharge imaging procedures at practitioner level, supported by education which does not require a previous degree (i.e. 'direct entry' to ultrasound). Such approaches would seem appealing if a defined scope of ultrasound practice can be agreed at practitioner level. This approach may help to address service capacity issues and release the advanced practice sonographer to discharge advanced practice activities with regard to all four pillars of practice. This idea is not without controversy since, in the absence of statutory regulation and a protected title, the role and scope of practice of the sonographer may vary between individual healthcare providers.

Similarly, a discussion on whether, for a diagnostic or therapeutic radiographer, mammography is advanced practice in its own right or a specialism within imaging is interesting, as within breast imaging there is no practitioner mammographer. Nevertheless, advanced practitioner mammographers do exist through the development of advanced clinical skill in areas of breast biopsy and image reporting, leading some of them to ask about career development and education within this area of imaging practice.

Elsewhere, a similar debate has arisen within the field of MRI imaging practice, including a reassessment of whether it is truly necessary only to educate MRI practitioners at postgraduate level subsequent to undergraduate diagnostic radiography training (Westbrook 2017). Westbrook also identifies the need to differentiate between specialism and advanced practice within this field of practice. For both ultrasound and MRI practice, it is evident that advanced practice roles historically linked to the development of technology and skill specialism are ripe for further scrutiny and evaluation to better reflect the pillars of advanced practice.

7.7 Future Developments and Opportunities

Technological advances in imaging and radiotherapy practices act as drivers for change within professional responsibilities and specialisms. As a group of professions, diagnostic radiographers, therapeutic radiographers, and sonographers are forced to constantly reassess and reposition their own professional status, in light of the fact that the adoption of innovative practices and role extension quickly metamorphose into routine practice and responsibility. For example, in radiotherapy, *image-guided radiotherapy* and *intensity-modulated radiotherapy* are now the acknowledged standard practices within treatment delivery, having previously been viewed as advanced techniques. These changes clearly provide a greater range of practice specialism for today's radiographer, with scope for transition to advanced practice within each of these roles. This said, such individual roles should ideally be adaptive to progress in practice developments and the rapid pace of change. These individuals should be prepared to innovate, lead, and evaluate new practices to the benefit of patient care, otherwise individual advanced practice roles quickly become unnecessary and outdated.

Advanced practice roles undoubtedly offer opportunities for increasing capacity and improving the efficacy of patient pathways. Field and Snaith (2013) also report enhanced multiprofessional communication as a consequence. Expansion of the scope of practice and professional development opportunities for radiographers has also realized opportunities to work toward assuming consultant practitioner status. This has been facilitated by a better understanding of where advanced practitioners sit within the continuum of practice, educational programs that underpin personal and professional development, and a clear articulation from the College of Radiographers regarding the defined features of consultant practice and how to achieve that position (CoR 2017). Experienced advanced practitioners may therefore be afforded further career opportunities and may consider themselves as notional trainee consultants, although this requires careful planning, costing, and managerial support for development of these individuals.

There remain a number of challenges to the adoption of such roles. Most significantly, there is very little research evidence that directly assesses the impact of such roles on patient outcomes and service quality. Hardy et al. (2016) have reported that examples of robust assessment of diagnostic radiographer advanced practice, as evaluated via service quality metrics such as patient mortality or cost savings, are extremely limited, and even therein, using financial savings as vicarious indicators of quality improvement is somewhat dubious. The majority of extant research into advanced practice in radiography is disproportionally skewed toward comparative analyses of the image-reporting skills of diagnostic radiographers versus those of their radiology colleagues (e.g. England et al. 2010). Such evidence only addresses one aspect of the espoused domains of ACP, namely expert clinical practice, and, as a result, there is scope to explore the impact of other advanced practitioner skills, including leadership qualities and service design more generally, so that wider assessment of service quality improvements might be made.

Fundamental to the development of advanced practice roles and those who aspire to undertake them is ongoing support from and involvement of the medical profession. Changes to skills mix and service pressure demands have resulted in aspects of imaging and treatment practice being ceded to radiographers. However, this is only possible with the involvement of the medical profession in the education, training, and continuing support of the advanced practitioner. Within the context of diagnostic imaging and particularly image reporting, both professional bodies of the radiographer and radiologist workforce recognize that effective interprofessional team working is important to enhance patient services (RCR/CoR, 2012; HEE, 2017a). Increased clinical responsibility for the advanced practice radiographer necessarily involves assuming responsibilities traditionally within the domain of the medical profession. Despite measurable benefits to the adoption of advanced practice roles, particularly with respect to increasing imaging capacity, recognition of the extended role of the radiographer is not necessarily a seamless process. Field and Snaith (2013) report some apprehension among supervising physicians. Traditional hierarchies of practice are still evident in many areas of imaging and oncology practice, and professional protectionism is being reported, although this issue varies greatly between different service providers. At the core of this disquiet appears to be the limit to which a radiographer may be up-skilled without recourse to extended training, similar to that seen within the field of medicine. The Royal College of Radiologists has reported little appetite among its members in Scotland for the role of radiographers in reporting of cross-sectional images, stating that only medical professionals may produce reports that can be truly "diagnostic and actionable," whilst they consider radiographers' reports to be "observational and descriptive" (RCR 2017). The College of Radiographers understandably has taken issue with this, and has sought to emphasize the importance of advanced practice radiography more widely.

7.8 Conclusion

This chapter has provided a discussion surrounding the current position of advanced practice for the diagnostic radiographer, therapeutic radiographer, and sonographer within the modern workforce. Recent drivers for change have led to a reassessment of the notion of advanced practice within the imaging and radiotherapy workforce, with aspects of education and levels of competence being the focus of interest. In particular, the many varied and complex differences that exist between individual advanced practice radiographers within their own defined job description has led to debate surrounding that which truly qualifies as advanced practice. Real gains with respect to efficiency and cost saving have been reported, particularly in the field of advanced practice diagnostic radiographer reporting, and the workflow within a radiotherapy department enabled by advanced practitioner therapeutic radiographers. Despite this, there is scope to gain more research evidence to assess the impact the advanced practitioner radiographer has within the context of measurable patient outcomes.

Key Questions

1. Suggest barriers to the adoption and implementation of the advanced practice radiographer role. Discuss how these might be overcome.
2. What are the key gains that may be achieved via the adoption of advanced practice roles by diagnostic radiographers, therapeutic radiographers, and sonographers?
3. What key metrics might be used to evaluate the impact of the role of the advanced practice radiographer?

Glossary

Brachytherapy: a form of radiotherapy whereby the source of radiation is positioned within or very close to the area that requires treatment.

College of Radiographers (CoR; https://www.sor. org/college-of-radiographers): the professional body for radiographers and all non-medical members of the workforce in diagnostic imaging and radiotherapy in the UK.

Computerized tomography (CT): X-ray imaging that produces detailed anatomical images in slices throughout the scanned subject.

Diagnostic radiographer: a Health and Care Professions Council–protected title for a specialist, non-medical imaging professional specializing predominantly in a broad range of X-ray imaging procedures.

Image-guided radiotherapy (IGRT): a form of radiotherapy in which frequent imaging is used before and during radiotherapy to ensure the planned treatment is administered accurately and safely.

Intensity-modulated radiotherapy (IMRT): a form of radiotherapy in which advanced technologies allow for the administration of X-ray beams of varying intensities, so that the radiation treatment administered may conform to the shape of the tumor.

Mammographer: a non-medical imaging professional specializing in breast imaging.

Magnetic resonance imaging (MRI): medical imaging using magnetic field and radio waves to generate anatomical and physiological images throughout the scanned subject.

Radiologist: a medical professional specializing in the field of medical imaging.

Radiotherapy: the use of ionizing radiation (e.g. high energy X-rays) to treat diseases including cancer.

Sonographer: a health practitioner specializing in the use of medical ultrasound for the purpose of clinical imaging. A sonographer is a nonregulated professional and the title is not protected.

Therapeutic radiographer: a Health and Care Professions Council–protected title for a specialist non-medical radiotherapy treatment professional responsible for the planning and delivery of accurate radiotherapy treatments.

References

Buskov, L., Abild, A., Christensen, A. et al. (2013). Radiographers and trainee radiologists reporting accident radiographs: a comparative plain film-reading performance study. *Clinical Radiology* 68: 55–58.

Cancer Research UK and NHS England (2014). *Vision for Radiotherapy 2014–2024*. London: CRUK, NHS England.

College of Radiographers (2009). *Radiotherapy Moving Forward: Delivering New Radiography Staffing Models in Response to the Cancer Reform Strategy*. London: College of Radiographers.

College of Radiographers (2010). *Education and Professional Development: New Directions*. London: College of Radiographers.

College of Radiographers (2013). *Education and Career Framework for the Radiography Workforce*. London: College of Radiographers.

College of Radiographers (2017). *Consultant Radiographer – Guidance for the Support of New and Established Roles*. College of Radiographers: London.

Cowling, C. (2008). A global overview of the changing roles of radiographers. *Radiography* 14: e28–e32.

Department of Health (2000). *The NHS Cancer Plan*. Department of Health: London.

Department of Health (2003). *Radiography Skills Mix: A Report on the Four-tier Service Delivery Model*. London: Department of Health.

Department of Health (2007a). *Modernising Allied Health Profession (AHP) Careers. A Competence Based Framework*. London: Department of Health.

Department of Health (2007b). *The Cancer Reform Strategy*. London: Department of Health.

Department of Health (2013). *Delivering High Quality, Effective, Compassionate Care: Developing the Right People with the Right Skills and the Right Values. A Mandate from the Government to Health Education England: April 2013 to March 2015*. London: Department of Health.

Eddy, A. (2008). Advanced practice for therapy radiographers – a discussion paper. *Radiography* 14: 24–31.

England, A., Best, A., and Friend, C. (2010). A comparison of radiographers and radiologists in CT based measurements of abdominal aortic aneurysms. *Radiography* 16: 321–326.

Field L. J and Snaith B. (2013) Developing radiographer roles in the context of advanced and consultant practice. *Journal of Medical Radiation Sciences* 60 (1): 11–15.

Griffiths, M. (2013). Advanced practice in radiography. Advanced Practice for Patient Benefit: Advanced Practice Conference, 12 March 2013. http://eprints.uwe.ac.uk/22065/1/Advanced%20practice%20in%20radiography_13.pdf (accessed January 8, 2019).

Hardy, M., Johnson, L., Sharples, R. et al. (2016). Does radiography advanced practice improve patient outcomes and health service quality? A systematic review. *British Journal of Radiology* 89 (1062): 20151066.

Health Education England. (2017a) Cancer Workforce Plan. Phase 1: Delivering the cancer strategy to 2021. https://www.hee.nhs.uk/sites/default/files/documents/Cancer%20Workforce%20Plan%20phase%201%20-%20Delivering%20the%20cancer%20strategy%20to%202021.pdf (accessed January 8, 2019).

Health Education England. (2017b). Multi-professional framework for advanced clinical practice in England. https://www.hee.nhs.uk/our-work/advanced-clinical-practice/multi-professional-framework (accessed January 8, 2019).

Henderson, I., Mathers, S., McConnell, J., and Minnoch, D. (2016). Advanced and extended scope practice of radiographers: the Scottish perspective. *Radiography* 22: 185–193.

McGee, P. and Cole, D. (2009). Advanced practice in allied health professions. In: *Advanced Practice in Nursing and the Allied Health Professions*, 3e (ed. P. McGee), 29–42. Oxford, UK: Wiley-Blackwell.

Milner, R. and Snaith, B. (2017). Are reporting radiographers fulfilling the role of advanced practitioner? *Radiography* 23 (1): 48–54.

Nightingale, J. and McNulty, J. (2016). Maximising the potential of the modern radiographer workforce. *Health Management* 16 (3): 230–233.

Rolfe, G. (2014). Understanding advanced nursing practice. *Nursing Times* 110 (27): 20–23.

Royal College of Radiologists (2017). The radiology crisis in Scotland: sustainable solutions are needed now. https://www.rcr.ac.uk/posts/radiology-crisis-scotland-sustainable-solutions-are-needed-now (accessed January 8, 2019).

Royal College of Radiologists, Society and College of Radiographers (2012). *Team Working in Clinical Imaging*. London: RCR/SCoR.

Westbrook, C. (2017). Opening the debate on MRI practitioner education – is there a need for change? *Radiography* 23: S70–S74.

Woznitza, N. (2014). Radiographer reporting. *Journal of Medical Radiation Sciences* 61: 66–68.

CHAPTER 8

Advanced Practice in Speech and Language Therapy

Susan Beaumont

Worcestershire Health and Care NHS Trust, Worcester, UK

Key Issues
- Advanced practice in speech and language therapy
- Facilitating the development of less experienced colleagues
- Treating swallowing difficulties in children with profound disabilities

LEARNING OBJECTIVES

By the end of this chapter you will be able to:

- Critically compare and contrast the advanced skills demonstrated by the advanced speech and language therapist with those required in your own field of healthcare practice.

- Discuss the role of the advanced speech and language therapist in promoting ethical practice with children and their families.

- Critically examine the leadership role of the advanced speech and language therapist.

8.1 Introduction

Speech, language, communication, and swallowing involve a complex combination of skills and systems in the body: neurological, cognitive, physical, respiratory, gastrointestinal, and psychological. These skills are

Advanced Practice in Healthcare: Dynamic Developments in Nursing and Allied Health Professions,
Fourth Edition. Edited by Paula McGee and Chris Inman.
© 2019 John Wiley & Sons Ltd. Published 2019 by John Wiley & Sons Ltd.

taken for granted, so problems, when they arise, can cause extreme stress for the individual and family, and have potentially serious consequences such as educational and literacy difficulties, unemployment, offending, bullying, social exclusion, and physical and mental health issues (Morris and Klein 2000; Royal College of Speech and Language Therapists [RCSLT] 2017). In the UK, speech and language therapists (SLTs) are the leading experts in dealing with these problems. Their pre-registration training and subsequent experience give them greater depth of knowledge and skill in the assessment, differential diagnosis, treatment, and management of these disorders (RCSLT 2018). Once competences are attained, SLTs act autonomously. The management of some disorders, such as dysphagia, however, requires postgraduate preparation and supervised clinical practice before individuals can take full responsibility (Boaden et al. 2006).

The advanced speech and language therapist (ASLT) role was defined in 2005 in preparation for the Agenda for Change (RCSLT 2005; RCSLT and Amicus 2005). Most of the role focused on the direct clinical care of patients and the key differences to other SLT roles related to the level of freedom to act, knowledge and skills, planning and organization, and research. In practice, few SLTs use the term "advanced" in their title. At the same time, principal and consultant SLT roles were also clearly defined (RCSLT and Amicus 2005). These definitions remain in place today. Since that time, however, a generic analysis of advanced and consultant roles across health professions has further clarified the distinction between these two levels of practice (Skills for Health 2014a, b). For example, an advanced practitioner "demonstrates leadership and innovation in work contexts that are unpredictable and that require solving problems involving many interacting factors" (Skills for Health 2014a, p. 2). In contrast, a consultant practitioner also "demonstrates leadership," but here the emphasis is on "novel situations" (Skills for Health 2014b, p. 2). An advanced practitioner works across professional boundaries, has a wide breadth of knowledge and experience, is creative, and develops others. Alongside these generic attributes are role/profession-specific competences. A consultant practitioner role carries more responsibility, particularly for extending the evidence base for practice, assuming a leadership position in service improvement, and extending the boundaries of the particular field in which the post is situated (Skills for Health 2014b). RCSLT now endorses the Multi-professional Framework for Advanced Clinical Practice in England (NHS Health Education England 2017).

The framework is to be welcomed in encouraging consistency across the professions. Currently, these SLT roles vary between organizations. Variations may be related to the context, for example the staffing structure within the service, the size of the service, or funding issues. In some, an advanced practitioner may be the lead clinician in the clinical area of the service, whilst in others there may also be a principal or consultant and the roles will differ accordingly.

This chapter focuses on the ASLT role, with particular reference to the management of dysphagia in children, the author's specialism. The management of dysphagia is a very sensitive area of practice; difficulties in swallowing can be life threatening (Colodny 2005). Referral to an SLT may be a major shock for parents (Beaumont 2012), many of whom are facing clinical uncertainty about their child (Calnan 1984). All SLTs need good communication skills and to be competent in processing and conveying complex, sensitive information, because speech and language treatments are routinely delivered to children through their parents. Skills are transferred so that treatments can take place at home.

A relationship between therapist and parent, involving mutually understood roles and goals, is therefore essential to successful treatment (Bazley 2000; Glogowska and Campbell 2000; Marshall et al. 2007; Morris and Klein 2000). ASLTs have more experience of complex situations and those where issues may be contentious. At such times it is appropriate for an SLT to seek support from an ASLT. This may take the form of clinical supervision to talk through the case, or it may be necessary for a joint assessment or consultation to take place.

CASE STUDY

Many children with long-term learning and/or physical difficulties are totally dependent on parents and healthcare professionals from many disciplines. The care of these children raises a number of challenges and ethical dilemmas, which are sometimes kept under the spotlight for extensive periods of time by the media and receive a great deal of public attention. Decision making regarding care is key to advanced practice in all specialties and the ethical dimensions inevitably cause debates and dilemmas for the public and healthcare practitioners. The hypothetical case study discussed here examines one aspect of the challenges that may arise, parental refusal of a change in treatment, but it is not based on any particular case. The intention is to generate debate around the advanced practice decision-making issues which are transferable to other disciplines.

Dale was a child diagnosed with sensorimotor dysphagia secondary to complex medical conditions. The speech and language therapy service provided treatment from soon after birth, alongside interventions from practitioners in numerous professions. Dale attended a special school for children who had profound and multiple learning and other disabilities (PMLD) and was fully dependent on adults for all aspects of daily living. This included feeding. Dale was usually fed orally but, following an acute illness, was left physically weakened, with reduced ability and desire to consume enough food and drink safely, which worsened an already severe risk of aspiration (Hibberd et al. 2004). Dale's mother, the SLT, the school nurse, and the school staff were all concerned about the child's inability to consume enough food and fluid and the risk of aspiration, especially as Dale lost weight. In addition, reports from the GP and hospital consultant revealed that Dale had recently suffered repeated upper respiratory tract infections, with simultaneous crackles in the chest on each occasion; both the GP and the consultant considered that these infections were viral in origin. Treatment techniques were trialled, but did not improve the situation. The

SLT considered that instrumental assessment was needed to provide additional information regarding Dale's swallow status and risk of aspiration. She therefore sought help and advice from the ASLT, who was competent to carry this assessment out. Now consider your answers to the following Exercise 8.1:

EXERCISE 8.1

What are the elements of the consultant role in advanced practice?

The SLT and ASLT jointly assessed Dale's ability to swallow and behaviour during a mealtime observation. The ASLT also carried out cervical auscultation (Frakking et al. 2013). They considered Dale's presentation holistically regarding health status, developmental skills, and environmental factors, and discussed the findings in the light of current knowledge regarding predictive factors for aspiration pneumonia (Hibberd et al. 2013). The SLT then met with Dale's mother and advised that the child met the criteria for a Videofluoroscopic Swallow Study (VFSS; Arvedson 2013). Pediatric VFSS was not available locally, so the ASLT negotiated access at the regional hospital and referral via the local pediatrician, who, under the Ionizing Radiation (Medical Exposure) Regulations 2000 (Department of Health 2017), could justify the procedure and authorize the expenditure. The SLT contacted the pediatrician and a VFSS was arranged.

VFSS is an instrumental procedure for which additional SLT competences are required. Although the SLT understood the procedure from her dysphagia training, she had only discussed it in role-play situations at that time. The ASLT, therefore, accompanied her to provide support and assess her competence when discussing the procedure with Dale's mother. The SLT explained the procedure, including the risks and benefits, seating, other feeding requirements, and the possible outcomes of the assessment, one of which might be non-oral feeding. Dale's mother expressed her opposition to non-oral feeding. She felt that mealtimes were the only time that Dale communicated with her and that oral feeding was important to quality of life. Even so, she wanted the VFSS to proceed due to concerns about possible dehydration, despite explanations by the SLT that the procedure would not directly address this. The SLT and ASLT accompanied Dale and the mother to the VFSS; the ASLT worked with the SLT to analyze the results and formulate a diagnosis, which they explained to Dale's mother. The VFSS revealed severe, overt, and silent aspiration, implying that continuing oral feeding would incur a serious risk of aspiration pneumonia (Tutor and Gosa 2012; Cass et al. 2005; Weir et al. 2007). Now consider your answers to the following Exercise 8.2:

> ### EXERCISE 8.2
>
> Dealing with professionals can be a daunting process for relatives. In your field of practice, how could you, as an advanced practitioner, provide help and support to a relative who has a difficult decision to make about a loved one?

Subsequent referral to a respiratory consultant determined that Dale's lung function and status were satisfactory. The consultant recognized that Dale was at severe risk of aspiration, had been unable to meet nutrition and hydration requirements, and could not consistently consume medication. Supplemental tube feeding with some limited oral feeding was recommended by the consultant to stabilize Dale's health and weight. The mother remained resistant to any tube feeding and refused consent to this plan, but she agreed to take part in a meeting with school staff and health and other professionals to consider the recommendations (Arvedson and Brodsky 2002). She also agreed that further information and preparation would be helpful prior to the meeting, and the SLT organized this with ASLT advice and support.

The first step was a discussion between Dale's mother, the SLT, and the deputy head teacher about the implications for feeding in school. Dale was normally fed by teaching assistants and lunchtime staff in school but, given the outcome of the assessment, this was no longer possible. In future, Dale's mother would feed her child at lunchtime. The SLT then asked the deputy head teacher to arrange for the mother to meet with the parents of a child with similar difficulties and the community nurses, for them to give information about the care involved in non-oral feeding.

As the situation was potentially contentious, the SLT asked the ASLT to explain the risks and benefits of non-oral versus oral feeding to Dale's mother. This included ways of incorporating communication strategies into non-oral feeding situations. The ASLT acknowledged that the implications for long-term aspiration have not yet been established through research. She also acknowledged that tube feeding is not risk free (Gantasala et al. 2013; NPSA 2005, 2011). They discussed the complexities of Dale's health status and the elements that have been found to be significant in predicting the risk of aspiration pneumonia (Hibberd et al. 2013). They also discussed the need for medication, as well as the provision of nutrition and hydration. The ASLT highlighted these aspects as contributing to the child's quality of life and, in so doing, gently challenged Dale's mother's thoughts regarding this. She also, however, reassured her that the time spent preparing tasty food would not be wasted and that Dale could continue to savour smaller amounts. The ASLT needed to raise the issue of Dale's refusal of food and drink beyond small amounts, and this was particularly difficult emotionally for the mother. Sensitivity was needed, as Dale's mother was worried about her child's inability to meet these requirements. The ASLT openly acknowledged these difficulties and listened to allow the mother to express her emotion and concerns.

Dale's mother later agreed that the meeting should go ahead and that she felt prepared. At the meeting, she took an active role in discussing the different aspects of the plan and the factors for consideration. She continued, however, to oppose the recommendation of supplemental tube feeding alongside limited oral feeding. Her stated reasons for disagreement remained the same.

Now consider your answers to the following Exercise 8.3:

> ### EXERCISE 8.3
>
> What are the ethical issues in this situation?

IMPLICATIONS

Parental refusal of treatment presents an ethical dilemma for health professionals. Parents are autonomous in their child's care, unless that autonomy is legally removed from them. They are also advocates for their children. Decisions regarding the need for non-oral feeding are led by the medical team, but include information from other health professionals and parents. Decisions regarding continued oral feeding for children with dysphagia and a known risk of aspiration and respiratory presentations are based on the child's presumed ability to tolerate the consequences of ongoing aspiration (Lefton-Greif and McGrath-Morrow 2007).

Parental refusal of non-oral feeding can create a complex situation with potentially serious consequences (Body and McAllister 2009). The child could suffer physical harm; all involved could suffer emotional harm; and parents and professionals could also be open to legal challenges. There is a high risk of conflict, which can escalate into protracted legal battles. SLT practice with adults who choose to continue with oral intake despite a recognized risk of aspiration, or for whom tube feeding is unsuitable, is guided by established risk feeding protocols (Hansjee 2013). When a child is involved, the situation is far less clear cut. Each child will have a different range of professionals involved in providing care, treatment, and education in community settings, and these may be locally, regionally, or even nationally spread. Gathering everyone together to try to find a way forward can be a challenging exercise, and in this case did not result in parental acceptance of the plan. Now consider your answers to the following Exercise 8.4:

EXERCISE 8.4

How far should parental autonomy extend and who should decide a child's best interests?

FURTHER DEVELOPMENT OF THE SERVICE

The ASLT led the multidisciplinary team in the development of pathways and protocols for children at risk of aspiration, to ensure timely intervention and referral for monitoring of their pulmonary, nutrition, and hydration status (Cass et al. 2005; National Institute for Health and Care Excellence [NICE] 2017). A routine annual review of nutrition, hydration, and swallow status by relevant professionals allowed a baseline to be established and tracking of progress by the pediatrician to occur. Triggers, such as unexplained weight loss and frequent chest infections, were identified for the involvement of different team members when needed, such as the dietician, SLT, or pediatrician. This allowed for the timely sharing of information and, wherever possible, prevention of problems from escalating. The aim is for decision making about nutrition and hydration to become much more team based. Agreed protocols ensure the involvement of parents and carers throughout the process, so that they are more informed and involved in discussions and more prepared as problems arise.

In cases where parents disagree with team recommendations, formal protocols can provide a framework for staff, so that they can continue to support families as appropriate. Such protocols should enable consideration of medical recommendations, patient and parent preferences, quality of life, contextual factors, capacity for decision making, and ethics (RCSLT 2018; Johnsen et al. 2010; Morrow et al. 2006). Consideration of these factors, open acknowledgment of differing opinions, and recognition of the limitations of current knowledge are essential in maintaining a respectful dialogue between professionals and parents in order to safeguard the interests of the child. Parents are advocates for their child and the child is reliant on their decision making. It often takes time and very detailed and sensitive communication for professionals and parents to understand one another's viewpoints. In some cases, however, more urgent medical intervention is needed to safeguard the child. Thresholds for a safeguarding referral in these situations, where there are no other unrelated concerns about the safety of children, need to be established. The involvement of a social worker for children with disabilities at an earlier stage in the pathway may support the dialogue between professionals and parents, and might prevent the need for the escalation of concern.

The challenge involves changing the culture of the teams around the child so that all understand and respect the limitations of each other's findings and roles in these situations, but continue to work collaboratively to support the child and family. Policies and protocols support the process, but take time to establish.

8.2 The Role of the Advanced Practitioner Speech and Language Therapist

The case presented here demonstrates the role of the ASLT in a range of activities. It highlights the complex decision making that can arise in treating a child with PMLD, and facilitating both the family and the professionals involved with the aim of negotiating an appropriate outcome. In addressing Dale's situation, the ASLT used her expertise to enable others rather than to take over their roles. This required the indirect application of expert practice, combined with coaching, guiding, and leadership. Each is discussed in the following sections.

8.2.1 Expert Practice

The case study demonstrates some aspects of the advanced practitioner's clinical expertise. On a practical level, this is evident in instrumental examination. The ASLT had undertaken further training and assessment to meet the requirements of RCSLT regarding competences for managing dysphagia (RCSLT 2013). She was competent to carry out cervical auscultation, to manage or support others to manage cases needing VFSS, and to train and support others in doing so. Other areas of competence in this field requiring additional training include neonates and children under 12 months of age (RCSLT 2014a), tracheostomy (RCSLT 2014b), and fiberoptic endoscopic evaluation of swallowing (RCSLT 2015). These skills are not limited to ASLTs, but training and supervision in acquiring them may not be easily available (RCSLT 2008). ASLTs are frequently the lead experts in their specialism in their own healthcare organizations and NHS Trusts. The assessment of their competence within their own organization, as they acquire these skills, can be challenging.

The ASLT's interpersonal skills are also evident in this case study. These were important in working effectively with the SLT, school staff, and Dale's mother, whose emotional journey in this situation cannot be underestimated (Gantasala et al. 2013; Cass et al. 2005; Guerrierre et al. 2003). Parents may resist non-oral feeding, particularly when, as in this case, mealtimes are perceived to present the only opportunity for some form of meaningful communication with their child. It is vital to maintain good communication with parents to ensure that they remain fully engaged with decision making. Communication in a situation such as Dale's is highly sensitive and is vulnerable to breakdown (Beaumont 2012). The ASLT was able to facilitate communication between the SLT and Dale's mother by remaining close to, rather than distant from, the situation.

Professional relationships that maintain closeness rather than detachment have been found to be valued by parents in similar situations (Beaumont 2012). Closeness can help to create an environment in which all those involved are able to voice their concerns and feel that they will be listened to with respect (Hamric and Delgado 2014). This is particularly important for parents, who may feel overwhelmed by both events and professionals. In remaining close, the ASLT can restore confidence and empower parents to take an active role in discussion and decision making (Beaumont 2012). The ASLT led preparation for the meeting with Dale's mother, which allowed her to actively discuss the factors involved with professionals and the ethical issues. Skills include separating feelings from the problem, but recognizing both as important, and acting as a broker, enabling the various parties to hear one another (Whiteing 2008; Hamric and Delgado 2014). Dale's mother did not accept the plan for supplemental tube feeding alongside limited oral feeding. By maintaining a respectful dialogue, however, the ASLT paved the way for future discussion.

8.2.2 Education

The case study shows the advanced practitioner engaged in educational activities with the SLT and Dale's mother. These were informal, allowing the ASLT's knowledge and skill to be shared in a conversational style and practical application rather than lectures. This approach is consistent with remaining close to a situation and using interpersonal skills to facilitate others. Thus, the ASLT's educational activities focused on *coaching and guiding* to help others make changes in their lives, adapt to new circumstances, or integrate new information. These changes are referred to as *transitions*, which are characterized by uncertainty and the experience of new needs that do not fit with one's current life. Transitions may be developmental or situational, and arise because of changes in one's state of health or because of organizational changes. An individual may experience one or several transitions at any one time (Hamric and Babine 2014).

For the SLT in this case, the transitions were related to the changes in Dale's swallowing and state of health, but may also have been related to her own professional development, because it was she who approached the ASLT. Thus, the need for coaching and guiding reflected an acknowledgment of the limitations of her expertise. In the case study, the ASLT worked alongside the SLT to assess Dale's swallow and the factors at play in this situation. The ASLT did not take over; rather, she enabled the SLT to use her own knowledge and then guided her through interventions that included investigations and explaining the findings and their implications to Dale's mother, with the aim of bringing about change. Underpinning this activity were the ASLT's interpersonal skills, her enhanced expertise, and her own assessment of the risks inherent in the situation.

For Dale's mother, the transitions were related to coping with new information and adapting to changes in her child's life. Here, the ASLT established and maintained communication, ensuring that Dale's mother understood the outcomes of the assessments her child required, and the risks and benefits of change versus a lack of change in Dale's care. The ASLT was not successful in enabling Dale's mother to accept change, but kept open the opportunity for further discussion. However, realistically, the risks and benefits of postponing change might have to be weighed against those relating to the child's well-being.

At a broader professional level, ASLTs have a responsibility to facilitate the development of colleagues. In addition to working with individual SLTs, an ASLT will also provide regular clinical supervision to individuals and groups alongside other experienced members of an SLT team. This allows the sharing of complex issues, benchmarking of services, and undertaking of projects. Membership of Clinical Excellence Network groups overseen by RCSLT nationally for continuing professional development is also encouraged. However, the provision of clinical supervision for ASLTs themselves can be more problematic. There may not be any provision within the employing organization and it may be necessary to arrange clinical supervision elsewhere. The ASLT's responsibilities also extend to participation in the clinical training of undergraduates, clinical tutoring, and support at postgraduate level. An ASLT needs to know service requirements and ensure training is targeted to provide value for money. Other training requirements may include the practical training of school staff who feed children with dysphagia to more academic talks to medical consultants and general practitioners (GPs). As ASLTs gain professional credibility and a reputation, requests to share their knowledge and experience present further opportunities, for example to speak at regional and national conferences. An ASLT's knowledge and skills are then open to peer review.

8.2.3 Leadership

The case study demonstrates the ASLT's role in providing clinical and professional leadership. The distinction between the two is that *clinical leadership* focuses on the patient and *professional leadership* on empowering fellow professionals (Tracy and Hanson 2014). In considering clinical leadership, it is evident that Dale's situation was complex. Swallowing was difficult and the desire to eat and drink diminished. Investigations revealed aspiration of food and fluid. This was a serious, potentially life-threatening situation, further complicated by Dale's other disabilities. Dale's mother, the SLT, and, no doubt, school staff all wished to do what was best for Dale, but could not find a satisfactory solution. In adopting a clinical leadership role, the ASLT focused on clarifying the salient points in the child's situation, investigating these further, and facilitating communication between the SLT, Dale's mother, the school, and the multidisciplinary team (Benner 1984). The ASLT's activities depend on a high level of clinical expertise in the management of dysphagia, particularly skill in the performance of VFSS, and a clear sense, a vision, of what is possible. An understanding of how to ensure that the healthcare system worked for Dale's benefit, for example by negotiating access to VFSS, was also essential. Sensitivity to the parent's feelings was very important. Heightened emotions among the various parties involved with Dale could easily have descended into acrimony and defensiveness alongside refusal of treatment (Body and McAllister 2009; Horner et al. 2016). The ASLT, however, worked closely with Dale's mother to understand her reasoning, ensure that it was fully informed and that she had considered all aspects of the situation. She also worked closely with the professionals involved to ensure that decision making took place in an open and supportive way, and that delay in proceeding with medical recommendations was safe for Dale.

Professional leadership was most evident in the ASLT's mentoring of the SLT, enabling her to continue in her professional role as Dale's therapist.

Coaching and guiding by the ASLT enabled the SLT to engage in constructive discussions with Dale's mother and ensure that her decisions were fully informed. Thus, the SLT remained in place as Dale's therapist and was empowered to develop her skills. Professional leadership facilitates the development of followers, enabling them to achieve in their own right (Tracy and Hanson 2014).

Throughout this case study there was an underlying thread of the ASLT's freedom to act. This is an important aspect of leadership in ASLT roles. Freedom to act here depended on multiple relationships between the ASLT, management, and the wider team involved in Dale's care. Without trust between the various parties, not only might changes in Dale's care not have been realized, but the potential development of the SLT service might have been jeopardized (Ballatt and Campling 2011). ASLTs need to gain respect for their clinical expertise and decision making so that managers can trust the calculated risks they must take in the interest of patients, innovation, or service advancement. Likewise, ASLTs need to have confidence that the team and managers will support them when they need to act. This is increasingly difficult in our risk-averse society and healthcare practice (Ballatt and Campling 2011).

At a wider level, an ASLT can provide leadership through the development of protocols and the provision of training to ensure that children with dysphagia receive safe care in the management of their feeding. Special schools are one such arena in which an ASLT can make a difference by contributing to the prevention of choking and aspiration. This helps to keep children out of hospital and promotes quality of life for the children and their families (RCSLT 2017). In the case study, it helped to enable both SLTs and school staff to fulfill their duty of care towards Dale (Health and Care Professions Council 2017).

8.3 Current Challenges in Advanced Speech and Language Therapy

Current organizational changes in the NHS, austerity measures, and competition with the independent sector demand the attention of ASLTs (Ballatt and Campling 2011). ASLTs need to be aware of proposed changes to services and contribute to consultations to ensure that quality and safety are maintained (NHS England 2017). The RCSLT Outcomes Project seeks to facilitate the gathering of data and comparison between services via an online tool (Gadhok et al. 2018). ASLTs need to be active in collecting data for service evaluation, clinical audit, and research to demonstrate to commissioners and budget holders the contribution to patient care made by SLT and ASLT services, allow them to predict trends and target training needs (Gadhok et al. 2018). Current trends, for example, indicate a need to be proactive in preparing staff to deal with increasingly complex conditions needing treatment in the community, for example children with conditions requiring long-term ventilation.

An additional issue is the retention of SLTs in post. Once trained in dysphagia, their skills are highly sought after, and opportunities for promotion in other healthcare organizations can result in high staff turnover. Staff need to feel valued and supported. They also need development opportunities to attract them to stay, and management and commissioner support may be needed to create these.

Changes in working practices are inevitable in a rapidly changing healthcare system. ASLTs need to be proactive, acting as leaders in developing new approaches. They need to be in the right place, talking to the right people, at the right time. Forging links with other services, such as neonatal and respiratory, could lead to a principal or consultant SLT negotiating contracts to ensure deeper integration in the care of children with dysphagia and more coherent service provision. A principal or consultant SLT holds responsibility for strategic planning, service development, and devising the policies needed to support these developments.

Measuring outcomes is also important for patients, their families, care settings, and commissioners at local, regional, and national levels (Moyse 2017; NHS England 2017). The RCSLT Outcomes Project has developed an online tool to improve outcome measurement, minimize the work involved in data collection, investigate the practicality of benchmarking, and assure quality across services (Gadhok et al. 2018). As dysphagia is most often co-morbid with other diagnoses and secondary to them, holistic multidisciplinary measurement of outcomes is likely to be more appropriate. This means, however, that there would not be a dysphagia outcome measure that is specific to SLT (Enderby 2016, p. 19). Outcome measurement in dysphagia is therefore complex and adaptations to the tool may need to be used (Enderby 2016, p. 19).

8.4 Conclusion

This chapter has discussed the effectiveness of ASLT in the management of dysphagia in a child with PMLD. This required the application of expertise in clinical practice, coaching and guidance, and leadership. In the current healthcare climate, advanced practitioners must be able not only to be of benefit to patients and their families, but also to produce evidence that is meaningful to service commissioners and budget holders. This requires ASLTs to be proactive in securing their future and in contributing to that of their profession.

Key Questions

1. How can you negotiate freedom to act in your field of practice?
2. What information would service commissioners and budget holders require to help them understand your contribution to patient care as an advanced practitioner?
3. What actions could managers take to encourage ASLTs to remain in a healthcare organization?

Glossary

Agenda for Change: the national pay system for National Health Service staff in the UK.

Aspiration: the passage of food or drink below the level of the vocal cords.

Aspiration pneumonia: inflammation of the lung caused by bacteria, in which the air sacs become filled with inflammatory cells and the lung becomes solid, and where aspiration is the suspected cause.

Cervical auscultation: listening to swallow sounds through a stethoscope strategically placed on the neck.

Clinical supervision: a means by which practitioners with different levels of experience can meet and reflect on practice.

Dysphagia: feeding, eating, drinking, and swallowing difficulty. This can include difficulties in the anticipatory, oral, pharyngeal, or esophageal stages of swallowing or a combination thereof.

Fiberoptic endoscopic evaluation of swallowing (FEES): an instrumental procedure in which a flexible telescope is inserted into the nose and used to view the swallow from the nasopharynx.

Health and Care Professions Council (HCPC; www.hcpc-uk.co.uk): the body that regulates 16 health and care professions in the UK, maintains a register of qualified individuals, sets standards, and approves training programs for those professions.

IR(ME)R: Ionising Radiation (Medical Exposure) Regulations 2000: regulations regarding the use of radiation.

Multidisciplinary team: the team of different professionals involved in a child's care. In the care of children with PMLD and dysphagia, key health professionals may include consultant pediatrician, speech and language therapist, dietician, school or community nurse, physiotherapist, and occupational therapist. Professionals from other agencies may include school staff and a social worker for children with disabilities.

National Institute for Health and Clinical Excellence (NICE; www.nice.org.uk): the body that provides evidence-based guidance, advice, resources, and information for health and social care professionals.

Non-oral feeding: see tube feeding.

Profound and multiple learning disabilities (PMLD): a combination of severe learning difficulty with other disabilities. There are often associated problems with motor, sensory, and communication skills. People with PMLD often have a severely compromised ability to live independently.

Royal College of Speech and Language Therapists (www.rcslt.org): the professional body for speech and language therapists in the UK.

Sensorimotor dysphagia: deficits in both the sensory (input division of the nervous system) and motor (output division of the nervous system) aspects of swallowing.

Silent aspiration: aspiration with no overt signs such as coughing.

Skills for Health (www.skillsforhealth.org.uk): an organization that supports employers in developing the workforce skills and procedures required for the provision of efficient, cost-effective, and flexible health services.

Special school: a UK term for a school providing education for children with additional needs, for example learning disabilities, behavioral problems, developmental issues, or physical disabilities. Special schools provide the facilities and individualized approaches that would not be possible in typical educational settings.

Supplemental tube feeding: when tube feeding is used alongside oral feeding to support the meeting of nutrition and hydration needs, which would otherwise not be maintained.

Tracheostomy: a surgical procedure in which a hole is made in the trachea and a tube inserted to bypass an obstruction to breathing in the airway.

Tube feeding: introducing a nutritionally complete formula via a tube through the nose and into the stomach (nasogastric tube feeding) or via a PEG (percutaneous endoscopic gastrostomy, an endoscopic procedure involving insertion of a tube through the stomach wall) to provide a means of feeding when oral feeding is not adequate to meet nutrition and hydration requirements.

Videoflouroscopic Swallow Study (VFSS): an instrumental dynamic radiographical study of swallowing. The procedure is performed by a radiologist, who helps the ASLT analyze the information gained. A radiographer and ASLT are also in attendance.

Acknowledgments

Heartfelt thanks to Judi Hibberd, Sarah Hanlon, and Karen Hayden for their helpful comments regarding this chapter and, along with Deb Whiting, for their continued support in clinical supervision.

References

Arvedson, J.C. (2013). Feeding children with cerebral palsy and swallowing difficulties. *European Journal of Clinical Nutrition* 67: 59–512.

Advedson, J.C. and Brodsky, L. (2002). *Paediatric Swallowing and Feeding: Assessment and Management*, 2e. Toronto: Singular Thomson Learning.

Ballatt, J. and Campling, P. (2011). *Intelligent Kindness: Reforming the Culture of Healthcare*. London: RCPsych Publications.

Bazley, R. (2000). Speech and language. In: *Working with Parents: Learning from Other People's Experience* (ed. A. Wheal). Dorset: Russell House Publishing.

Beaumont S. (2012) What are a parent's expectations and experiences of an initial appointment with an advanced speech and language therapist with regard to their child's feeding? MSc dissertation. Birmingham City University.

Benner, P. (1984). *From Novice to Expert: Excellence and Power in Clinical Nursing Practice*. Boston, MA: Addison-Wesley.

Boaden E., Davies S., Storey L. on behalf of the National Dysphagia Competence Steering Group (2006). Interprofessional Dysphagia Framework. https://www.rcslt.org/-/media/Project/RCSLT/framework.pdf (accessed January 20, 2019).

Body, R. and McAllister, L. (2009). *Ethics in Speech and Language Therapy*. Chichester: Wiley.

Calnan, M. (1984). Clinical uncertainty: is it a problem in the doctor-patient relationship. *Sociology of Health and Illness* 6 (1): 74–85.

Cass, H., Wallis, C., Ryan, M. et al. (2005). Assessing the pulmonary consequences of dysphagia in children with neurological disabilities: when to intervene? *Medicine and Child Neurology* 47: 347–352.

Colodny, N. (2005). Dysphagic independent feeders' justifications for noncompliance with recommendations by a speech-language pathologist. *American Journal of Speech-Language Pathology* 14: 61–70.

Department of Health (2017). Ionising Radiation (Medical Exposure) Regulations 2000. http://www.legislation.gov.uk/uksi/2000/1059/contents/made (accessed January 8, 2019).

Enderby P. (2016). Outcome measures in acute dysphagia. RCSLT Bulletin February. 19.

Frakking, T.T., Chang, A.B., O'Grady, K.-A.F. et al. (2013). Cervical auscultation in the diagnosis of oropharyngeal aspiration in children: a study protocol for a randomised controlled trial. *Trials* 14 (Nov 7): 377.

Gadhok K., Farrell J., Moyse K .(2018). Are you ROOT ready? The value of the RCSLT Online Outcome Tool. Webinar and presentation. https://www.rcslt.org/past-events-and-webinars/are-you-root-ready-the-value-of-the-rcslt-online-outcome-tool (accessed January 20, 2019).

Gantasala, S., Sullivan, P.B., and Thomas, A.G. (2013). Gastrostomy feeding versus oral feeding alone for children with cerebral palsy. *Cochrane Developmental, Psychosocial and Learning Problems Group* 31 (7): CD003943. https://doi.org/10.1002/14651858.CD003943.pub3.

Glogowska, M. and Campbell, R. (2000). Investigating parental views of involvement in pre-school speech and language therapy. *International Journal of Language and Communication Disorders* 35 (3): 391–405.

Guerrierre, D.N., McKeever, P., Llewellyn-Thomas, H., and Berall, G. (2003). Mothers' decisions about gastrostomy insertion in children: factors contributing to uncertainty. *Developmental Medicine and Child Neurology* 45: 470–476.

Hamric, A. and Babine, R. (2014). Guidance and coaching. In: *Advanced Nursing Practice. An Integrative Approach*, 5e (ed. A. Hamric, J. Spross and C. Hanson), 183–212. St. Louis: Elsevier Saunders.

Hamric, A. and Delgado, S. (2014). Ethical decision making. In: *Advanced Nursing Practice. An Integrative Approach*, 5e (ed. A. Hamric, J. Spross and C. Hanson), 328–357. St. Louis: Elsevier Saunders.

Hansjee D. (2013). A safer approach to risk feeding. RCSLT Bulletin February. 20–21.

Health and Care Professions Council (HCPC) (2017). Standards of conduct, performance and ethics https://www.hcpc-uk.org/standards/standards-of-conduct-performance-and-ethics (accessed January 8, 2019).

Hibberd, J., Fraser, J., Chapman, C. et al. (2013). Can we use influencing factors to predict aspiration pneumonia in the UK? *Multidisciplinary Respiratory Medicine* 8: 39. https://doi.org/10.1186/2049-6958-8-39.

Hibberd J., Silk I., Taylor J. (2004). Ascribing a risk of aspiration for dysphagia In children. Course by Quest Training UK, 3 March 2004, Birmingham.

Horner, J., Modayil, M., Roche Chapman, L., and Dinh, A. (2016). Tutorial: consent, refusal, and waivers in patient-centred dysphagia care: using law, ethics and evidence to guide clinical practice. *American Journal of Speech-Language Pathology* 25: 453–469. November.

Johnsen, A.R., Siegler, M., and Winslade, W.J. (2010). *Clinical Ethics: A Practical Approach to Clinical Decisions in Medicine*, 7e. New York: McGraw-Hill.

Lefton-Greif, M.A. and McGrath-Morrow, S.A. (2007). Deglutition and respiration: development, coordination, and practical implications. *Seminars in Speech and Language* 28 (3): 166–179.

Marshall, J., Goldbart, J., and Phillips, J. (2007). Parents' and speech and language therapists' explanatory models of language development, language delay and intervention. *International Journal of Language and Communication Disorders* 42 (5): 533–555.

Morris, S.E. and Klein, M.D. (2000). *Pre-feeding Skills: A Comprehensive Resource for Mealtime Development*, 2e. Annandale, VA: Therapy Skill Builders.

Morrow, A.M., Quine, S., and Craig, J.C. (2006). Health professionals' perceptions of feeding-related quality of life in children with quadriplegic cerebral palsy. *Child Care, Health and Development* 33 (5): 529–538.

Moyse, K. (2017). *Outcomes and SLT: Interpretations and Context.* London: RCSLT.

National Health Service England (2017). *Allied Health Professions into Action. Using Allied Health Professionals to Transform Health, Care and Wellbeing.* London: NHS England.

National Institute for Health and Care Excellence (2017). Guideline NG 62: Cerebral palsy in under 25s: assessment and management. https://www.nice.org.uk/guidance/ng62 (accessed January 8, 2019).

National Patient Safety Agency (2005). Reducing the harm caused by misplaced nasogastric feeding tubes – Patient Safety Alert – 90 KB 0180-2005-02-21-V1. https://www.plymouthhospitals.nhs.uk/download.cfm?doc=docm93jijm4n2687 (accessed January 19, 2019).

National Patient Safety Agency (2011). Learning from patient safety incidents. http://www.nrls.npsa.nhs.uk/resources/?entryid45=94851 (accessed January 8, 2019).

NHS Health Education England (2017) *Multi-professional framework for advanced clinical practice in England.* https://www.hee.nhs.uk/our-work/advanced-clinical-practice/multi-professional-framework (accessed 9 May, 2019).

Royal College of Speech and Language Therapists (2005). *Agenda for Change: Guidance for Speech and Language Therapy Staff for Developing KSF Outlines.* London: RCSLT.

Royal College of Speech and Language Therapists (2008). *Policy Statement: Evolving Roles in Speech and Language Therapy.* London: RCSLT.

Royal College of Speech and Language Therapists (2013). *Videofluoroscopic Evaluation of Oropharyngeal Swallowing Function (VFS): The Role of Speech and Language Therapists. RCSLT Position Paper 2013.* London: RCSLT.

Royal College of Speech and Language Therapists (2014a). *Eating, Drinking and Swallowing Disorders (Dysphagia): Recommendations for Knowledge, Skills and Competency Development across the Speech and Language Therapy Profession.* London: RCSLT.

Royal College of Speech and Language Therapists (2014b). *Tracheostomy Competency Framework.* London: RCSLT.

Royal College of Speech and Language Therapists (2015). *Position Paper: Fibreoptic Endoscopic Evaluation of Swallowing (FEES): The Role of Speech and Language Therapy.* London: RCSLT.

Royal College of Speech and Language Therapists (2017). Giving Voice Factsheets. https://www.rcslt.org/speech_and_language_therapy/docs/factsheets/children (accessed January 8, 2019).

Royal College of Speech and Language Therapists (2018). Clinical Resources: Dysphagic overview. https://www.rcslt.org/clinical_resources/dysphagia/overview (accessed January 8, 2019).

Royal College of Speech and Language Therapists and Amicus (2005). *Agenda for Change: Supplementary Guidance.* London: RCSLT.

Skills for Health (2014a). *Transferable Role Template: Career Framework Level 7.* Bristol: Skills for Health.

Skills for Health (2014b). *Transferable Role Template: Career Framework Level 8.* Bristol: Skills for Health.

Tracy, M. and Hanson, C. (2014). Leadership. In: *Advanced Nursing Practice. An Integrative Approach,* 5e (ed. A. Hamric, J. Spross and C. Hanson), 266–298. St. Louis: Elsevier Saunders.

Tutor, J.D. and Gosa, M.M. (2012). Dysphagia and aspiration in children. *Pediatric Pulmonology.* 47: 321–337.

Weir, K., McMahon, S., Barry, L. et al. (2007). Oropharyngeal aspiration and pneumonia in children. *Pediatric Pulmonology* 42: 1024–1031.

Whiteing, N. (2008). Domain 7: monitoring and ensuring the quality of health care practice. In: *Competencies for Advanced Nursing Practice* (ed. S. Hinchliff and R. Rogers), 92–119. London: Hodder-Arnold.

PART 3

The Advanced Practitioner in Direct Patient Care

CHAPTER 9

Prescribing and Advanced Practice

Andrew Campbell

Dudley & Walsall Mental Health Partnership NHS Trust, Dudley, UK

Key Issues

- The background to non-medical prescribing practice in the UK
- The entry requirements for training to become a non-medical prescriber
- Principles of safe and effective prescribing

LEARNING OBJECTIVES

By the end of this chapter you will be able to:

- Identify the historical context of non-medical prescribing in the UK.
- Understand the recent developments in non-medical prescribing for differing professional groups.
- Understand the principles of safe and effective prescribing and apply these to your practice.

9.1 Introduction

This chapter presents an overview of the prescribing of medicines by Non-Medical Prescribers (NMPs) in the UK. NMPs is a term used to refer to nurses, pharmacists, optometrists, and members of the allied health professions who are qualified to prescribe medication and medical products for patients. Many, but not all, of these professionals will be advanced practitioners. This chapter examines aspects of prescribing practice for these professionals. It begins by outlining the historical context of non-medical prescribing in the UK and some of the associated legal issues involved. The chapter then moves on to explain the process of becoming an NMP, who

Advanced Practice in Healthcare: Dynamic Developments in Nursing and Allied Health Professions,
Fourth Edition. Edited by Paula McGee and Chris Inman.
© 2019 John Wiley & Sons Ltd. Published 2019 by John Wiley & Sons Ltd.

may prescribe what, for whom, and the circumstances in which they may do so. This is followed by the principles of good prescribing as outlined by the Royal Pharmaceutical Society (RPS), and the importance of clinical governance. The chapter closes by briefly considering the potential future for non-medical prescribing, both in the UK and elsewhere. Any discussion about non-medical prescribing requires the use of terminology with which some readers may be unfamiliar; the key terms are therefore explained in the glossary.

9.2 The History of Non-medical Prescribing in the UK

NMP in the UK had its inception in 1992; legislation which permitted nurse prescribing followed in 1994 (Department of Health and Social Security 1992). Following the successful implementation of non-medical prescribing in pilot sites, a national rollout of nurse prescribing began in 1998 and was completed by March 2001. In 2003, pharmacists were the second group of health professionals to become eligible to train to become NMPs (Baqir et al. 2012) and since then there has been an increase in the number of healthcare professionals who are eligible to become NMPs, the number of NMPs, and the range of medicines they are legally able to prescribe (Cope et al. 2016).

The first independent prescribing courses were launched in 2002 and, in 2006, the formulary was expanded to include all general sales list medicines, pharmacy medicines, and about 240 prescription-only medicines (Department of Health [DH] 2006). Although this was a great move forward, nurses were still limited in their ability to provide complete episodes of care. Consequently, following further consultation with the Medicines and Healthcare Products Regulatory Agency (MHRA) (2005), it was recommended that suitably qualified nurses and pharmacists would be able to prescribe any licensed medicine, excluding some controlled drugs, for any medical condition within their competence. In May 2006 these new regulations came into effect and had a huge impact on the prescribing practice of independent prescribers (DH 2006). This was particularly beneficial for advanced practitioners, who had been frustrated at being unable to complete episodes of care for their patients.

In growing recognition of the role of allied healthcare professionals as primary healthcare providers, the DH introduced supplementary prescribing rights for physiotherapists, radiographers, and chiropodists/podiatrists (DH 2005). This was followed two years later by optometrists, who joined the ranks of healthcare professionals able to independently prescribe medicines (DH 2007), and more recently physiotherapists and podiatrists were given the right to prescribe medicines independently (DH 2013). All allied health professional NMPs may prescribe only within their area of competence, for example specific ocular conditions for optometrists or movement disorders for physiotherapists. During 2016, NHS England announced new legislation permitting independent prescribing by therapeutic radiographers (NHS England 2016a) and supplementary prescribing by dietitians (NHS England, 2016b).

9.3 Registered Non-medical Prescribers in England

NMPs are a growing workforce (Table 9.1). They play an increasing role in supporting the clinical commissioning program for the National Health Service (NHS; Weeks et al. 2016). In total, there are 67 521 registered NMPs in England. However, it is recognized that, in real terms, this figure does not reflect the active NMP workforce, as not all qualified and registered NMPs are in fact using their NMP qualification. For example, a survey of NMPs in England revealed that 15% of nurses and pharmacists took longer than six months to issue their first prescription. In addition to a delay in issuing a prescription, changes in job role following training can sometimes have implications for continued prescribing practice (Latter et al. 2010).

9.4 Preparing for Prescribing

There are currently four routes to becoming an NMP:

1. Bachelor's degree–level courses for nurses, midwives, and pharmacists wishing to become independent and supplementary prescribers.
2. Master's degree–level courses for nurses and midwives wishing to become independent and supplementary prescribers.
3. Bachelor's degree–level courses for allied health professionals wishing to become supplementary prescribers.
4. Separate courses for community nurse practitioners: district nurses, health visitors, and school nurses.

The criteria for training to become an NMP vary between healthcare professions (Table 9.2).

TABLE 9.1

Numbers of registered Non-Medical Prescribers in England, 2018.

Professional group	Number of registered NMPs	% of the non-medical workforce
Nurses and midwives	59,657[a]	88.3
Pharmacists	4990[b]	7.4
Optometrists	613[c]	0.9
Allied health professionals	2261[d]	3.3
Total	67 521	

[a]Data obtained from the Nursing and Midwifery Council, February 2018.
[b]Data obtained from the General Pharmaceutical Council, January 2018.
[c]Data obtained from the General Optical Council, February 2018.
[d]Data obtained from the Health and Professions Council, February 2018.

> **TABLE 9.2**
>
> **Criteria for training to become a Non-Medical Prescriber.**
>
> Prospective trainees must:
> - Be a registered member of a healthcare professional group with a legal framework governing prescribing practice.
> - Intend to practice in an area of clinical need which will be beneficial to patient care.
> - Have the approval and support of a relevant manager and organizational non-medical prescribing lead.
> - Have practiced for a minimum of two years after qualifying in their profession.
> - Provide evidence of their ability to study at degree level.
> - Be able to identify a doctor or, where relevant, practicing prescriber who (for those undertaking V100/150 programs) will act as their practice supervisor.

9.4.1 Nurses

Community nurses are only allowed to prescribe from a limited formulary, which contains prescription-only medicines, some pharmacy medicines, and general sales list medicines, plus a list of dressings and appliances (British National Formulary and the Royal Pharmaceutical Society of Great Britain 2015–2017). The separate courses for community nurses may be undertaken either as part of a specialist practitioner program or as standalone modules for those who do not hold a specialist practitioner qualification.

All prescribing courses for nurses in other fields of practice must be validated by the Nursing and Midwifery Council (NMC; 2015) and students must meet all requirements of this body and the DH. To be accepted on a course for independent and supplementary prescribing, nurses must be registered with the NMC, have recent (within three years) Disclosure and Barring Service clearance, and three years' experience as a practicing nurse, midwife, or specialist community public health nurse. Of these three years, the year prior to application must have been in the field in which they intend to prescribe (Dowden 2016). Additionally, nurses must be sponsored and supported by their employers. Many educational institutions also stipulate that the nurse should have undertaken post-qualifying courses in history taking and health assessment, although there is a wide variation across the country regarding this.

9.4.2 Pharmacists

All pharmacist prescribers must undertake studies at an educational establishment approved by the General Pharmaceutical Council (GPhC 2017). At present there are over 40 approved programs for training to become an NMP across the UK. In 2006 regulations came into effect which allowed pharmacists to prescribe independently. Prior to this, pharmacists were able to train and practice as supplementary prescribers, and were limited to prescribing under a clinical management plan. Typically the independent prescribing program is run over a six-month period and includes face-to-face teaching and self-directed study.

9.4.3 **Allied Health Professionals**

Training to undertake independent prescribing is available to some allied health professionals, including chiropodists, podiatrists, radiographers, and physiotherapists. They are also able to train as supplementary prescribers, which means that they are not allowed to diagnose, but may plan and prescribe current and future treatments in conjunction with an independent prescriber, who may be a doctor or dentist (DH 2005). The cornerstone of the working arrangement between supplementary and independent prescribers in this situation is a clinical management plan. This is a formal, legal document developed by the independent and supplementary prescribers for an individual patient (DH 2011). The plan includes the names of the two prescribers and the patient, and details of any allergies or sensitivities to medication. The patient's condition and the aim of treatment are clearly set out. This information is followed by a list of the medication and dosage that the supplementary prescriber may prescribe and in what circumstances. The criteria for referral back to the independent prescriber must also be clearly stated. The plan should include details of how the patient will be monitored and the procedure to be followed if that person has an adverse reaction to any of the medication prescribed. Both prescribers must sign and date the plan. Allied health professionals must comply with the requirements of the Health Professions Council and the DH. These requirements reflect those for nurses, midwives, optometrists, and pharmacists.

9.4.4 **Optometrists**

Optometrists may undertake non-medical prescribing training at universities which are approved by the General Optical Council. At present there are five approved programs for training to become an NMP. The focus of the training reflects the specialty of optometry. All optometrists are able to administer and supply medication, within an existing framework, to manage simple conditions such as conjunctivitis, blepharitis, minor eye trauma, and dry eye. Optometrists who have undertaken additional accredited training can issue signed orders for an extended range of medicines. Training to become an NMP widens the scope of practice further still, enabling the prescribing of any licensed medicines for ocular conditions.

9.5 Who May Prescribe What?

All non-medical prescribing practitioners are expected to prescribe within their sphere of competence, subject to accepted good clinical practice.

9.5.1 **Nurses**

Nurses who have undertaken independent and supplementary prescribing are able to prescribe, administer, and give directions for the administration of Schedules 2, 3, 4, and 5 controlled drugs and unlicensed medicines.

9.5.2 **Pharmacists**

Pharmacist independent prescribers can prescribe any medicine for any medical condition. This includes unlicensed medicines and the autonomy to prescribe, administer, and give directions for the administration of Schedules 2, 3, 4, and 5 controlled drugs.

9.5.3 **Optometrists**

Optometrist independent prescribers are able to prescribe any licensed medicine for ocular conditions, affecting the eye and the tissues surrounding the eye, except controlled drugs or medicines for parenteral administration.

9.5.4 **Physiotherapists**

Physiotherapist independent prescribers can prescribe any medicine for any medical condition. This includes "off-label" medicines. They are also allowed to prescribe a limited range of controlled drugs.

9.5.5 **Chiropodists/Podiatrists**

Chiropodist and podiatrist independent prescribers can prescribe any licensed medicine for any condition within their competence and relevant to the treatment of disorders affecting the foot, ankle, and associated structures. Similar to physiotherapists, they are allowed to prescribe "off-label" medicines and a limited range of controlled drugs.

9.5.6 **Therapeutic Radiographers**

Therapeutic radiographer independent prescribers can prescribe any medicine for any medical condition, including "off-label" medicines. At present they are not allowed to prescribe controlled drugs.

9.5.7 **Independent or Supplementary Prescribing Considerations**

There may be occasions when an independent prescriber may choose to act as a supplementary prescriber. An example might be new or inexperienced prescribers who need the safety net of a clinical management plan until they develop their expertise. Healthcare providers can sometimes stipulate that independent prescribers undertake post-qualification supervision of a supplementary prescriber, to develop the individual's confidence and competence in prescribing practice. Thus, supplementary prescribing can be used as a means of developing competence or as a vehicle for evaluating the safety, efficacy, and acceptability of non-medical prescribing (Dawoud et al. 2011).

9.5.8 Controlled Drugs

The use of controlled drugs for medicinal purposes is allowed under the Misuse of Drugs Regulations 2001. This Act was amended in 2012 to allow nurses, midwives, and pharmacists who are qualified as independent prescribers to prescribe all controlled drugs listed in Schedules 2, 3, 4, and 5, where clinically appropriate and within their competence. The amendment to the Act excludes the use of cocaine, diamorphine, and dipipanone for the treatment of addiction. Chiropodist, podiatrist, and physiotherapist independent prescribers can prescribe from a limited group of controlled drugs.

9.5.9 Patient Group Directions

Patient group directions are written instructions that allow the supply or administration of a licensed medicine in an identified clinical situation for a specified group of patients without individual prescriptions being written (National Prescribing Centre [NPC] 2004). A patient group direction is drawn up locally by doctors, pharmacists, and other health professionals and must meet minimum legal criteria (DH 2000). In 2013, the National Institute for Health and Care Excellence (NICE) published guidance supporting good practice for the development and use of patient group directions, as well as advice on determining their need (NICE 2013).

In practice, an individual patient group direction must be signed by a doctor, a pharmacist, and a representative of the NHS Trust. Professionals using patient group directions do not have to become prescribers or obtain any specific qualification, but their employers must assess them to ensure that they are fully competent, qualified, and trained. More recently, patient group directions have been developed nationally in the UK for use by community pharmacists as part of a seasonal influenza vaccination program.

9.5.10 Emergency Situations

Exemptions provided by Article 7 of the Prescription Only Medicines (Human Use) Order 1997 mean that patient group directions are not required for the following countermeasures when given by anyone in an emergency, to save life: atropine sulfate injection, dicobalt edetate injection, glucose injection, and pralidoxine chloride injection.

CASE STUDIES

Melanie is a 27-year-old engineer; she is 10 weeks pregnant and presented to you in a clinic setting complaining of urinary urgency, polyuria, and a burning sensation on micturition.

You suspect that she is suffering with a urinary tract infection.

1. What additional information would you require before confirming the suspected diagnosis?

2. What are the patient-related factors that would influence your choice of treatment?

Barbara is a 35-year-old mother of two. She is currently being treated for bipolar affective disorder with lithium carbonate 600 mg nocte and has been on lithium for the past three years. Recently, Barbara has noticed that she is feeling tired, and has marked constipation and cold extremities.

1. What could be the cause of these symptoms?

2. How could you confirm this?

9.6 The Principles of Effective Prescribing

Optimizing the use of medicines is based on the four principles outlined by the RPS (2013). The principles underpinning medicines optimization are patient focused and aligned with getting the best from investment in and use of medicines. Effective prescribing requires a holistic approach, an enhanced level of patient-centered care, and a focus on partnership working between healthcare professionals and the recipients of care. These principles are underpinned by a holistic assessment and diagnosis of the patient's presenting complaint. This assessment should follow a structured model and take into account the patient's past medical history, current co-morbidities, any allergies, and a full medication history, as well as the patient's perspective on the available treatment options.

9.6.1 Principle 1: Understanding the Patient Experience

The patient is at the heart of prescribing and once a diagnosis has been confirmed the NMP must consider the most appropriate strategy; issuing a prescription may not always be in the patient's best interests. Many significant factors need to be considered to aid the prescriber in making the decision as to whether medication is the best course of action to take. The decision to prescribe or deprescribe medicines must reflect an ongoing, open dialog with the patient and/or their carer about the patient's choice and experience of using medicines to manage their condition, recognizing that the patient's experience may change over time, even if the medicines do not.

Prescribing a medicine requires far more than completing a prescription. What is important is individual choice; the patient is asked to agree to decide whether to accept the medication, based on appropriate and understandable information. In some instances, negotiating with a patient may require further action. Taking medication may have to be incorporated into a particular individual's lifestyle to ensure maximum effect; one example is the introduction of insulin injections to someone newly diagnosed with Type 1 diabetes. Other considerations may apply where a patient has a notifiable disease such as tuberculosis, where regularly taking medicines is linked to ensuring the health of others.

In essence, the principle of understanding the patient experience reinforces the need to move toward shared decision making, with an inherent assumption that there are two professionals, the patient and the practitioner, who are engaged in determining the optimal treatment (Corrigan et al. 2012). This principle is intended to facilitate:

- Engagement and improved understanding leading to informed decision making, including choices about illness prevention and healthy living.
- Shared decision making in which the patient is considered the expert in their own well-being and in which the professional understands their beliefs and preferences about medicines.
- Adherence to prescribed medication.
- Patients feeling confident enough to share openly their experiences of medication-taking behaviors and the impact on their quality of life.

Before reading on, consider Exercise 9.1.

> **EXERCISE 9.1**
>
> What steps will you take to develop patient-centered prescribing?
>
> What are some of the indicators of good communication during the consultation?
>
> How will you seek to empower patients as part of your routine practice?

9.6.2 Principle 2: Evidence-based Choice of Medicines

Once the decision to prescribe medication has been made, the NMP must identify the most appropriate preparation. This decision is dependent on understanding the most clinically appropriate and cost-effective medicine(s). This in turn is informed by the best available evidence, which must be understood by the NMP to meet the needs of the patient.

To explain this further, a patient may be planning to become pregnant; in other circumstances, some medicines may not be suitable for the very young or the elderly. Further, a patient may have a history of adverse reactions to particular medicines. Some medicines are safe and effective when used singly, but cannot be used in combination with others because of the risk of unwanted side effects. This is a particularly problematic issue where patients have more than one clinical condition requiring treatment; in this context, decisions about medication involve balancing the demands of different conditions and trying to avoid prescribing too many medicines at the same time. This principle is intended to ensure that:

- Optimal patient outcomes are obtained from choosing a medicine using best evidence, for example following local formulary recommendations or NICE guidance.
- Treatments of limited clinical value are not prescribed and medicines which are no longer required are discontinued.
- Decisions about access to medicines are transparent and in accordance with the NHS Constitution.

The cost of medicines is an important issue. Depending on the circumstances, it may be wiser to begin treatment with a less expensive medicine and progress to more expensive alternatives if the patient's problems continue. Furthermore, in the UK some medicines such as paracetamol are available in high-street pharmacies and supermarkets at a lower price than if they are prescribed. In these instances, the NMP may advise the patient on the cheaper alternative. Before reading on, consider Exercise 9.2.

> **EXERCISE 9.2**
>
> How will you ensure that you keep abreast of the emerging evidence underpinning your area of prescribing competence?
>
> What is the relevance of evidence on prescribing practice?
>
> How will you use evidence to inform your practice?
>
> What are the patient-related factors that must be taken into consideration when prescribing in specific patient groups, e.g. the elderly, pregnant women, children?

9.6.3 Principle 3: Ensure Medicines Use Is as Safe as Possible

The harm arising from the use of medication is well documented and it is estimated that 6% of emergency readmissions to hospital are caused by avoidable adverse reactions to medicines (Pirmohamed et al. 2004), with approximately 1.7 million serious prescribing errors occurring in general practice during 2010 (Avery et al. 2012). The NMP is responsible for informing the patient about the potential side effects, how long to take the medication for, and who to contact in the case of an adverse reaction.

Once the patient has agreed to take the medication, the name of the medicine, the dose, and the date should be entered in the patient's records. If the patient has agreed to take the medication as prescribed, it may be appropriate to arrange a review, particularly where the patient has a long-term condition or complex health issues. Even in seemingly straightforward situations, such as the treatment of a chest infection in an otherwise healthy person, a review may be advisable to check that the medication prescribed has worked. Feeling better may not always reflect a complete recovery and further treatment may still be needed.

If an adverse event is thought to be linked with prescribed medication, the NMP has a responsibility to document this clearly in the patient's records and to complete a report via the MHRA yellow card reporting system. This principle is intended to ensure that:

- Incidents of avoidable harm from medicines are reduced.
- Patients have more confidence in taking their medicines.
- Patients are empowered to ask healthcare professionals when they have a query or a difficulty with their medicines.
- Patients receive benefits from treatment, with a reduction in admissions and readmissions to hospitals related to medicines usage.
- Patients discuss potential side effects and there is an increase in reporting to the MHRA.

Before reading on, consider Exercise 9.3.

> **EXERCISE 9.3**
>
> What are the steps that you will take to ensure that your prescribing practice is safe?
>
> How will you engage with the patient to ensure the safe and effective use of medicines?
>
> How does the National Reporting and Learning System support the safe and effective use of medicines?
>
> How can you support the safe and effective use of medicines when patients are transferred across healthcare settings?

9.6.4 Principle 4: Make Medicines Optimization Part of Routine Practice

The NMP has a range of legal and professional responsibilities, which require reflection on practice to ensure safety. This means that NMPs can only prescribe within their area of competence and must keep up to date with the current evidence relating to their prescribing practice. Like medical prescribers, NMPs are likely to attract the attention of pharmaceutical marketing departments. An objective approach to such attention, balanced with an ability to critically appraise information, is essential in maintaining both the independent integrity of NMPs and the safety of their practice. In addition, NMPs must ensure that their practice is consistent with the law and workplace policies (Beckwith and Franklin 2007). This principle is intended to ensure that:

- Patients feel able to discuss and review their medicines with anyone involved in their care.
- Patients receive consistent messages about medicines because the members of the healthcare team liaise effectively.
- It becomes routine practice to signpost patients to further help with their medicines and to local patient support groups.
- Interprofessional and interagency communication about patients' medicines is improved.
- Medicines wastage is reduced.

Before reading on, consider Exercise 9.4.

EXERCISE **9.4**

How will you ensure that your practice reflects the principle of medicines optimization and what are the key considerations?

What are the key considerations when considering continuity of care for individuals with long-term conditions?

What is the scope for expanding non-medical prescribing in the changing healthcare landscape?

9.7 Safety and Clinical Governance

Clinical governance is a system in which healthcare organizations strive continuously to improve the quality of healthcare and safeguard standards by creating an environment in which high-quality clinical care can flourish (Avery et al. 2012). Quality issues and standards apply to non-medical prescribing and responsibility is shared between the individual practitioner and the healthcare organization. In 2016, the RPS published a revision to the single prescribing competence framework which includes all prescribers. The framework identifies a common set of competences that underpin prescribing, and provides a framework that can be used by all, supporting safe, effective prescribing (RPS 2016).

Individual prescribers are accountable for their own prescribing practice and should adhere to the principles of good prescribing and their professional codes (NMC 2008; NPC 2012; RPS 2016). Alongside these individual responsibilities are those of the employing organization, which has a duty to ensure that prescribers are suitably trained and that prescribing practice is audited and monitored regularly. Moreover, the organization must ensure that appropriate indemnity insurance is in place for all prescribers. However, the individual NMP should ensure that appropriate indemnity arrangements have been made prior to undertaking prescribing (NMC 2014). Even with the best standards of prescribing practice, mistakes can and do happen. Patients do not always present their symptoms in the expected way; individuals may experience the same illness quite differently. Consequently, in formulating a diagnosis, the professional is faced with a range of options on which to base a decision and may, occasionally, select the wrong one. In addition, even where the diagnosis is correctly chosen, patients may have adverse reactions to treatment, sometimes with serious results. Indemnity insurance against non-negligent harm is, therefore, essential for all prescribers.

Safety and clinical governance present a number of opportunities and challenges for the advanced practitioner. As a prescriber working directly with patients, the advanced practitioner is able to identify the extent to which prescribing practice is safe and appropriate for patients' needs. Direct contact with patients will facilitate monitoring of the wanted side effects of medication and patients' preferences in the management of their conditions. The emphasis is on safe prescribing and concordance with treatment (National Health Safety Executive 1998; RPS 2013). Where changes are needed, the leadership and interpersonal skills of the advanced practitioner can be used to promote constructive dialog between the different professionals involved in prescribing and interorganizational working. The research skills of the advanced practitioner may be used to monitor and evaluate prescribing practice; these skills can also contribute toward the investigation of specific problems. The key point of clinical governance is to ensure that all parties collaborate to create a working environment in which practice is based on the best available evidence. Best practice also reduces the likelihood of recurrent mistakes and ensures that there is wider learning from incidents. This means, from the advanced practitioner's perspective, fostering a no-blame culture in which individuals can be honest about their mistakes and supported in their efforts to improve, which is consistent with the recommendations of the Francis Report (2013). In this context, advanced practitioners may draw on their coaching and guiding skills to enable prescribers to adopt new or safer ways of working.

9.8 The Future of Non-medical Prescribing

Within the context of an increasingly elderly population and providing care to individuals with complex needs, there may be a requirement to expand the training of nursing and pharmacist NMPs to prescribe across a range of conditions for patients with co-morbid disease states. With the focus of healthcare provision on the integration of health and social care across the UK, there is a potential gap in the adult social care setting, in which care homes could benefit from non-medical prescribing input. The prescribing skills of NMPs could also be utilized if there were sufficient resources to enable training and ongoing support for prescribers akin to those employed by the NHS.

The next evolutionary step in non-medical prescribing could lead to the development of training programs at undergraduate level, which would lead to "prescribing-ready" practitioners at the point of qualification. With an expanding non-medical prescribing workforce, it is possible in the future that supervision of training NMPs would be extended to experienced NMPs. It is advocated that such a move would facilitate the sharing of experiences among NMPs and would also create scope to train more NMPs.

As part of a wider strategy to expand the non-medical prescribing workforce, there is a desire to extend independent prescribing rights to other healthcare professional groups such as paramedics. The extension of prescribing to a wider group of healthcare professionals creates the potential for shared learning in new and different ways. However, there remains the challenge of how the educational needs of the differing professional groups can be met.

Non-medical prescribing has the potential to improve the lives of patients by enabling advanced practitioners and other health professionals to provide complete episodes of care. Patients only have to recount their signs and symptoms once; the increased number of prescribers means that access to healthcare is improved and that patients have more choice. In some instances, a single episode may be all that is needed to solve a particular patient's health problem. Even when a follow-up session is required, there is the potential for greater continuity in care and better relationships between patients and professionals. From the advanced practitioner's perspective, independent prescribing is consistent with the scope of expert practice. The expert practitioner is able to home in very quickly on the most important aspects of a patient's clinical condition and take appropriate action. This is particularly important in emergency situations and when working with patients who have complex needs. The advanced practitioner has the skills required to promote safe and effective prescribing, both at an individual level and across the healthcare organization as a whole.

Evaluations demonstrate that nurses and pharmacists are cautious and safe in their prescribing practice (Weeks et al. 2016), but they need to integrate this with comprehensive, accurate assessment and diagnostic skills (Latter et al. 2010). This can be challenging, because prescribing courses tend to be generic. More work is needed in helping prescribers apply their learning within their specialties. Advanced practitioners have the skills required to facilitate the investigation of the many current concerns about non-medical prescribing, to promote dialog between the various different points of view. Skills in communication, leadership, and ethical reasoning can be harnessed to create working environments in which individuals feel able to express their opinions and be listened to with respect and enabled to participate in bringing about change.

Internationally, non-medical prescribing raises other possibilities for the advanced practitioner. For example, there are wide variations in the development and practice of nurse prescribing. In Australia, nurse non-medical prescribing is still evolving and until 2010 legislation prevented nurse prescribers from prescribing under subsidized schemes which were available to medical prescribers; thus, the patient would pay more for medication if prescribed by a nurse compared with a doctor (Nissen and Kyle 2010). Furthermore, despite the progress with nurse prescribing, there has been significant medical resistance to its evolution (MacLellan et al. 2015). In the USA, there are variations across the country as to what and when nurses can prescribe (Cope et al. 2016). Other non-medical prescribing roles also differ in terms of what the law in each country will allow. Advanced practitioners have the skills to involve themselves in addressing these issues at both national and international levels.

9.9 Conclusion

The extent to which non-medical prescribing develops in the UK will largely depend on the emerging healthcare landscape and the drive to deliver cost-effective, patient-centered care. As independent and supplementary prescribers, advanced practitioners can do a great deal to promote confidence by demonstrating their competence in safe and effective prescribing practice. They are also well placed to identify the needs of patients and enable healthcare providers to bring about change. However, despite the emerging growth in non-medical prescribing, further research is needed to determine the impact of non-medical prescribing in relation to the principles of effective prescribing as outlined by the RPS.

Acknowledgment

This chapter is a revised version of 'Prescribing and advanced practice' by Sue Shortland and Katharine Hardware, in P. McGee (ed.), *Advanced Practice in Nursing and the Allied Health Professions*, 3rd edn, 2009. pp. 70–80. Oxford: Wiley Blackwell. Part of their text is reproduced here with their permission.

Key Questions

1. How could non-medical prescribing enhance care for specific patients in your field of practice?
2. How will you evaluate the impact of your prescribing practice on patient care?
3. Look at your local formulary/prescribing guidance for a condition for which you prescribe. Summarize the evidence underpinning the recommendations for the given condition. Do the local recommendations differ from national guidance? If yes, is there any justification?
4. When prescribing, how will you balance the needs of the individual against the wider economic constraints governing prescribing practice?
5. What might be the implications to your profession of introducing non-medical prescribing training at the undergraduate level?

Glossary

Clinical management plan (CMP): written or electronic details of an individual patient, that person's clinical condition, and the range of medicines which can be used to treat the specific condition. Before supplementary prescribing can take place, it is obligatory for a CMP to be agreed between a supplementary prescriber and an independent prescriber (doctor or dentist), and the plan must be placed on the patient record.

Disclosure and Barring Service (DBS; https://www.gov.uk/government/organisations/disclosure-and-barring-service): acts on behalf of employers to conduct checks of criminal records to ensure that unsuitable applicants are not appointed to positions requiring work with children or vulnerable adults.

General Optical Council (www.optical.org): professional body responsible for the regulation of optometrists and dispensing opticians.

General Pharmaceutical Council (www.pharmacyregulation.org): regulates pharmacists, pharmacy technicians, and pharmacy premises. The Council maintains a register of qualified individuals, sets standards, and approves training programs.

General sales list medicines: medicines that can be sold or supplied through general retail outlets, including pharmacies.

Independent prescriber: a practitioner, e.g. doctor, dentist, nurse, or pharmacist, responsible and accountable for the assessment of patients with undiagnosed or diagnosed conditions, and for decisions about the clinical management required, including prescribing.

Medicines and Healthcare Products Regulatory Agency (MHRA; https://www.gov.uk/government/organisations/medicines-and-healthcare-products-regulatory-agency/about): responsible for ensuring that medicines, medical devices, and blood components meet current standards. The yellow card scheme enables the MHRA to collect information about adverse reactions to drugs and medical devices and other safety issues.

Misuse of drugs regulations: covers the prescription, storage, and dispensing of medicines. Within these regulations, medicines are classified in groups called schedules according to the risks involved in their use.

NHS Constitution (https://www.gov.uk/government/publications/the-nhs-constitution-for-england): sets out the guiding principles of the NHS, including patients' rights and responsibilities.

Non-medical prescriber (NMP): suitably qualified nurse, pharmacist, or allied health professional.

Off-label medicines: the use of medicines outside the terms of their license, for example prescribing them for a different illness or age group.

Patient group directions: written instructions that allow the supply or administration of a licensed medicine to patients, in an identified clinical situation, such as coronary care. Patient group directions do not require individual prescriptions for each patient.

Pharmaceutical preparations: medicines intended for human or veterinary use, presented in their finished dosage form, including the materials used in the preparation and/or formulation of the finished dosage form.

Pharmacy medicines: medicines that can be sold or supplied through registered pharmacies under the personal supervision of a pharmacist.

Prescription-only medicines: medicines that are available only through a prescription from a supplementary or independent prescriber.

Royal Pharmaceutical Society (RPS; https://www.rpharms.com/about-us): the professional body for pharmacists.

Supplementary prescriber: a practitioner qualified to prescribe a limited list of medicines, voluntarily agreed with a doctor or dentist, and within the context of an agreed patient-specific clinical management plan.

References

Avery, A.J, N Barber, M Ghaleb, B Dean-Franklin, S Armstrong, S Crowe et al. (2012). Investigating the prevalence and causes of prescribing errors in general practice: The Practicle study. A report for the GMC. General Medical Council and University of Nottingham, May. http://www.gmc-uk.org/about/research/12996.asp (accessed November 2017).

Baqir, W., Miller, D., and Richardson, G. (2012). A brief history of pharmacist prescribing in the UK. *European Journal of Hospital Pharmacy: Science and Practice* 19 (5): 487–488.

Beckwith, S. and Franklin, P. (2007). *Oxford Handbook of Nurse Prescribing*. Oxford: Oxford University Press.

British National Formulary and the Royal Pharmaceutical Society of Great Britain (2015–2017). *The Nurse Prescriber's Formulary for Community Practitioners*. London: BNF and RPSGB.

Cope, L.C., Abuzour, A.S., and Tully, M.P. (2016). Nonmedical prescribing: where are we now? *Therapeutic Advances in Drug Safety* 7 (4): 165–172.

Corrigan, P.W., Angell, B., Davidson, L. et al. (2012). From adherence to self-determination: evolution of a treatment paradigm for people with serious mental illnesses. *Psychiatric Services* 63 (2): 169–173.

Dawoud, D., Griffiths, P., Maben, J. et al. (2011). Pharmacist supplementary prescribing: a step toward more independence? *Research in Social and Administrative Pharmacy* 7 (3): 246–256.

Department of Health (2000). Patient Group Directions (England only). Health Service Circular 2000/026. https://webarchive.nationalarchives.gov.uk/20120503110635/http://www.dh.gov.uk/en/Publicationsandstatistics/Lettersandcirculars/Healthservicecirculars/DH_4004179 (accessed January 11, 2019).

Department of Health (2005). *Supplementary Prescribing by Nurses, Pharmacists, Chiropodists/Podiatrists, Physiotherapists and Radiographers within the NHS in England.* London: DH.

Department of Health (2006). *Improving Patients' Access to Medicines: A Guide to Implementing Nurse and Pharmacists Independent Prescribing within the NHS England.* London: DH.

Department of Health (2007). *Optometrists to Get Independent Prescribing Rights (Press Release).* London: DH.

Department of Health (2011). Clinical Management Plans (CMPs). https://webarchive.nationalarchives.gov.uk/+/http://www.dh.gov.uk/en/Healthcare/Medicinespharmacyandindustry/Prescriptions/The Non-MedicalPrescribingProgramme/Supplementaryprescribing/DH_4123030 (accessed January 11, 2019).

Department of Health (2013). *The Medicines Act 1968 and the Human Medicines Regulations (Amendment Order).* London: DH.

Department of Health and Social Security (1992). *Medicinal Products; Prescriptions by Nurses etc. Act.* London: HMSO.

Dowden, A. (2016). The expanding role of nurse prescribers. *Prescriber* 27 (6): 24–27.

Francis, R. (2013). *Report of the Mid Staffordshire NHS Foundation Trust Public Inquiry.* London: Stationery Office.

General Pharmaceutical Council (2017). *Accreditation of Independent Prescribing Programmes: Guidance for Providers for 2017/18 Academic Year.* London: GPhC.

Latter, S., Blenkinsopp, A., Smith, A. et al. (2010). *Evaluation of Nurse and Pharmacist Independent Prescribing.* London: DH.

MacLellan, L., Higgins, I., and Levett-Jones, T. (2015). Medical acceptance of the nurse practitioner role in Australia: a decade on. *Journal of the American Association of Nurse Practitioners* 27 (3): 152–159.

Medicines Healthcare Products Regulatory Agency (2005). *Consultation on Proposals to Introduce Independent Prescribing by Pharmacists.* London: MHRA.

National Health Service Executive (1998). *Clinical Governance. Quality in the NHS.* London: DH.

National Institute for Health and Care Excellence (2013). Patient Group Directions. www.nice.org.uk/guidance/mpg2 (accessed July 17, 2017).

National Prescribing Centre (2004). *Patient Group Directions: Practical Guide and Framework of Competencies for All Professionals Using Patient Group Directions*

Incorporating an Overview of Existing Mechanisms for the Supply and Prescribing of Medicines. Liverpool: NPC.

National Prescribing Centre (2012). *A Single Competency Framework for all Prescribers.* London: NICE.

NHS England Allied Health Professions Medicines Project (2016a). Consultation on proposals to introduce independent prescribing by radiographers across the United Kingdom. https://www.engage.england.nhs.uk/consultation/independent-prescribing-radiographers/user_uploads/pat-pub-summ-radiographers-mar.pdf (accessed January 11, 2019).

NHS England Allied Health Professions Medicines Project (2016b). Consultation on proposals to introduce supplementary prescribing by dietitians across the United Kingdom. https://www.england.nhs.uk/ourwork/qual-clin-lead/ahp/med-project/dietitians (accessed September 27, 2017).

Nissen, L. and Kyle, G. (2010). Non-medical prescribing in Australia. *Australian Prescriber* 33 (6): 166–167.

Nursing and Midwifery Council (2008). *The Code. Standards of Conduct, Performance and Ethics for Nurses and Midwives.* London: NMC.

Nursing and Midwifery Council (2014). *Professional Indemnity Arrangement: A New Requirement for Registration.* London: NMC.

Nursing and Midwifery Council (2015). *Standards for Proficiency of Nurse and Midwife Prescribers.* London: NMC.

Pirmohamed, M., James, S., Meakin, S. et al. (2004). Adverse drug reactions as cause of admission to hospital: analysis of 18 820 patients. *BMJ* 329: 15–19.

Royal Pharmaceutical Society of Great Britain (2013). *Medicines Optimisation: Helping Patients to Make the Most of Medicines Good Practice Guidance for Health Care Professionals in England.* London: RPSGB https://www.rpharms.com/Portals/0/RPS%20document%20library/Open%20access/Policy/helping-patients-make-the-most-of-their-medicines.pdf (accessed January 11, 2019).

Royal Pharmaceutical Society of Great Britain (2016). *A Competency Framework for All Prescribers.* London: RPSGB https://www.rpharms.com/Portals/0/RPS%20document%20library/Open%20access/Professional%20standards/Prescribing%20competency%20framework/prescribing-competency-framework.pdf (accessed January 11, 2019).

Weeks, G., George, J., Maclure, K., and Stewart, D. (2016). Non-medical prescribing versus medical prescribing for acute and chronic disease management in primary and secondary care. *Cochrane Database Systematic Review* (11): CD011227. https://doi.org/10.1002/14651858.CD011227.pub2.

CHAPTER 10

The Advanced Clinical Nurse Practitioner and Direct Care

Mary Hutchinson

Birmingham City University, Birmingham, UK

Key Issues

- The principles of assessment required in the direct care of patients
- Critical thinking and decision making
- Holism and fragmentation of care

LEARNING OBJECTIVES

By the end of this chapter you will be able to:

- Evaluate two systematic approaches to history taking.
- Critically discuss the process of formulating a differential diagnosis.

10.1 Introduction

Direct care is a clinical, social, or public health activity concerned with the prevention, investigation, and treatment of illness and the alleviation of individuals' suffering (NHS England 2013). From the patients' perspective, as participant in or recipient of direct care, the requirement is for a knowledgeable practitioner who brings to their situation clinical acumen coupled with genuine concern for their well-being, so that their experience is one of being cared for (National Institute for Health and Care Excellence [NICE] 2012). Clinical care demands knowledge not only of health and pathophysiology, diagnoses, and treatment, but of statutes, policies, systems, organizations, environments, equipment, teams, and individuals. To provide meaningful direct care, the clinician requires person-centric professional curiosity to discover who their patient is, and

Advanced Practice in Healthcare: Dynamic Developments in Nursing and Allied Health Professions,
Fourth Edition. Edited by Paula McGee and Chris Inman.
© 2019 John Wiley & Sons Ltd. Published 2019 by John Wiley & Sons Ltd.

emotional intelligence coupled with self-awareness in order to establish an effective therapeutic relationship.

Direct clinical care is the foundation of advanced nursing practice. It requires a breadth and depth of expertise that transcend qualified nurse practice. As an autonomous practitioner, the advanced clinical practitioner (ACP) facilitates a holistic approach to physical and mental health. Good communication skills are essential to this approach; listening to the patient's account and expectations of the problem, taking a history, and carrying out an examination (Matthys et al. 2009). Alongside these skills are decisions about further investigations, where appropriate, such as X-rays, magnetic resonance imaging (MRI), or computed tomography (CT) scans, which the ACP requests and interprets. Finally, the ACP synthesizes the information gained, explains this to the patient, and, if appropriate, prescribes treatment. Thus, the suitably prepared ACP is able to provide a complete episode of care, but may also refer the patient to another healthcare professional if necessary.

This chapter examines the advanced practitioner's provision of direct clinical care through the medium of a case study divided into four parts. Between each part there is a description and an analysis of the ACP's history taking, physical examination of the patient, critical thinking, and actions, plus activities to prompt readers to think through their own responses to related questions. The case study does not relate to any individual patient; it is based on the author's experience in working in emergency departments (EDs), minor injuries units, and nurse-led urgent care/out-of-hours services.

CASE STUDY

Mrs. Green was a 70-year-old woman who had celebrated her birthday earlier in the Christmas holiday week. She presented to the ED with a two-day history of worsening abdominal pain. At triage, ED staff gave Mrs. Green two tablets of co-codamol, a compound analgesic containing codeine phosphate 30 mg and paracetamol 500 mg. The nurse then carried out a dipstick urinalysis test which revealed:

- a large amount of ketones
- a medium amount of leucocytes
- a small amount of blood
- nitrites.

Mrs. Green was referred to the adjacent out-of-hours service for further management, where she was assessed by the ACP.

Before reading on, consider Exercise 10.1.

EXERCISE 10.1

What are the positive and negative aspects of Mrs. Green's management in the ED?

What further information is needed about her condition?

PART 1 – MEETING THE PATIENT AND TAKING A HISTORY

The ACP introduced herself and checked with Mrs. Green that the information she had received about her was correct. Inviting the patient to sit down and make herself comfortable makes eye contact easier, as both parties are seated at the same level; having the patient lie on the examination couch may reduce ease of communication and increase power issues between the ACP and the patient.

First impressions are important: they help to put the patient at ease and enable the ACP to begin utilizing the "diagnostic, prognostic, and humanistic tool" of inspection during the initial encounter with the patient (Gupta et al. 2017). Does the patient look well, or unwell? Do they stand, walk, and sit with ease? Do they share eye contact? Do they return your smile? What does their facial expression, or voice, tell you? Checking information is also important in ensuring patient safety, which, in turn, is dependent on the skills, attitudes, and actions of healthcare professionals and the systems and processes in place to support their work (National Patient Safety Agency 2010). Lessons learned from aviation safety training have led to a greater understanding of the role of human factors in clinical errors; self and situational awareness are critical elements in ensuring patient safety (Mitchell 2013; Krasner et al. 2009).

After checking that the co-codamol has helped relieve the pain, the ACP may then begin to take a formal history from Mrs. Green (Turk and Melzack 2011). This is an activity in which the ACP utilizes academic and experiential knowledge to creatively explore the patient's health problem. A holistic approach requires the ACP to be truly present in the process, because "process alone is empty without presence. Presence alone is insufficient without process" (Potter and Frisch 2007).

A comprehensive history has several strands that include the current problem, past medical history, medication and allergies, social circumstances, and family history. Reassessment of patient comfort throughout the history taking and gaining their consent to continue will assist in strengthening rapport. Assessment should be based on a systematic approach to the collection, summarizing and recording of data (Tables 10.1 and 10.2). The two examples of a systematic approach shown here are concerned with the assessment of pain, its location, severity, duration, quality, and associated factors. The SOCRATES approach (Table 10.1) was developed as part of a staff development package at the Northwestern Memorial Hospital in Chicago. The questions form a prelude to the hospital's own procedures for pain management (Clayton et al. 2000; Briggs 2010). In contrast, OPQRST (Table 10.2) seems to be simply a mnemonic to aid the assessment of pain. Both approaches will provide useful information about Mrs. Green but, as with all such tools, the information should be synthesized with understanding of other issues such as culture, which may influence how she both experiences and expresses pain. It is also wise to be alert to the possibility that any medicine she has taken at home, including illicit or street drugs, may be a contributing factor to, or indeed the cause of, her presenting symptoms. For example, conditions such as sickle cell disease and some analgesics, such as codeine, may actually cause abdominal pain. Similarly, checking past medical history, including injuries, operations, and common serious illnesses, may also provide an indication about the cause of Mrs. Green's pain or the presence of another condition (Table 10.3). For example, her urine sample contained a lot of ketones; one possible explanation of this result is that Mrs. Green has undiagnosed diabetes. Any known allergies such as medications, insect stings, or other substances need to be explored to identify the nature, severity, and extent of the reaction and determine if it is a true allergy.

TABLE 10.1

SOCRATES.

Site	Where exactly is the pain?
Onset	When did it start? Today; this week etc.? How did it start – suddenly or gradually?
Character	Sharp; aching etc.
Radiation	Does it stay in one place or does it spread? If so how and where to?
Associations	Any other signs or symptoms associated with the pain?
Time course	Does the pain follow any pattern or vary throughout the day?
Exacerbating/relieving factors	Does heat; cold; movement; pressure etc., alter the pain?
Severity	On a scale of 1 (very mild) to 10 (intolerable pain), how severe is it?

TABLE **10.2**	
OPQRST.	
Onset	"Did your pain/symptom start suddenly or gradually get worse and worse? What were you doing when the pain/symptom started?"
Provokes or Palliates	"What makes it better or worse?"
Quality	"What words would you use to describe your pain?" or "What does your pain feel like?"
Radiates	"Point to where it hurts the most. Where does your pain move/spread from there?"
Severity	Remember, pain is subjective and relative to each individual patient you treat. Ask about and record their pain score, e.g. using a 10-point pain scale.
Time	This is a reference to when the pain started or how long ago it started.

TABLE **10.3**
Quick guide to history taking about past injuries, operations, and common serious illnesses.
Jaundice
Anemia or other hematological condition
Myocardial infarction
Tuberculosis
Hypertension or heart disease
Rheumatic fever
Epilepsy
Asthma or chronic obstructive pulmonary disorder
Diabetes
Stroke

Before reading on, consider Exercise 10.2.

EXERCISE 10.2

Critically examine the systematic approach you use when taking a patient's history.

Mrs. Green's daily life and circumstances, including her current and/or past occupation, are relevant. Information about her normal diet and fluid intake and any changes that have occurred should be noted, including eating away from home. In celebrating her birthday she may have consumed something new or may have contracted an infection. Travel abroad can also increase the risk of exposure to diverse pathogens/parasites, which could be linked to her abdominal pain; she should be asked about dates of travel and any immunization program undertaken.

Certain subjects require some extra sensitivity. The ACP will have to ask questions about whether Mrs. Green smokes, how many cigarettes, and for how long, whether she has given up, and if so how long ago. Questions about alcohol intake will attempt to ascertain the number of units consumed per day in wine, beer, and/or spirits. CAGE is a validated screening tool composed of four questions related to alcohol consumption (Ewing 1984; Table 10.4). The ACP should not alert the patient to the fact that there are going to be questions about their use of alcohol, but simply ask the

---

TABLE 10.4

Assessing alcohol intake – CAGE.

Have you ever felt you should **C**ut down on your drinking?
Have people **A**nnoyed you by criticizing your drinking?
Have you ever felt bad or **G**uilty about your drinking?
Have you ever had a drink first thing in the morning to steady your nerves or to get rid of a hangover (**E**ye opener)?
Score = 1 for each positive response.

TABLE 10.5

Guide to assessing social circumstances – the BATHE technique.

Background	What is going on in your life?
Affect	How do you feel about that?
Trouble	What troubles you the most?
Handling	How are you handling that?
Empathy	That must be very difficult

This is a model of inquiry which assures that the clinician listens to the patient and responds empathically, while the patient maintains personal responsibility for their health and well-being.

---

questions using a low key, matter-of-fact approach and record the response. A total score of 2 or more has been proven to have greater sensitivity for alcohol dependence than a laboratory gamma-glutamyl transpeptidase (GGT) liver function test (Bernadt et al. 1982). Finally, Mrs. Green's living arrangements, relationship status, and sexual history are further potentially sensitive issues. It is not wise to assume that, simply because of her age, she is/may not be sexually active; questioning may indicate urogenital problems or infections which may or may not be related to her current symptoms.

Before reading on, consider Exercise 10.3.

EXERCISE 10.3

How do you feel about discussing intimate issues like sexual activity with patients?

How do you phrase questions about this?

In gathering these data, the ACP remains alert to Mrs. Green's emotional state and the ways in which pathophysiology, some medicines, and emotional distress can manifest differently across the age spectrum (McEwen et al. 2015). In this context, the ACP enquires sensitively about how she is feeling and coping with her life at this time (Stuart and Lieberman 2015; Table 10.5). If depression and possible suicidal ideation are possibilities, there are simple tools that can assist the clinician in establishing risk. The most commonly used in primary care is the Patient Health Questionnaire-9 (PHQ-9); this is a screening tool which consists of nine questions and takes about three minutes to complete. The outcomes can be linked to the Diagnostic and Statistical Manual of Mental Disorders (DSM) criteria, and so provide a useful starting point for further discussion and assessment of any possible mental health issues using more detailed frameworks such as the Hospital Anxiety and Depression Score (HADS) and Beck Depression Inventory (BDI-II). The PHQ-9 has been criticized because some patients feel that it does not fit well with their experiences of low mood and other difficulties (Malpass et al. 2016). Inaccuracies have also been detected in the HADS and BDI-II when tested against the Hamilton Rating Score for Depression (HRSD-17; Cameron et al. 2011). Consequently, it is wise to bear in mind that "that the interpretation of scores alone should not be relied upon when assessing an individual with possible depression, but that other factors, including functional impairment, history, family history, and presence of other comorbid conditions, should also be considered" (NICE 2015).

Outcome

While taking the history, the ACP noted that Mrs. Green looked tired and pale but essentially well, and she was able to give a clear and comprehensive history. She had developed back pain and abdominal bloating on December 26, plus difficulty in passing wind, which, she thought, had caused central abdominal pain that had settled in her right pelvic area, radiating to her back. She had felt hot and then cold. The pain came in spasms, which she estimated as 8 out of 10, where 10 is the highest score. The pain occasionally caused her to double up, but it had resolved with the co-codamol given in the ED. Her appetite was reduced, but she was purposefully drinking plenty of water. She had nausea, but had not vomited. She experienced frequency of micturition and dysuria, and stated that she could only pass about a teaspoon of urine at any time. She had never experienced any of these symptoms in the past. She had passed a small soft stool that morning, but did not notice any blood or mucus. She had not traveled abroad recently.

The day before her visit to the ED, she had consulted her general practitioner (GP), who had suggested she had "been living it up too much," diagnosed a flare-up of diverticulosis, and prescribed colofac to reduce muscle spasm. She had taken colofac before bed and paracetamol 1 g at 0400 that morning, with no relief. Mrs. Green said that her GP thought that she had had irritable bowel syndrome (IBS) for some years. She was not taking any prescribed medicines and had no known allergies. She had never smoked and rarely drank alcohol.

Before reading on, consider Exercise 10.4.

EXERCISE 10.4

Is this enough information to make a diagnosis? If not, what else would you need to know?

PART 2 – PHYSICAL EXAMINATION

Remember the importance of always washing and cleaning hands prior to and after physically examining the patient. The ACP should explain what the physical examination involves, gain the patient's consent, and offer the patient the opportunity to ask any questions during the examination.

Measuring relevant vital signs provides a baseline of the patient's physiological status at that point, and it may influence the clinician's direction in the physical examination. For example, evidence of fever may prompt examination of the lymphatic system, whereas hypothermia should always trigger assessment of distal limb circulation and sensation. Low oxygen saturation in the well-perfused patient can be challenged by asking the patient to take a few deep inspirations; if the reading increases, there is satisfactory respiratory exchange of gases.

Persistent respiratory distress in the patient who has normal vital signs (and is not hyperventilating) may indicate a metabolic acidosis, and the urgent need for measurement of blood gases. Peak expiratory flow measurement, if technique is satisfactory, gives a quick snapshot of the patient's ability to expel air from their lungs, and provides evidence of airway flow. Extremes of pulse or blood pressure may point to the need for a comprehensive cardiovascular or neurological examination, regardless of the presenting complaint.

Examination of one or more body systems is not always required if the history and near-patient investigations, such as urine testing, lead to a diagnosis. However, signs of clinical significance can be missed if the patient is not examined properly. In this case, Mrs. Green should be asked to remove some of her clothes in order to expose her abdomen; the ACP should assure patient dignity and privacy, and that she is made comfortable in the optimum position for and following the examination. Examination of the torso involves the four standard elements, normally in the sequence of:

- Inspection: observing for normal and abnormal variants.
- Palpation: touching and feeling anatomical sites.
- Percussion: tapping of a part of the body to discern the underlying tissue density.
- Auscultation: listening for heart, respiratory, or bowel sounds, usually with a stethoscope. Before reading on, consider Exercise 10.5.

EXERCISE 10.5

Make a list of the possible differential diagnoses you might consider for Mrs. Green.

How would you discuss the items in your list and your clinical reasoning with her?

What steps would you take next?

Outcome

Mrs. Green's vital signs were:

- Temperature: 36.5 °C
- Pulse: 75/minute regular
- Oxygen saturation: 98% on air
- Respirations: 16/minute
- Blood pressure: 150/68

Her consent was gained to examine her abdomen, and she moved to lie down on the couch with relative ease. There was no sign of jaundice or conjunctival pallor; her hands, fingers, and nails were normal; there was no palmar erythema nor asterixis. She was a slender woman, but her abdomen appeared rounded and bloated; there were no visible lesions, scars, or any rash. Normal bowel sounds were discerned in all quadrants, and, though there was no obvious guarding of her abdomen, percussion (dull) and gentle palpation did elicit tenderness up to her epigastria. There was no hard palpable mass, but every suggestion of a fully stretched bladder. Mrs. Green had no renal angle tenderness on palpation of her costo-vertebral angles; Murphy's sign was negative.

PART 3 – CRITICAL THINKING AND CLINICAL DECISION MAKING

Critical thinking is an objective stance in which information is analyzed and judged. In healthcare, critical thinking requires a clear understanding of the patient's situation based on synthesis of the evidence provided by the history, physical examination, and clinical investigations. Critical thinking processes enable the practitioner to examine competing diagnoses of what has happened to the patient and select the best one. It also requires the emotional intelligence to articulate the selected diagnosis and negotiate an outcome that is in the patient's best interest. Inherent in critical thinking processes is the concept of evidence-based practice (EBP; Gambill 2012). A founding ethical principle of EBP is that clinicians should base their decisions and actions on the best available evidence. This means critically appraising research findings and, where these do not exist or are not deemed robust, other sources, and applying the outcomes to patient care and treatment. Critical thinking is essential in enabling the ACP to diagnose Mrs. Green's problem correctly and develop a patient-centered plan of action.

Outcome

Mrs. Green's vital signs were generally within the normal adult range. The co-codamol given in the ED could have reduced any fever she may have had. It had effectively quelled her pain at this point. There was no convincing evidence of a kidney stone; a stone would have induced renal colic, arising in waves of severe and intractable pain. Her systolic blood pressure was elevated, which can be induced by simply being in a hospital or clinic environment, and her diastolic pressure was satisfactory given her present malaise. There was no left-sided abdominal pain, no left iliac fossa tenderness, nor any history of blood per rectum, which are common symptoms of diverticulitis. She had no renal angle tenderness on firm palpation, which reduced the likelihood of an upper urinary tract infection. Her bladder was more than full, which suggested there was no ureteric compromise, though by now there could be some reflux of urine. There was no evidence of any spinal neurological or pelvic plexus compromise. There was no sign of gastrointestinal obstruction nor any evidence of a pelvic mass (feces, tumor) obstructing outflow of urine from her bladder; it appeared that the acuity of inflammation in her bladder and urethra was prohibiting any adequate micturition.

PART 4 – CLOSING THE EPISODE OF CARE

The ACP decided that Mrs. Green had a lower tract urinary infection with signs of urinary retention and explained this to the patient, ensuring that she understood the information. The ACP then negotiated for her to have a bladder scan, which was carried out in her consulting room by a healthcare assistant from the ED. This revealed that the bladder contained over 1000 ml. The ACP prescribed antibiotics, according to regional microbiological guidelines, and analgesia and advised Mrs. Green about self-care measures, including adequate hydration, how to self-manage her symptoms, and what to do if these escalated. The ACP thanked the patient for her participation in the consultation and offered to assist with anything she may require, for example where she would find an open pharmacy during a holiday period. Mrs. Green was then referred back to the ED, because the out-of-hours service did not provide urinary catheterization. This would be carried out in the ED and appropriate follow-up arranged.

10.2 Holistic Health Assessment

Mrs. Green's case demonstrates the importance of holistic health assessment at the outset of an episode of care. The GP she consulted probably felt pressured to provide time-limited consultations, and so hurriedly applied a form of pattern recognition to reach an incorrect diagnosis, which resulted in ineffectual treatment. The ED triage nurse may have been influenced by the dipstick result to assume the patient had an uncomplicated urinary tract infection and so referred Mrs. Green to the out-of-hours service. Whatever the drivers, this episode does not indicate that cost-effective, seamless care occurred, as Mrs. Green was seen by five different clinicians (GP, triage nurse, ACP, healthcare assistant, and ED nurse) in three different environments (GP surgery, ED, out-of-hours service) before she had an adequate history taken, a physical examination with further investigation, and appropriate treatment.

The case also draws attention to the experience and expertise of the ACP. Newly qualified practitioners may feel very conscious of their lack of knowledge and have insufficient confidence to formulate a diagnosis; they may even feel the need to focus on this at the expense of caring for their patient. This can easily lead to missing the patient's individual qualities and needs as the clinician struggles to perform in a challenging role. Advanced clinical practice at its best allows patient-centric attributes to subtly move the focus from diagnosis and treatment, important as these are, to patient enablement, passing control back to the patient. In preparing this chapter, I spoke with diverse advanced practitioners about what their patients told them that they, the patients, had appreciated about their care. Listening was a major factor, even in pressured clinical environments, and speaking to patients in words and ways that they could understand, explaining the value and pros and cons of healthcare interventions. Taking action, "you did something about it," was an additional response, perhaps reflecting both the advanced practitioner's efforts and the feelings of patients in a setting in which they can feel lost. These views are supported by Lowe et al. (2012), who argue that advanced practitioners provide patient care equal to that of doctors, "with high levels of patient satisfaction, combined with increased advice on education, health promotion, and follow-up advice."

The competitive marketplace of UK primary care provision that has gradually evolved and increased over the past two to three decades, plus relentless demands on hospital and community services, creates internal pressures that can get in the way of patient-centric care and increase risk for patients (Roland and Rosen 2011). It is exactly in this environment that advanced practitioners must give of themselves and demonstrate their professional attributes: keeping a clear mind, retaining a patient-centered focus, maintaining active listening, and engaging in critical thinking in their clinical reasoning and decision making. Through mindful communication, advanced practitioners can promote their patients' well-being and use their fluency in the language of health and healthcare systems to negotiate outcomes that are in those patients' best interest.

In Mrs. Green's case, it is the ACP who plugs the gap in service provision by listening to her and doing something about her problem. However, the ACP is unable to provide a complete episode of care on this occasion because of organizational constraints. In this case, another healthcare worker has the relevant equipment and has been trained to perform the bladder scan. Likewise, it is another department, the ED, that has a stock of urinary catheters plus the communication system in place to arrange suitable "trial without catheter" (TWOC) clinic follow-up. So, in this instance, despite having the nursing skills to intervene by simply catheterizing Mrs. Green, the ACP must function within service parameters and, having effectively assessed her and made the clinical decision regarding her immediate care, refer the patient back to the ED for the practical interventions needed prior to closure of this episode of care.

This raises concerns about the ACP's role. If the ACP is a nurse with enhanced knowledge, skill, and experience, then it seems appropriate to use those to perform the procedure. Alternatively, if the ACP is simply regarded by the organization as a substitute doctor, then nursing expertise is relegated to a subordinate position because the role is focused on getting through the medical workload. Organizational policies, priorities, and boundaries may, therefore, push clinicians and healthcare toward a management-led rather than professional approach (Greenhalgh et al. 2014). In contrast, advanced practice education and development focus on quality of care rather than quantity and speed of patient throughput. Nevertheless, in their retrospective review of ACPs who had been employed purposefully as doctor substitutes in the ED, Cooke et al. (2014) discovered that the ACP saw more patients per hour than the middle-grade doctors.

10.3 Conclusion

Health assessment and direct care are influenced by the clinical domain in which they occur. ACPs adapt and apply the principles of advanced practice in their realm of work, taking action across traditionally established professional boundaries to provide whole episodes of care for the individual where possible. As clinicians in diverse disciplines develop their vision and see how the principles of advanced practice can be applied to provide their patients with seamless care and improve service quality, the ACP model has the potential to yield improved health outcomes while ensuring cost-effective care. The attributes and qualities of the ACP are similar to those of any other knowledgeable, caring, and compassionate clinician when caring for their patient. What is unique is the ACP's responsiveness to the ever-changing demands of healthcare, manifested through creatively employing the four pillars of advanced practice (Jones et al. 2015). ACPs value the key role of clinical audit in terms of good governance and professional protection for the individual, and utilize this to reflect on their own performance, as well as disseminate audit findings to others in the team. These findings, as well as a quality assurance metric, can often provide the foundation for service change and improvement.

Key Questions

1. In your field of practice, what factors contribute to fragmentation of care?

2. As an advanced practitioner, to what extent are you able to use your nursing skills?

Glossary

Asterixis: flapping of the hands, a symptom of liver disease.

Costo-vertebral angle: angle formed between the 12th rib and the vertebral column.

Diagnostic and Statistical Manual of Mental Disorders (DSM): defines and classifies mental health disorders. It is published and updated by the American Psychiatric Association (www.psychiatry.org).

Murphy's sign: a test for gall bladder inflammation.

Out-of-hours care: the provision of urgent medical care outside of normal GP opening hours. Out-of-hours services are provided between 1830 and 0800 during the week and throughout weekends and bank holidays on a 24-hour basis. Staff may be GPs or nurses. Urgent (nonemergency) medical care refers to health problems and illnesses that cannot wait until the GP surgery reopens.

Patient Health Questionnaire (PHQ-9): a freely available questionnaire that can be self-administered, which is widely used by health professionals to assess and monitor depression. It is linked to the Diagnostic and Statistical Manual of Mental Disorders. See Spitzer et al. (1999) and Kroenke et al. (2001).

References

Bernadt, M.W., Taylor, C., Mumford, J. et al. (1982). Comparison of questionnaire and laboratory tests in the detection of excessive drinking and alcoholism. *The Lancet* 319 (8267): 325–328.

Briggs, E. (2010). Assessment and expression of pain. *Nursing Standard* 25 (2): 35–38.

Cameron, I.M., Cardy, A., Crawford, J.R. et al. (2011). Measuring depression severity in general practice: discriminatory performance of the PHQ-9, HADS-D, and BDI-II. *British Journal of General Practice* 61 (588): e419–e426.

Clayton, H.A., Reschak, G.L.C., Gaynor, S.E., and Creamer, J.L. (2000). A novel program to assess and manage pain. *MEDSURG Nursing* 9 (6): 318–321.

Cooke, M., Swann, G., Chessum, P. *et al* (2014). Substituting doctors in emergency departments with non-medical practitioners. Unpublished paper presented to the International Conference of Emergency Medicine, Hong Kong. In Williams, K. (2017) Advanced practitioners in emergency care: a literature review. Emergency Nurse 25(4), 36–41.

Ewing, J.A. (1984). The CAGE questionnaire. *Journal of the American Medical Association* 252 (14): 1905–1907.

Gambill, E. (2012). *Critical Thinking in Clinical Practice*, 3e. Hoboken, NJ: Wiley.

Greenhalgh, T., Howick, J., and Maskrey, N. (2014). Evidence based medicine: a movement in crisis? *British Medical Journal* 348: 3725.

Gupta, S., Saint, S., and Detsky, A.S. (2017). Hiding in plain sight—resurrecting the power of inspecting the patient. *JAMA Internal Medicine* 177 (6): 757–758.

Jones, A., Powell, T., Watkins, D., and Kelly, D. (2015). Realising their potential? Exploring interprofessional perceptions and potential of the advanced practitioner role: a qualitative analysis. *BMJ Open* 5 (12): 1–8.

Krasner, M.S., Epstein, R.M., Beckman, H. et al. (2009). Association of an educational program in mindful communication with burnout, empathy, and attitudes among primary care physicians. *Journal of the American Medical Association* 302 (12): 1284–1293.

Kroenke, K., Spitzer, R.L., and Williams, J.B. (2001). The PHQ-9: validity of a brief depression severity measure. *Journal of General Internal Medicine* 16 (9): 606–613.

Lowe, G., Plummer, V., O'Brien, A.P., and Boyd, L. (2012). Time to clarify the value of advanced practice nursing roles in health care. *Journal of Advanced Nursing* 68 (3): 677–685.

Malpass, A., Dowrick, C., Gilbody, S. et al. (2016). Usefulness of PHQ-9 in primary care to determine meaningful symptoms of low need: a qualitative study. *British Journal of General Practice* 66 (643): e78–e84.

Matthys, J., Elwyn, G., Van Nuland, M. et al. (2009). Patients' ideas, concerns, and expectations (ICE) in general practice: impact on prescribing. *British Journal of General Practice* 59 (558): 29–36.

Mazer-Poline, C. and Fomari, V. (2009). Anorexia nervosa and pregnancy: having a baby when you are dying to be thin - case report and proposed treatment guidelines. *International Journal of Eating Disorders* 42 (4): 382–384

McEwen, B.S., Gray, J.D., and Nasca, C. (2015). Recognizing resilience: learning from the effects of stress on the brain. *Neurobiology of Stress* 1: 1–11.

Mitchell, P. (ed.) (2013). *Safer Care: Human Factors for Healthcare. Trainer's Manual.* Argyll and Bute: Swan and Horn.

National Patient Safety Agency (2010). *Medical Error. What to Do if Things Go Wrong: A Guide for Junior Doctors.* London: NPSA.

NHS England (2013). *The Information Governance Review.* London: Williams Lea for the Department of Health.

National Institute for Health and Care Excellence (2012). Patient experience in adult NHS services: improving the experience of care for people using adult NHS services. Clinical Guideline 138. https://www.nice.org.uk/guidance/cg138 (accessed January 11, 2019).

National Institute for Health and Care Excellence (2015). Depression in adults: recognition and management. Clinical Guideline 90. https://www.nice.org.uk/guidance/cg90 (accessed January 11, 2019).

Potter, P.J. and Frisch, N. (2007). Holistic assessment and care: presence in the process. *Nursing Clinics* 42 (2): 213–228.

Roland, M. and Rosen, R. (2011). Health policy report. English NHS embarks on controversial and risky market-style reforms in health care. *New England Journal of Medicine* 364 (14): 1360–1366.

Spitzer, R., Kroenke, K., and Williams, J. (1999). Validation and utility of a self-report version of PRIME-MD: the PHQ primary care study. *Journal of the American Medical Association* 282: 1737–1744.

Stuart, M.R. and Lieberman, J.A. III (2015). *The Fifteen Minute Hour: Therapeutic Talk in Primary Care,* 5e. London: Radcliffe Publishing.

Turk, D.C. and Melzack, R. (eds.) (2011). *Handbook of Pain Assessment.* New York: Guilford Press.

CHAPTER 11

The Advanced Critical Care Practitioner

Paula McGee[1] and Jonathan Downham[2]

[1]Birmingham City University, Birmingham, UK
[2]Warwick Foundation NHS Trust, Warwick, UK

Key Issues

- The nature and scope of practice of the advanced critical care practitioner
- Proning a patient with acute respiratory distress syndrome
- The inter-relatedness of advanced practice competences

LEARNING OBJECTIVES

By the end of this chapter you will be able to:

- Critically discuss the processes that may contribute to the development of a specialty.

- Examine current issues in advanced critical care practice with reference to your own professional field

11.1 Introduction

Critical care is a highly specialized field of healthcare in which multidisciplinary teams provide continuous monitoring, treatment, and care for patients with life-threatening conditions. It is a field that is constantly evolving in response to new knowledge and technological developments, and requires a highly skilled workforce able to interpret changes in complex physiological data and provide appropriate interventions. Critical care teams are led by medical practitioners and include a range of professionals who have specialized in the field: nurses, physiotherapists, pharmacists, dieticians, psychologists, and occupational therapists. This field requires adaptability and new ways of working which,

Advanced Practice in Healthcare: Dynamic Developments in Nursing and Allied Health Professions,
Fourth Edition. Edited by Paula McGee and Chris Inman.
© 2019 John Wiley & Sons Ltd. Published 2019 by John Wiley & Sons Ltd.

over time, have led nurses and members of allied health professions to develop advanced levels of practice that blend normal professional practice, new activities, and work previously within the medical domain. These advanced roles themselves are not static. Continued evolution, the constantly changing context of both healthcare generally and critical care in particular, and "the inherently unpredictable nature of working with people" have all contributed to the need for additional new roles that facilitate certain aspects of patient care delivery (Ramis Wu and Pearson 2013, p. 178). The advanced critical care practitioner (ACCP) is one of these roles. This chapter begins with a discussion of the ACCP role in the UK and the nature of the scope of practice. This is followed by a case study that demonstrates aspects of the role in direct patient care. The chapter then moves on to present an analysis of the processes involved in the development of advanced critical care practice, and closes with a discussion of current issues in this field.

11.2 The Advanced Critical Care Practitioner Role

In the UK, the ACCP role is to "provide care that is focused on patients and their needs, save life, recognise acutely ill patients, initiate early treatment, support patients through critical illness and, where appropriate, enable a dignified death ... and enhance continuity and quality of care" (Department of Health [DH] 2008, p. 1). A critical care nurse "has the right knowledge, skills, and competences to meet the needs of a critically ill patient without direct supervision. The knowledge, skills and competences they require to nurse critically ill patients should reflect the level of patient need, rather than being determined by the patient care environment (for example, a high dependency or intensive care unit)" (RCN 2003, www.rcn.org.uk). Thus, the provision of critical care and advanced critical care roles are primarily about patient need and the level of care required. The aim is to "support patients through critical illness," toward recovery, or if this is not possible "a dignified death" (DH 2008, p. 1).

Determining patient need inevitably involves selection. Critical resources are directed toward the treatment and care of seriously ill patients who, it is anticipated, will recover and, eventually, be discharged. Whilst it is recognized that some may deteriorate further and not prove responsive to treatment, critical care is emphatically neither a measure of last resort nor an attempt to avoid an inevitable death. Current guidance on selection divides patients into three levels of need. At level 1, patients are admitted to hospital because they require interventions and closer observation than can be carried out at home. Examples may include a patient with asthma who needs oxygen, chest physiotherapy, and antibiotics. These patients do not need critical care expertise unless they deteriorate. At level 2 are patients who may need critical care, either because they cannot, at that time, manage a vital function unaided or are deemed at risk of deterioration in their ability to do so. Examples may include patients who need a high level of postoperative care following complex surgery and who may require respiratory and cardiovascular assistance as part of their recovery.

At level 3 are patients who definitely require critical care because they cannot maintain two or more vital systems unaided or require respiratory support (Intensive Care Society 2009). The level of patient need also takes precedence over "the patient care environment" (DH 2008, p. 1). Whilst many ACCPs do practice in intensive care and high-dependency units in hospitals, where it is more efficient to gather the required resources and expertise together, critical care practice can and does take place in other settings.

11.3 Scope of Practice

Critical care is an "intellectually and emotionally challenging" arena that requires the ability to act with speed and accuracy and in which there is "little margin for error" (Benner et al. 2011, p. 1). ACCPs are required to develop the "theoretical knowledge, practical skills and an understanding of professional judgement" to enable them to work autonomously as members of a critical care team (DH 2008, p. 11; Table 11.1). This means that they must be competent to conduct a rapid physical assessment of a patient who is either seriously ill or in an unstable condition and make a diagnosis. They must then be able to initiate and manage a treatment plan, which often incorporates invasive procedures that were previously only in the medical domain (Table 11.1).

ACCPs have the knowledge, skill, and expertise to function autonomously, providing leadership and coordination in the direct care of patients who are critically ill with compromised respiratory and/or cardiovascular systems, sepsis, or other serious conditions that require close monitoring. This level of practice demands "thinking in action," a term used by Benner et al. 2011, p. 10) to denote full, active engagement and clinical reasoning in managing the patient's situation. In their view, thinking in action "conveys the innovative and productive nature of the clinician's active thinking." This differs from Schön's (1987) "reflection in action," which implies "stepping back or being outside the situation." Thinking in action goes beyond what is learned in class. It integrates theoretical knowledge with experiential learning to create an "embodied way of knowing" that cannot be acquired in any other way, because it cannot be formally taught. This embodied way of knowing transcends both theoretical and practical knowledge. It facilitates clinical reasoning in what can be rapidly changing situations, in which the ACCP must be able to accurately identify and focus on the most important elements, draw quickly on a range of possible solutions, and act appropriately (Benner et al. 1996, 2011, p. 22).

Communication is a particularly important competence in critical care (Table 11.1). The high level of technological and clinical expertise at play in critical care has the potential to obscure psychological human needs for comfort and reassurance. Knowing how to speak to people in different roles and circumstances, what to reveal, when and to whom, and the level of detail needed is not easy. Patients and their relatives are likely to be very concerned and anxious, both about events leading to the need for critical care and about what this care may entail. Listening and responding to their concerns require skill and compassion, but also some degree of judgment about how much information individuals under stress can absorb. Nevertheless, explanation may not only

TABLE 11.1

ACCP scope of practice.

Utilize nursing skills in history taking, physical examination, and assessment to identify patient need.

Interpret clinical and laboratory data and respond in a timely manner.

Diagnose, initiate, and modify treatment of critical illness based on the best available evidence.

Prescribe and modify medication and intravenous fluids.

Perform specialist procedures which may be within the medical domain, e.g. insert venous lines for dialysis, perform intubation.

Monitor patient progress.

Rapid response to and wide repertoire of strategies for patients with changing and fluctuating conditions.

Communicate effectively with patients, colleagues, families, and others to ensure understanding of continuity in care and treatment.

Provide clinical and professional leadership.

Practice within an ethical and legal framework.

Ensure patient dignity and privacy.

Ensure that personal care (e.g. washing, mouth care, bowel and bladder care) are carried out.

Support patients and families in understanding care and treatment, possible future requirements such as rehabilitation, and other areas.

Work as a member of a multiprofessional and multidisciplinary team.

Provide training and supervision for other staff including junior doctors. Delegate to others as appropriate.

Participate in research, service audits, and evaluations.

Engage in continuous professional development.

Show respect for cultural and religious beliefs and practices.

Prevent hazards and ensure patient safety.

Manage the provision of dignified end-of-life care.

Discharge planning and support staff outside the critical care environment, for example as patients recover and are discharged into their care.

Ensure safe patient transport.

Manage organ tissue donation.

Source: Summarized from Benner et al. (2011), Department of Health (2008), Kleinpell (2005).

help to relieve their anxiety, but also reveal information that may be of use in treatment; discussion about recovery and long-term outcomes may also be broached. Communication with professionals requires a different approach depending on the experience and roles of the personnel involved; clarity, conciseness, courtesy, and speed matter more than usual in this environment. As an expert practitioner, the ACCP is able to recognize the challenges inherent in communicating effectively with diverse individuals with different needs and preferred communication styles (Lenz 2013).

Acute respiratory distress syndrome (ARDS) is a life-threatening condition of acute onset, "characterized by inflammatory pulmonary edema resulting in severe hypoxemia" (Fan et al. 2017, p. 1254). According to the *Berlin definition*, which is the gold standard developed by the European Society of Intensive Care Medicine, there are three factors in diagnosing ARDS: timing, chest imaging, and pulmonary edema (Ranieri et al. 2012). Onset must occur within a week as the result of trauma and/or infection and a range of other conditions which require treatment alongside that related to ARDS. The presence of pulmonary edema cannot be explained by other causes, and chest imaging shows bilateral opacities (Ranieri et al. 2012). Symptoms may develop very quickly or slowly over a few days. The condition is often fatal. The presence of edema increases lung weight and interferes with the action of both surfactant and gaseous exchange, as alveoli collapse or fill with fluid. This in turn may lead to poor oxygenation with consequent implications for the circulation and the potential of multiple organ failure. The severity of ARDS varies and assessment depends largely on the ratio of the partial pressure of oxygen (PaO_2) to the fraction of inspired oxygen (FiO_2; Ranieri et al. 2012). As ARDS is a syndrome, there is no specific diagnostic test. In addition to the Berlin definition, there are several unvalidated scales for measuring severity such as the Lung Injury Score, but the outcome is difficult to predict; mortality is estimated at between 24% and 48% depending on severity (Faculty of Intensive Care Medicine and Intensive Care Society 2018).

Mrs. K, aged 71, experienced increasing shortness of breath over a three-day period. This has worsened gradually overnight and paramedics have brought her to the Emergency Department via ambulance. Mrs. K is very dyspneic; pulse oximetry shows oxygen saturation levels fluctuating between 80% and 85%. Even when the O_2 is increased to 15L/M via a non-re-breathable mask, saturation continues to remain below 90%. Her skin feels clammy and she has a mild tachycardia. She can speak only in short sentences. The medical registrar calls the ACCP from the critical care unit to review Mrs. K.

Before you read on, consider Exercise 11.1.

EXERCISE 11.1

As the ACCP, outline the initial assessment you would make. Include any tests or investigations you would consider necessary.

What data would give you cause for concern?

The ACCP acts quickly, performing auscultation, which reveals widespread chest crackles consistent with the presence of pulmonary edema. Chest imaging shows bilateral fluffy opacities. There are no pleural effusions. These factors, in addition to Mrs. K's poor oxygen saturation, are consistent with a diagnosis of ARDS by the ACCP and the medical consultant. The ACCP decides that Mrs. K requires intubation and mechanical ventilation. She is sedated and the ACCP performs intubation whilst supervised by the intensive care consultant. Mrs. K is then transferred to the critical care unit for mechanical ventilation; sedation is continued. Unfortunately, Mrs. K's oxygen saturations do not improve, but remain at 80% and 85% despite her receiving 100% oxygen.

Before reading on, consider Exercises 11.2 and 11.3.

EXERCISE 11.2

What diagnosis would you make and why?

What immediate action would you take?

EXERCISE 11.3

As the ACCP, what further actions could be taken to improve Mrs. K's condition and why?

Current guidance indicates that, in this type of situation, there are some interventions which might make a difference. Proning the patient, turning them onto their front, is one such method. There are two reasons for this. First, when Mrs. K lies on her back, her ventral lungs will be ventilated more favorably than her dorsal lungs. Second, blood supply at the back of the lungs is normally better than at the front. Gravity causes fluid to flow downward to the lowest level and so, if Mrs. K lies on her back, fluid will accumulate at the back of her lungs and obstruct gaseous exchange in that area. Placing her on her front will redistribute the fluid toward the front, allow new areas to be aerated, and facilitate gaseous exchange (Gattinoni et al. 2013). Proning a critically ill patient with ARDS is potentially hazardous, either because of the procedure itself or because of problems arising from staying prone. In addition, any trauma associated with the onset of ARDS, such as spinal damage or abdominal wounds, would be a contraindication for this procedure (Gattinoni et al. 2013).

The ACCP is the sole member of staff with experience of performing proning in the management of ARDS and so offers to lead the procedure. The situation requires urgent action. The ACCP prepares staff, including the intensive care consultant, at the bedside, outlining the procedure and explaining the steps required. Mrs. K remains sedated. A team of at least six staff is needed. Two staff at one side of the bed use the bottom sheet to gently roll Mrs. K toward the other side, where two more staff receive her and ease her into the prone position. Care must be taken to ensure that her limbs are correctly positioned to avoid damage to joints, that her head is turned to one side, and that her eyes are protected. The other two or more staff are responsible for ensuring that tubes and lines are not disconnected (Hudack 2012). Mrs. K responds very well to the turn. Her oxygen saturation improves to 100% within a couple of hours; the oxygen concentration is then reduced to 60%. The ACCP explains to the staff that she should remain in the prone position for 16 hours, as guidance advises, at which point she is to be turned back onto her back using the same procedure as before. If her progress is slow over the next few days, she may be proned again up to a maximum of three times (Fan et al. 2017; FICM and ICS 2018). Mrs. K makes slow but positive progress and is eventually discharged from critical care.

11.4 Competences for the Advanced Critical Care Practitioner Role

This case study demonstrates some of the competences required in the advanced practice role generally and how these apply in advanced critical care practice. First, the ACCP was called as a *consultant*; that is, as someone regarded by others as having specialist expertise. In the Emergency Department the medical registrar had responsibility for Mrs. K but, by implication, acknowledged the limitations either in their own experience or the ability of the department to meet this patient's needs.

There are several types of consultant activity, most of which are forms of indirect care, for example working at organizational level to improve a service or providing advice to practitioners to help them develop their skills or cope with a difficult situation (Vosit-Steller and Morse 2014). However, in the case study, the ACCP was asked, as a clinical expert, to engage directly with Mrs. K, to conduct an assessment and diagnose her exact problem, and then initiate a treatment plan. Thus, in the case of a patient with complex and urgent needs, the consultant has to be able to work across traditional boundaries between care settings and, if necessary, may act as a demonstrator of what needs to be done. Inherent in being consulted is the recognition and value placed, by others, on the consultant's expertise and the anticipation that a particular situation may be resolved. Exercising competence as a consultant also depends on valuing one's own specialist expertise, and feeling realistically confident in one's own clinical competence. No one will value the ACCP's expertise if that person does not value themselves as possessing specific knowledge and skill, whilst also recognizing their limitations. Lack of confidence in themselves will affect how the ACCP acts and communicates with patients and colleagues. In this case study, Mrs. K needs decisive action based on a high level of specialist knowledge, and the medical registrar needs to have confidence that the patient is safe (Barron and White 2009; Lenz 2013).

Second, the ACCP implemented two more advanced competences: *leadership* and *coaching and guiding* (Spross and Babine 2014; Tracy and Hanson 2014). This is particularly evident in relation to the decision to prone Mrs. K. No other member of staff had experience of performing this procedure, so the ACCP was able to act as clinical leader, combining leadership with coaching and guiding colleagues by quickly explaining to them how to prone the patient safely. Of particular interest here is the way in which this case study demonstrates the inter-relatedness of advanced practice competences. Most text books on advanced practice tend to present each competence in a silo. This is appropriate as an exercise in examining the nature and attributes of individual competences in detail, but real-life practice is not like this: it is messy. Competences are rarely applied singly; there is constant interaction and overlap between them. For example, an advanced practitioner may be providing *direct, evidence-based care* to a patient alongside *coaching and guiding* that person to cope with newly diagnosed diabetes, whilst at the same time ensuring that this coaching is *ethically* appropriate. Similarly, in the case study, *leadership* and *teaching and guiding* overlapped; it was not enough to tell colleagues what to do, they had to be led through the procedure as a team. In addition, competence as a *consultant* overlapped with providing *direct care, ethical decision making* regarding Mrs. K's suitability for critical care, and *collaboration* with medical staff. This case study demonstrates the high level of knowledge, decision making, and practical skill that underpin the ACCP's role, but it also reveals something of the breadth and depth of the advanced practice role in general.

Before reading on, consider Exercise 11.4.

EXERCISE 11.4

As an ACCP, critically reflect on a short and recent period of your practice. An hour would be ample time to select.

How many advanced competences did you employ? How and why did you do so?

11.5 Processes in the Development of the Advanced Critical Care Practitioner Role

The emergence of ACCP roles is widely attributed to a combination of multiple factors, such as reductions in the number and availability of doctors as a result of changes in medical education, the increasing costs of healthcare, and new knowledge and technologies that increase patients' chances of survival. However, the development of new roles and specialties in healthcare can also be seen as a growing trend throughout the twentieth century, as health professions and occupations sought to move from "a simple division of labor" in order to "forward and control their own development" (Bucher 1988, pp. 131 and 132). In this context, ACCP roles can be seen as the product of processes through which development has taken place. This analysis draws on Bucher's (1988) examination of these processes through which new professional groups in healthcare emerge and relates them to advanced critical care practice. The focus on processes is based on the recognition that developments are fluid, and may progress forward, backward, sideways, or not at all. There is no fixed or clear pathway and acceptance of this facilitates exploration beyond causation. Identifying causes does contribute to an understanding of events; causes are often complex and do not necessarily help in grappling with the present. What follows here is a discussion of four processes which may occur in any order or even at the same time.

11.5.1 **Internal Processes**

Every profession delineates its sphere of work, the standards to which this work should be done, the criteria for entry, the values espoused, and so on. In nursing these are enshrined in a code of practice, which states that all nurses must prioritize people, practice effectively, preserve safety, and promote professionalism and trust (Nursing and Midwifery Council [NMC] 2018). This is complemented by a statement of the standards of proficiency that must be attained and retained by every nurse (NMC 2018). These documents are necessarily sufficiently broad, because the work of nurses is constantly undergoing changes. Some of these changes have occurred as medicine itself has changed. For example, the British Cardiac Society was formed in 1946 when cardiology emerged as a medical specialty and, from 1972 onward, nurses began pursuing their own education in this field (Joint Board of Clinical Nursing Studies 1990). Gradually, other clinical specialties emerged, but remained under the umbrella of nursing, which has continued to act as the sole gatekeeper. However, changes have also occurred because nurses have expanded their sphere of practice into places where doctors are in short supply: remote and rural areas in parts of Scotland and Wales, patient education, and support in diabetes care; and where doctors may be absent or not readily available: among street dwellers, at workplaces, and with charitable organizations such as Macmillan Cancer Support (www. macmillan.org.uk). Organizations may also encourage and create expansion of roles. The NHS Plan (DH 2000) and the Five Year Forward View (NHS England 2014) actively encouraged new ways of working. The introduction of nurse practitioners led to the development of new roles to suit local purposes, through the performance of specific tasks such as staffing night duty rotas in hospitals and conducting preadmission clinics (Kendall et al. 1997).

ACCP roles seem to have developed in response to a combination of factors. The impact of the Working Time (Amendment) Regulations 2002 limited the availability of doctors by reducing the working hours of junior doctors and consultants; the availability of junior doctors was also limited by changes in medical education. New knowledge and the "increasing complexity of care pathways and technology" also had an impact. Consequently, health service organizations sought to develop new roles that 'extended the scope of practice of nurses, technicians, physiotherapists and clinical pharmacists" (DH 2008, p. iii). Internal processes therefore reflect disruption of the status quo, a challenge to the established way of operating. Initial responses may focus on tinkering with the system, moving resources, or changing staff roles, but in time it becomes clear that this is not enough. Moreover, the practitioners caught up in these processes may begin to question what is happening to them and seek out like-minded others.

11.5.2 "Finding a Niche" Processes

Over time interest groups begin to form, gatherings of practitioners working in a particular field or setting and initiated by a small number of individuals with a common interest. Informal and unfunded, these groups facilitate the discovery of "colleagueship," and of being, in some way, separate from or different to other members of the profession (Bucher 1988). They provide space in which to share matters of common interest and concern, to seek advice, share news, network, and create a sense of belonging to something and somewhere in which discussion of a concern does not always have to be prefaced by a detailed explanation of the background. Facebook, Twitter, WhatsApp, and other internet-based fora, alongside more traditional communications such as publications, newsletters, and conferences, serve to extend the reach of these groups. Their activities expand, but remain inner directed. Leaders emerge. Groups begin to refine their purpose by developing their own ideologies with specific aims, definitions, procedures, and records; formal membership arrangements and subscriptions define insiders and outsiders. These activities confirm a sense of separateness, that "we are different because …," and form a base for outward-focused processes that are devoted to trying to establish a territory, a domain in which a group's members can feel they belong and which they can begin to articulate to outsiders, particularly those powerful enough to accept the new group's claims as legitimate. Development and control of training mark a significant step, because it requires negotiating space in university and clinical domains, the development of standards, competences, and curricula, and the acquisition of resources.

The development of advanced nursing practice in the UK has followed these processes, first in developing special interest groups such as the Association of Advanced Practice Educators and the Royal College of Nursing Advanced Nurse Practitioner Forum. Second, advanced nurses sought, unsuccessfully, to legitimate their status through registration of their additional qualifications with the Nursing and Midwifery Council (McGee 2009). ACCPs have pursued slightly different processes in aligning themselves with the Faculty of Intensive Care Medicine. The Faculty offers membership to ACCPs who have successfully completed training as set out in the National Competency Framework in units approved for stages 1 and 2 intensive care medicine training (DH 2008) and hold substantive posts in either the NHS or Defence Medical Services (www.ficm.ac.uk). This membership allows ACCPs to participate in faculty events, committees, and further training. How many will take up this membership remains to be seen.

Finding a niche processes are, therefore, primarily about the challenges of separating from established professional practice, taking on a new role that differs from those of fellow professionals, and finding new "colleagueship" among others in the same situation. New groups evolve from informal collections of a few like-minded individuals into formal organizations whose members are accepted as possessing specific expertise that requires formal training. There is a sense of "maturity," of having "turned a corner and passed beyond the emerging stage" (Bucher 1988, p. 141).

11.5.3 **Consolidation Processes**

Turning the corner reveals that there is still a great deal to do: "a major feature of an occupation or occupational segment's maturity is an elaboration of institutional forms and arrangements" (Bucher 1988, p. 141). The new groups are still called societies, associations, or some other term, but they continue to evolve. Issues that were not previously even thought of, such as maintaining the website, office space, securing funding, and developing policies, now have to be addressed; responsibilities have to be delegated to subgroups. It may even be necessary to employ staff to manage some roles, because members now want timely responses to their inquiries and to be able to see what they get in return for their subscriptions. Externally, the specialty, for this is now what it is, also changes; what the original group defined as territory is not constant, and so what was believed to have been settled has to be regularly revisited and reappraised. It is possible that new groups may start to form as a result. Leaders, therefore, have to be constantly aware and informed about both what is happening and what may happen. They need to be flexible, to be able to negotiate, and to plan strategically (Bucher 1988).

Having aligned themselves with the Faculty of Intensive Care Medicine, ACCPs appear to be reaching a stage of consolidation. This is evident in the work of the Faculty's ACCP Advisory Group, which has published "a CPD and Appraisal Pathway by which trained and qualified Advanced Critical Care Practitioners (ACCPs) can plan, institute, maintain and evidence their ongoing clinical, academic, and professional learning" (www.ficm.ac.uk). This detailed pathway is thought to be essential because so much of ACCPs' work is within the medical domain, but it is an adjunct to, rather than a replacement for, statutory revalidation with the individual's professional body. This pathway is significant for several reasons. First, it sets out the competences to be addressed in the annual appraisal and encourages practitioners to think about their own career development. Second, it potentially allows individuals wishing to relocate to other critical care units to take with them tangible, up-to-date evidence of their competence and level of competence, and to know that this will be recognized in their new place of work. Finally, it provides a basis for exclusivity. Practitioners who do not successfully complete a training course that meets the Faculty's specification may not be able to become a member and might then find it hard to gain employment as an ACCP. However, the uptake of this continuing professional development (CPD) and appraisal pathway is not yet clear, and the success of the scheme will need to be evaluated.

11.5.4 **Transformation Processes**

There are now two possible ways forward as the new specialty becomes more established. The first is the "decimated field," a situation in which the original problems are deemed unsolved and possibly unsolvable, or where what they really represent are "general principles" rather than a specialty in its own right. Bucher (1988, p. 144) cites general surgery as an example. There are general principles of surgery that apply across many varied fields, each of which is a specialty in itself. The second is the "rejuvenated field," in which the specialty is reconfigured. New knowledge and technology are embraced and "there is a fundamental redefinition of the nature of the field, of the underlying paradigm, of the territory, of the mission, or all of these" (Bucher 1988, p. 145).

In joining the Faculty of Intensive Care Medicine, advanced critical care practice has the opportunity to undergo transformational processes. How these unfold is yet to be decided, but there are several possibilities, one of which is becoming a separate, direct-entry profession whose members no longer have to be registered practitioners in other health professions. If this occurs, then advanced critical care would have continued to follow the pattern established in the twentieth century as health professions developed specialties, with the support of government and society. However, the current economic climate may be less supportive of the establishment of new professions and the costs of regulation (Professional Standards Authority 2015).

11.6 Current Issues in Advanced Critical Practice

The Faculty of Intensive Care Medicine's CPD and appraisal pathway for ACCPs accepts applicants who are either registered nurses or physiotherapists (www. ficm.ac.uk). However, it is possible that members of other allied health professions may, in time, also wish to develop ACCP roles. There is already some evidence of this. For example, in the UK the Royal Pharmaceutical Society is developing advanced practitioners in critical care using the Advanced Pharmacy Framework (Royal Pharmaceutical Society 2013). Competences outlined in this framework are similar to those for advanced nursing and include expert practice, leadership, management, working as a member of a team, and research; it is the application of them that varies. The critical care group of the UK Clinical Pharmacy Association claims over 350 members, so there is clearly an interest in this area of practice. This mix of professional expertise raises some issues about the ACCP role. Practitioners from diverse professional roles will bring different expertise to critical care. It is easy to identify the contribution of nurses, physiotherapists, pharmacists, and paramedics to critical care work, but, whilst their expertise may overlap, it may not be interchangeable. Moreover, there may be members of other allied health professions, such as dieticians and operating department practitioners, who may also see critical care as a field into which they might expand. The question that then arises is whether all direct-entry ACCPs will be the same, able to deliver the same type and level of care, or whether there will be different branches of advanced critical care practice, each with its own particular skills.

Alternatively, preparation as an ACCP may act as a stepping stone to another professional role. The Emergency Retrieval Service in Scotland developed a pilot scheme to enable five staff with either nursing or paramedic experience to become ACCPs. In the absence of a tailored course, development was initially through on-the-job training, but this was later replaced by a Postgraduate Certificate (PGCert) course in Advanced Clinical Practice Retrieval Medicine. The service now has seven retrieval practitioners, three nurses and four paramedics, who are able to replace registrars in the team if needed (Sinclair and Curatolo 2014). This example suggests that becoming an ACCP may not be an end in itself. This is in line with career frameworks for a number of health professions, such as paramedic practice (College of Paramedics 2015) and physiotherapy (Chartered Society of Physiotherapists 2016), in which the advanced level of practice is below that of consultant. Thus, advanced practice, including that in critical care, may be a stage rather than the pinnacle of a professional career.

The National Education and Competence Framework for ACCPs indicates that, in future, recruitment could include individuals who are not members of established health professions and who may not even have a background in healthcare (DH 2008). This raises questions about the nature of the preparation required before embarking on advanced critical care training. There must also be some additional concerns about whether the expertise that trainee ACCPs currently bring and incorporate into critical care can be learned, in courses of the same length, by health students from outside healthcare. For example, current trainees have prior experience of communicating with and giving comfort to patients and families who are very anxious and distressed, for example as a result of delirium. They are equipped to provide what is often referred to as "basic care" as part of their critical care practice, but they have also learned the importance of focusing on patients as human beings rather than as a collection of physical systems (Benner et al. 2011). Moreover, ACCPs carry a high level of responsibility, which can be challenging because "the steep learning curve in transitioning from being a facilitator of care to becoming a director of care can be daunting due to knowledge deficits, high expectations, and most importantly, the pressures of being responsible for time-sensitive, high impact decisions" (Paton et al. 2013, p. 440). Consequently, it has yet to be seen whether recruits from outside healthcare actually become a reality. There is some evidence to support these concerns from the introduction of physicians' assistants (PAs) into an intensive care unit in New York. These PAs had little prior experience of critical care and, perhaps naively, there was initially a lack of understanding among staff of "the significant educational and experiential disparities" when PAs were compared to critical care nurse practitioners (CCNPs). There were also difficulties in developing good working relationships between the PAs and the CCNPs. A review of the situation led to the PAs being required to work under CCNP supervision during an extended mentorship period to allow them more time to develop their skills (Paton et al. 2013, p. 442).

An additional issue is that, whilst ACCPs work collaboratively with members of different professions, their role crosses professional boundaries. This is inevitable if they are to provide timely and effective care, but it can be immensely challenging and a source of conflict. ACCPs, therefore, have to learn to navigate the interfaces between their own and other's roles, as well as the spaces between the different professional groups. One particular interprofessional space is that between ACCPs and junior doctors. ACCPs play an important role in orienting and teaching new medical staff and can be an important resource in enhancing doctors' education. However, it is also possible that both ACCPs and junior doctors may be competing for similar learning opportunities, which may make it difficult for the ACCPs to gain sufficient experience (Paton et al. 2013). In addition, if ACCPs are replacing more senior doctors in staffing rotas, then there is also a potential for medical deskilling at that level.

11.7 Conclusion

Advanced critical care practice fulfills a much-needed role, in a variety of settings, in the care and treatment of seriously ill and/or injured patients who require close monitoring but who are expected to recover. Meeting the needs of these patients requires practitioners with high levels of knowledge and skill, and the ability to respond appropriately to rapid changes in a patient's condition. ACCPs are well equipped to take on the responsibilities that this involves and seem to have found a niche. Their numbers incorporate nurses, physiotherapists, and paramedics, and may in time include members of other allied health professions. In this they may be unusual, in that so much of advanced practice tends to be construed as profession specific. ACCPs seem to be exploring and venturing beyond this into new fields in which direct entry, if properly managed, may become a reality. If this happens, they will have undergone a complete transformation, from the early *internal* processes that challenged the status quo, through *finding a niche* processes in which they became valued and essential members of the critical care team, to *consolidation* processes. A complete paradigm shift will have been effected, but there is then the possibility of beginning a new stage in their professional evolution.

Key Questions

1. To what extent do the four processes discussed in this chapter relate to the development of advanced practice in your field?
2. In your field of practice, to what extent are advanced practitioners drawn from different health professions and what impact does this have on patient care?
3. To what extent is there potential in your field for advanced practice to become a direct-entry profession?

Glossary

Acute respiratory distress syndrome (ARDS): a life-threatening condition which develops within seven days of trauma and/or infection. There are three levels of severity depending on the ratio of PaO_2 to FiO_2. In mild ARDS, the PaO_2/FiO_2 ratio is ≤300 mmHg. In moderate ARDS, this drops to ≤200 mmHg, and in severe ARDS to ≤100 mmHg (Ranieri et al. 2012).

Faculty of Intensive Care Medicine (www.ficm.ac.uk): a body that provides training and assessment for doctors and other professionals working in intensive/critical care.

Intensive Care Society (www.ics.ac.uk): a multidisciplinary organization providing resources for health professionals working in intensive/critical care.

Lung Injury Score: one of several unvalidated tools for assessing ARDS. See https://www.mdcalc.com/murray-score-acute-lung-injury.

Professional Standards Authority (www.professionalstandards.org.uk): an independent body that works with professional regulators to ensure public protection.

References

Barron, A. and White, P. (2009). Consultation. In: *Advanced Practice Nursing. An Integrative Approach*, 4e (ed. A. Hamric, J. Spross and C. Hanson), 191–216. St Louis: Elsevier Saunders.

Benner, P., Kryiadis, P.H., and Stannard, D. (2011). *Clinical Wisdom and Interventions in Acute and Critical Care*, 2e. New York: Springer.

Benner, P., Tanner, C., and Chesla, C. (1996). *Expertise in Nursing Practice. Caring, Clinical Judgement and Ethics*. New York: Springer.

Bucher, R. (1988). On the natural history of health care occupations. *Work and Occupations* 15 (2): 131–147.

Chartered Society of Physiotherapy (2016). Advanced practice in physiotherapy. Understanding the contribution of advanced practice in physiotherapy to transforming lives, maximising independence and empowering populations. https://www.csp.org.uk/publications/advanced-practice-physiotherapy (accessed January 11, 2019).

College of Paramedics (2015). *Paramedic Career Framework*, 3e. Bridgwater: College of Paramedics.

Department of Health (2000). *The NHS Plan. A Plan for Investment. A Plan for Reform.* London: DH.

Department of Health (2008). *The National Education and Competence Framework for Advanced Critical Care Practitioners.* London: DH.

Faculty of Intensive Care Medicine and Intensive Care Society (2018). *Guidelines on the Management of ARDS.* London: FICM and ICM.

Fan, E., Sorbo, L.D., Goligher, E. et al. (2017). An official American Thoracic Society/European Society of Intensive Care Medicine/Society of Critical Care Medicine clinical practice guideline: mechanical ventilation in adult patients with acute respiratory distress syndrome on behalf of the American Thoracic Society, European Society of Intensive Care Medicine, and Society of Critical Care Medicine. *American Journal of Respiratory and Critical Care Medicine* 195 (9): 1253–1263.

Gattinoni, L., Taccone, P., Carlesso, E., and Marin, J. (2013). Prone position in acute respiratory distress syndrome. Rationale, indications, and limits. *American Journal of Respiratory and Critical Care Medicine* 188 (11): 1286–1293.

Hudack, M. (2012). Prone positioning for patients with ARDS. *Nursing Critical Care* 7 (2): 20–24.

Intensive Care Society (2009). Levels of critical care for adult patients. https://www.ics.ac.uk/ICS/guidelines-and-standards.aspx (accessed January 11, 2019).

Joint Board of Clinical Nursing Studies (1990). Minutes and papers. http://discovery.nationalarchives.gov.uk/details/r/C95 (accessed January 11, 2019).

Kendall, S., Latter, S., and Rycroft-Malone, J. (1997). *Nursing's Hand in the New Deal: Nurse Practitioners and Secondary Health Care in North Thames.* Chalfont St Giles: Buckinghamshire College.

Kleinpell, R. (2005). Acute care nurse practitioner practice: results of a 5-year longitudinal study. *American Journal of Critical Care* 4 (3): 211–219.

Lenz, S. (2013). *Advanced Practice Nursing. Setting a New Paradigm for Care in the 1ˢᵗ Century.* Bloomington, IN: Author House.

McGee, P. (2009). *Advanced Practice in Nursing and the Allied Health Professions*, 3e, 11–12. Oxford: Wiley-Blackwell.

NHS England (2014) Five Year Forward View. https://www.england.nhs.uk/wp-content/uploads/2014/10/5yfv-web.pdf (accessed January 11, 2019).

Nursing and Midwifery Council (2018). *The Code. Professional Standards of Practice and Behaviour for Nurses and Midwives.* London: NMC.

Paton, A., Stein, D., Pastores, S.M. et al. (2013). Critical care medicine advanced practice provider model at a comprehensive cancer center: successes and challenges. *American Journal of Critical Care* 22 (5): 439–443.

Professional Standards Authority (2015). *Right Touch Regulation. Revised.* London: PSA.

Ramis, M., Wu, C., and Pearson, A. (2013). Experience of being an advanced practice nurse within Australian acute care settings: a systematic review of qualitative evidence. *International Journal of Evidence-Based Health Care* 11: 161–180.

Ranieri, V.M., Rubenfeld, G.D., Thompson, B.T. et al. (2012). Acute respiratory distress syndrome. The Berlin definition. *JAMA* 307 (23): 2526–2533.

Royal College of Nursing (2003). Critical care and flight nursing. https://www.rcn.org.uk/library/subject-guides/critical-care-and-in-flight-nursing (accessed January 20, 2019).

Royal Pharmaceutical Society (2013). *Advanced Pharmacy Framework.* London: RPS.

Schön, D. (1987). *Educating the Reflective Practitioner: Toward a New Design for Teaching and Learning in the Professions.* San Francisco, CA: Jossey-Bass.

Sinclair, N. and Curatolo, L. (2014). The evolving role of the emergency medical retrieval service critical care practitioner. *Journal of Paramedic Practice* 6 (1): 40–43.

Spross, J. and Babine, R. (2014). Guidance and coaching. In: *Advanced Practice Nursing. An Integrative Approach*, 5e (ed. A. Hamric, C. Hanson, M. Tracy and E. O'Grady), 183–212. St Louis: Elsevier Saunders.

Tracy, M. and Hanson, C. (2014). Leadership. In: *Advanced Practice Nursing. An Integrative Approach*, 5e (ed. A. Hamric, C. Hanson, M. Tracy and E. O'Grady), 266–298. St Louis: Elsevier Saunders.

Vosit-Steller, J. and Morse, A. (2014). Consultation. In: *Advanced Practice Nursing. An Integrative Approach*, 5e (ed. A. Hamric, C. Hanson, M. Tracy and E. O'Grady), 213–236. St Louis: Elsevier Saunders.

CHAPTER 12

The Interface between Advanced Nursing and Medical Practice

Lesley Kavi[1] and Paula McGee[2]

[1]*Birmingham, UK*
[2]*Birmingham City University, Birmingham, UK*

Key Issues
- The nature of general practice in the UK
- Current issues in general practice in the UK
- Competences for advanced nurse practitioners in general practice
- Developing good working relationships in general practice

LEARNING OBJECTIVES

By the end of this chapter you will be able to:

- Discuss the challenges facing general practice.

- Summarize the specific competences required by advanced nurse practitioners in general, and identify those relating to your own field of practice.

- Critically examine issues in developing good working relationships between advanced nurse practitioners and their medical colleagues.

12.1 Introduction

This chapter addresses the interface between medical practice and advanced nursing practice. This appears to be an unusual topic in the current advanced practice literature, which tends to focus more heavily on the advanced scope of

Advanced Practice in Healthcare: Dynamic Developments in Nursing and Allied Health Professions,
Fourth Edition. Edited by Paula McGee and Chris Inman.
© 2019 John Wiley & Sons Ltd. Published 2019 by John Wiley & Sons Ltd.

practice and work activities. The chapter begins with an overview of the nature of general practice in the UK. This is followed by an outline of some of the current issues in providing this service. The chapter then moves on to present the competences, agreed by the respective Royal Colleges, for advanced nursing practice in general practice. These are discussed first in relation to the core competences for advanced nursing practice that have been agreed by the various nursing organizations and theorists, and second in comparison with those for doctors. The chapter closes with some recommendations for good working practices. Exercises and questions for discussion are included as the chapter unfolds.

12.2 General Practice in the UK

In the UK, the general practitioner (GP) is a community-based doctor who acts as the first point of contact for people of all ages, who are seeking help with a wide range of acute illnesses and long-term physical and mental health conditions that vary in severity. There are approximately 52 000 GPs working in the UK. They normally work in teams that incorporate members of other health professions (British Medical Association [BMA] 2017). GPs provide over 300 million consultations each year, either face to face or via telephone, at a fraction of the cost of hospital services. GP services enable many patients to manage their health problems as part of their normal daily lives; those with more complex needs may be referred to specialists in hospitals. Most GP practices operate as businesses; individual doctors, nurses, and managers may be business partners, whilst other staff, including some doctors, may be salaried employees. Practices may function alone or as part of a group in order to maximize expertise and resources. Practices also liaise with other services such as social care and the voluntary sector.

GP services provide a very broad and constantly expanding range of services in response to the impact of both health service reforms aimed at reducing hospital usage and admissions, and changes in the population. These changes include the rising number of older adults who are living longer than in previous generations and who are more likely to develop complex health problems. The increasing incidence of Type 2 diabetes across all age groups presents major challenges in managing the disease process and preventing complications. The development of new knowledge of disease processes, better medical interventions, new clinical guidelines, regular screening programs, and modern pharmaceutical products have all contributed to improvements in diagnosis and care for all age groups. As a result, children and adults with long-term conditions such as heart disease, cancer, and end-stage renal failure, who might not previously have survived, are also experiencing extended lifespans and require care. Added to the services provided by GPs for these patient groups is a portfolio of health screening, vaccination programs, clinics focused on infant and child health, and clinics dealing with specific health problems such as hypertension and asthma and anticoagulation therapy. In addition, other work previously provided by hospital services, such as minor surgery, can now be undertaken in primary care as part of GPs' responsibilities.

12.3 Current Issues in General Practice

The increasing range of GP services has had a marked effect on GP workload, which has in turn raised concerns about patient safety (Baird et al. 2016; BMA 2016). The budgetary reallocation required to support the increased responsibilities of GPs has not been fully addressed, and disparities in funding contribute to the considerable strain on current services (Baird et al. 2016; NHS Health Education England and Royal College of General Practitioners 2016). As a result, many practices are experiencing considerable financial strain. Recruitment has not kept pace with demand and, as GPs retire, vacancies are more difficult to fill. The impact of withdrawal from the European Union has created added uncertainty about the potential for recruitment from other member states.

12.3.1 Increased Regulation and Bureaucracy

The General Practice Forward View (NHS Health Education England and Royal College of General Practitioners 2016) was intended to address the key issues affecting general practice by finding new ways of managing demand. These included tackling the complex bureaucracy which controls how GP practices are paid and regulated, and communications between GPs and hospitals. Patients who have queries about, or who miss, their hospital appointments are supposed to resolve these directly with the hospital, but some find this difficult and will, inappropriately, seek help from their GP. The introduction of new software to manage information and communication more effectively is an essential part of this process. Reducing the number of unnecessary GP appointments is also crucial. Clay and Stern (2015) found that 27% of 5000 consultations did not require a GP; patients could have been seen by a nurse or pharmacist, or could even have looked after themselves if they knew how to do so. Caring for and treating those patients who do not need a GP appointment requires members of other professions, who are specially trained, to prescribe and to educate patients about self-care. It is envisaged that GP practices of the future will have more doctors and nurses with expanded skills to provide comprehensive care and work more effectively across boundaries within the health service as a whole (Royal College of General Practitioners 2013). The introduction of locality hubs in some areas can also reduce pressure on individual practices by managing "demand across a number of practices and their respective patient lists, ensuring that patients in excess of safe working limits can still be seen by a GP or the wider primary health care team" (BMA 2016, p. 5).

GP workloads are also influenced by patients' expectations. The NHS Plan set out a series of targets aimed at ensuring timely access to health services. These targets included a promise that "by 2004 patients will be able to have a GP appointment within 48 hours." Those with urgent needs would be given an appointment within 24 hours (Department of Health [DH] 2000, p. 13). Whilst the 48-hour target was eventually scrapped by the incoming Conservative/ Liberal Democrat coalition government of 2010, public expectations rose. People were led to expect rapid access and were, understandably, unhappy when it was not forthcoming. Thus, the availability of appointments became politicized. The coalition government promised that GP services would be available

8 a.m. until 8 p.m. every day by 2020, including Saturdays and Sundays, to accommodate people who had jobs. However, a general election is scheduled for 2020, so it is uncertain whether this target will actually be achieved.

The availability of appointments is only one aspect of patients' expectations. Baird et al. (2016) reported that patients also want quick results. They want their problems resolved in a single consultation, treatment that is immediately effective and, if that is not possible, quick referrals to specialists. The NHS Constitution has set out patients' legal rights; as consumers they want action now and are not prepared to wait (NHS Health Education England 2015). Patients may be pleased to see any doctor when they are very ill and in urgent need of help, but, for the most part, they want more than an appointment. They want rapid access to someone they trust, who knows them, and who has time for them (Boyle et al. 2010). Patients want continuity in care. They want to see their "own" doctor and would rather wait to consult that person rather than anyone else (Boyle et al. 2010). Unfortunately, patients' expectations are not always realistic. The ideal of the single-handed family doctor has been replaced by team-based practice; seeing one's "own" doctor at every appointment is no longer an option.

Patients' reasons for consulting a GP have also undergone some changes. For example, there appears to be a decline in self-care, which in turn has increased demand for both face-to-face and telephone consultations. Reasons for this decline are unclear. Traditionally, families have passed on simple remedies for common ailments, and it is possible that they are now less likely to do this. Families whose members do not live nearby may not be able to offer advice and support; younger members may be less accepting of what they see as old-fashioned. It is also possible that some traditional remedies did not work as well as people liked to believe. The introduction of telephone consultations with GPs may encourage contact from patients, with the GP being expected to replace advice from family members about minor, often self-limiting illnesses (Baird et al. 2016). The availability of information via the internet, mobile phone usage, and social media may also play a part. People now want immediate results; a telephone conversation with someone at the local GP practice may be regarded as a quick way to fix a problem.

The NHS Constitution (NHS Health Education England 2015) states that patients have a responsibility to look after their own health and to seek advice about improving it. However, the ability and desire to do this depend on several factors: individual beliefs about the likelihood and consequences of developing health problems; perceptions of the advantages and disadvantages of taking action; and the ability to do what is needed (Ogden 2001). Simply allocating responsibility is not enough. Patients also need encouragement, education, and support to manage their own health and to know when to seek professional advice.

12.4 Advanced Nursing Practice

Advanced practice is nursing at a much higher level than basic training. Advanced nurse practitioners are more autonomous and accountable in clinical practice, management, research, and teaching. The introduction of advanced nursing practice in general practice is an essential development, because what society needs a GP to do is changing and will continue to evolve. The old model in which the GP did everything, from check-ups for women taking contraceptive pills to end-of-life care, is no longer appropriate. The practice of medicine is now more complex and team-based working means that GPs are far more involved in management. Consequently, they can no longer do everything that is needed for every patient in every circumstance.

The nature of current GP practice has created opportunities for advanced nurses to plug gaps in service provision, develop new skills, and pioneer new forms of practice. Meeting the challenges in current GP practice requires new ways of working that incorporate the skills of nurses and other health professionals. Advanced nurses who are educated at Master's level and have the qualifications required to prescribe medication could provide a single service for some of the more common health problems and the day-to-day needs of patients without referral to a doctor. This could leave more time for GPs to focus on patients with more complex needs.

The Royal College of General Practitioners (RCGP; 2015) and the Royal College of Nursing (RCN) recognize the potential of the advanced nurse practitioner as "an experienced and autonomous registered nurse who has developed and extended their practice and skills, guided by The Code in unpredictable situations. This may include managing patients with undiagnosed health care problems and is shaped by the context of their clinical practice. This advanced level is underpinned by the essence of nursing, and the values of caring. It applies the principles of knowledge of the patient as a distinct person and individual whilst respecting and working with their culture and diversity" (RGCP 2015, p. 6). The Colleges' position also takes account of the definitions of advanced nursing practice issued by the International Council of Nurses (ICN 2008), the four countries in the UK, and the DH (2010).

Before reading on, consider Exercise 12.1.

EXERCISE 12.1

How does this definition fit with advanced practice in your field of practice?

What would you change?

Write a statement to explain the nature of advanced practice in your field of practice.

In order to practice safely, the advanced nurse practitioner must meet the standards required not only in the four elements of direct patient care, leadership, education, and evidence/research-based practice, but also in the 15 competences set out by the Colleges (Table 12.1). Each of the competences for advanced nurse practitioners contains multiple subsections. For example, in the competence for pediatrics, there are seven subsections that address topics such as the provision of information to parents and children, health promotion, cultural differences, and end-of-life care. Each section requires self-assessment and workplace assessments conducted using a taxonomy based on Benner's (1984) theory of developing proficiency in nursing. This taxonomy is used to grade performance from a score of 1, indicating novice level, to a score of 5, reflecting expert practice. The overall aim is for the advanced nurse practitioner to demonstrate the ability to practice safely and autonomously (RCGP 2015). Alongside this assessment, the advanced nurse practitioner must

---

TABLE 12.1

Competences for advanced nurse practitioners in GP practice.

Direct clinical care

Leadership and collaborative practice

Improving quality and developing practice

Developing self and others

Care of patients with long-term conditions

Mental health and psychological care

Acute presentations

Men's health

Women's health

Family planning and sexual health

Public health and well-being

End-of-life care

Information technology and clinical practice

Pediatrics

Learning disability

Source: Summarized from Royal College of General Practitioners (2015), pp. 14–29.

---

develop a "portfolio of evidence" (RCGP 2015, p. 10), which can be used in discussion with mentors as well as for revalidation with the Nursing and Midwifery Council. Before reading on, undertake Exercise 12.2.

EXERCISE 12.2

List the specific competences required for advanced nursing practice in your field of practice.

How do these relate to the core competences?

Comparison of the competences required for nursing in general practice shows that these go beyond the core elements of advanced nursing practice specified by nursing organizations and theorists (DH 2010; ICN 2008; NMC 2005; RCN 2012). They are also necessarily broad and do not preclude the development of more focused expertise (Table 12.2). Bringing together the general and specific elements of an advanced nursing practice role is a useful step in articulating that role more precisely. This is important not only in formulating the role from a management perspective, but also in explaining it to patients and colleagues.

Before reading on, consider Exercise 12.3.

EXERCISE 12.3

Compare and contrast the specific competences for advanced nursing practice in your field with those of a doctor.

Do the roles overlap? In what way?

TABLE 12.2

Comparison of core and specific competences for advanced nurse practitioners in general practice.

Core competences	NMC (2005) UK	ICN (2008)	RCN (2012) UK	DH (2010)	RCGP AP
Expert practice	Assessment and management of the patient in health and illness √	√	Assessment of patients with undiagnosed problems and management of patients' illnesses √		Direct clinical care
Leadership	√	√ and management	√ as part of the professional role		Leadership
Collaboration	√	√	√ but as part of other competences		Collaborative practice
Cultural competence	√ As part of other competences	√ As part of other competences	√		
Guidance and coaching	√	Role not explicitly stated	√	Developing the self and others	Developing the self and others
Ethical practice	√	√	Not explicitly stated	Not explicitly stated	Aspects included in subsections
Interpersonal skills	√	√	Not explicitly stated		Aspects included in subsections
Acting as a consultant for others			√ As part of the professional role		
Evidence-based practice	Evidence-based practice	Evidence-based practice	Evidence-based practice		Aspects included in subsections
Evaluation, monitoring, and quality issues	√	√	√	Improving quality and developing practice	Improving quality and developing practice

Source: Summarized from Department of Health (2010); International Council of Nurses (2008); Nursing and Midwifery Council (2005); Royal College of Nursing (2012); Royal College of General Practitioners (2015), pp. 14–29.

Comparison of competences for trainee GPs can also help in clarifying similarities and differences between advanced nursing and GP roles (Table 12.3). In terms of clinical practice, both the advanced nurse practitioner and the GP assess patients, collect relevant information through examination and investigations, diagnose, and prescribe treatment. They both have to understand the health problems and needs of the locality in which they are based and the impacts cultural issues may have on patients' views and decisions about their health. However, the GP role requires a broader and deeper range of knowledge and skill in managing patients with complex needs, including those who may have multiple health problems. Both act as clinical leaders; they have responsibilities to maintain high standards and address quality issues; but the GP is often also running a business, which has to meet the demands and targets set by the NHS and remain financially viable. Both have to work effectively in teams and collaborate with other health professionals. However, advanced nurse practitioners may experience some difficulties in achieving this, because members of other professions and doctors outside the GP practice have been known to refuse referrals from nurses, an issue which prompted the development of

---

TABLE 12.3

Comparison of competences for advanced nurse practitioners and GPs.

Advanced practitioner competences	GP competences
Clinical practice: assessing, ordering investigations, diagnosing, prescribing, and treating patients Screening patients Making referrals Promoting health Practicing holistically	Identifying common conditions Examining patients, ordering, and interpreting investigations, diagnosing, decision making Managing patients with complex needs and/or co-morbidities Promoting health Practicing holistically Community orientation
Leadership	Management of change Organizational and clinical leadership skills
Collaborative working	Working effectively in teams
Development of the self and others	Development of the self and others
Ethical practice	Ethical practice
Interpersonal skills	Communication and consultation skills
Fitness to practice	Fitness to practice
Evidence-based practice	Understanding and applying the principles of evidence-based practice
Improving quality and developing practice	Improving quality and developing practice
Cultural competence	Understanding of impact of culture on health
Guiding and coaching	Teaching

Summarized from Royal College of Nursing (2012); Royal College of General Practitioners (2015), pp. 14–29, (2016).

guidance on referrals for clinical imaging (Radford 2011; RCN, Society and College of Radiographers et al. 2008). Fitness to practice is an essential issue for both the advanced nurse practitioner and the GP. This includes meeting the requirements for current registration, engaging in continuous professional development, practicing safely, and, where appropriate, recognizing the limitations of individual expertise. Both have responsibilities with regard to enabling others to develop their knowledge and skills. However, there may be situations in which the GP provides supervision and teaching for the advanced practitioner, especially for someone new in post.

12.5 The Advantages and Disadvantages of Advanced Nursing Practice in General Practice

Advanced nurse practitioners bring a range of expertise to the GP practice, which can be helpful in redistributing workloads and developing new approaches to patient care. However, much depends on the knowledge and skills of the individual nurse. For instance, an advanced nurse practitioner who has specialized in respiratory care will be able to provide day-to-day care for patients with chronic obstructive pulmonary disorder (COPD), enabling many to stay at home and avoid the need for frequent hospital admissions. Similarly, most patients with Type 2 diabetes may be cared for by a nurse with the required knowledge and expertise. This is not simply a case of replacing one type of professional with another, as advanced nurses have skills in areas such as asthma care, wound care, and coaching and guiding, in which they may be more knowledgeable than GPs. Whilst they use their medical knowledge, advanced nurse practitioners also draw on their nursing skills; they tend to work in ways that reduce social distance between them and patients, which encourages more informal interactions and allows different types of information to be gathered (Paniagua 2011). The result is not unlike a blend of Carper's (1978) ways of knowing. Used effectively, the knowledge and skills of advanced nurse practitioners allow much-needed time for GPs to concentrate on those patients with complex needs, for example those with brittle asthma or with diabetes who have issues in maintaining control or who are experiencing the effects of drug interactions. Good working relationships between advanced nurse practitioners and GPs depend on respect for one another's expertise, trust, and a willingness to collaborate for patients' benefit.

However, there are some potential disadvantages to consider. First, handing over the care of patients with specific health problems may mean that the GP sees noncomplex patients less often, which could, potentially, have a deskilling effect. A second and very real factor is the lack of uniformity in advanced nurse practitioners' breadth of experience, knowledge, and skill base. For instance, adult-trained nurses may have limited experience of working with infants and small children. This contrasts with GPs, whose training will have encompassed a very wide range of health needs, from pregnancy to end-of-life care. Advanced nurse practitioners with a more limited range may, inadvertently, increase the GP's workload, for example by needing to check the accuracy of a diagnosis, confirm the best course of action, or refer patients to the doctor. GP practice is characterized by an element of unpredictability and, whilst the extra time spent supporting an advanced practitioner can improve the nurse's skills and lead to better knowledge of their abilities, it may sometimes adversely affect the amount of time GPs have for their own patients. Consequently, much depends on individual advanced nurse practitioners, and it may take time to build up trust among both GP colleagues and patients (Jakimovoc et al. 2017).

CASE STUDY | **Working Well Together**

Advertisement – a vacancy for an advanced nurse practitioner in general practice

You will have responsibility for the day-to-day management of patients with long-term conditions, especially diabetes, and for assessing, diagnosing, prescribing, implementing, and evaluating treatments for patients with a wide variety of health needs. You will work with patients to improve adherence to treatment, and provide patient education and health promotion for a diverse local population with high levels of deprivation. You will work effectively as a member of the practice team and take on leadership roles within the practice. Good computer skills are essential.

1. What issues should the GP partners consider in setting up this post?

2. As an advanced nurse practitioner, what factors would be important to you in considering this post?

FACTORS TO CONSIDER IN SETTING UP AN ADVANCED NURSING PRACTICE POST

In deciding whether to employ an advanced nurse practitioner, the partners will need to identify why they think an advanced nurse practitioner is needed, what they expect the advanced nurse practitioner to do, how much the appointment will cost, and how the success of the post will be evaluated (Table 12.4). Identifying a problem clearly is not always easy. Feelings and specific events can create a distorted picture of what is really happening, so, whilst it is important to air and acknowledge the emotional dimensions of the problem, these should not be allowed to dominate decisions. Considering alternatives may reveal that the problem can be resolved among existing staff. It may even reveal that the problem is not actually the practice's problem at all, but actually arises elsewhere. Examining the benefits will highlight the extent to which the partners really understand what an advanced practitioner can be expected to do. This is important as a step toward creating a job description. Determining what may go wrong is also important. The cost may be prohibitive. An advanced nurse practitioner may not prove a good match for the problem.

TABLE 12.4

Is an advanced nurse practitioner really needed?

1. What is the problem?
What information do we have about the problem?
Is this problem affecting patient outcomes?
Is this problem preventing us from meeting specific targets?
How do we feel about this problem?
2. Are there alternatives?
What actions could we take?
Could we resolve the problem by changing how we do things?
Could we resolve the problem by changing how other practice staff do things?

3. What are the potential benefits of creating an advanced nurse practitioner post?

What do we know about this role?

What information do we have about it and what else do we need?

What clinical and other functions would this post fulfill?

4. What could go wrong?

How much would the post cost? Can we afford it?

Would it be value for money?
Could patient safety be compromised?

5. How can we make this happen?

Who will be responsible for this post and the postholder?

How should the post be evaluated? What are the criteria for success? How often should this be done?

How should we tackle overlap between advanced nursing and GP roles?

How should we prepare staff and patients for change?

FACTORS TO CONSIDER WHEN APPLYING FOR AN ADVANCED NURSE PRACTITIONER POST

There are a number of points to consider when applying for any advanced nurse practitioner post, and these may also be useful in developing a new role (Table 12.5). Identifying what the post is intended to achieve is not always easy. A template for a job description for an advanced nurse

---

TABLE 12.5

Applying for advanced practitioner posts.

1. What is the remit of the post?

What information is provided about the post?

What is the postholder expected to do?

Is there a probationary period? How long is this?

2. What are the benefits of this post?

How will this post help patients?

Will I need training to perform any of the work? Who will provide this (internal or externally provided training)? Will additional supervision be needed? Who will provide this and how?

What opportunities does the post offer?

3. What could go wrong?

How could I tackle overlap between advanced nursing and GP roles?

4. How can I make this happen?

How should the post be evaluated? What are the criteria for success? How often should this be done?

How should I prepare staff and patients for change?

practitioner in general practice is available from Health Education England (www.hee@nhs.uk) and a profile is available from NHS Employers (www.nhsemployers.org). Information about the post should make clear to whom the postholder will be responsible and accountable. The salary and annual leave entitlements should be stated.

The initially intended benefits to patients should be clear, but it must be recognized that these will change over time. The advanced nurse practitioner role will change as the post becomes established, and it is advisable to review work activities on a regular basis. This is to ensure that these remain within the nurse's scope of practice, a particularly important issue when developing a completely new role. Regular meetings between the postholder and the GP responsible for the post

are essential, at least every three months. These not only help in monitoring performance, but also in keeping abreast of the nature of work activities, competence, and legal issues, particularly if the nurse is pioneering new approaches or services. Like any other form of advanced nursing practice, advanced practice in general practice can offer opportunities to be creative, but it would be naive to assume that it is safe to do so without checking first on the risks. This is not to say that risks should never be taken, but that it is wise to consider what might not go according to plan. An additional factor to consider here is the overall effect on the nurse's career. There is, at present, a lack of career structure for advanced nurse practitioners working in general practice, so it is wise to think about where you might wish to be in, say, five years' time.

12.6 Conclusion

The interface between advanced nursing and GP practice is dynamic and will continue to evolve. Advanced nurses have a range of knowledge and skills to offer general practice, but they also have variations in experience, which may affect the degree to which GPs feel able to hand over responsibility for patients. Collaborative partnerships between doctors and advanced nurses take time to develop and, at present, much depends on the working relationships between particular individuals. Advanced nurse practitioners moving on from such a setting may find that they have to begin all over again to gain the trust and respect of their new colleagues. More work is needed to develop career pathways for advanced nurse practitioners and secure their future in general practice.

Key Questions

1. How might the interface between advanced nursing and GP practice be researched?
2. How could the impact of an advanced nurse practitioner in a GP surgery be assessed?

3. How could advanced allied health practitioners contribute to patient care in a GP surgery?

Glossary

British Medical Association (BMA; www.bma.org.uk): the trade union and professional body for doctors in the UK.

Department of Health and Social Care (DHSC; https://www.gov.uk/government/organisations/department-of-health-and-social-care): a government

department responsible for overseeing NHS policy on health and adult social care in England, and some aspects in Scotland, Wales, and Northern Ireland.

Healthcare Education England (HEE; www.hee.nhs.uk): a government-funded body that works across England to deliver education to the healthcare workforce.

National Health Service (**NHS**): launched in 1948, it provides healthcare services within the UK that are free to patients at the point of access and available to all. It is funded out of taxation.

NHS Constitution (https://www.gov.uk/government/publications/the-nhs-constitution-for-england): sets out the guiding principles of the NHS, including patients' rights and responsibilities.

Nursing and Midwifery Council (www.nmc.org.uk): the professional regulator for nurses and midwives in the UK.

Royal College of Nursing (www.rcn.org.uk): a trade union and professional body for nurses, midwives, and healthcare assistants in the UK.

Royal College of General Practitioners (www.rcgp.org.uk): the professional body for GPs in the UK, providing support throughout their careers.

References

Baird, B., Charles, A., Honeyman, M. et al. (2016). *Understanding Pressures in General Practice*. London: King's Fund.

Benner, P. (1984). *From Novice to Expert: Excellence and Power in Clinical Nursing Practice*. Menlo Park, CA: Addison Wesley.

Boyle, S., Appleby, J., and Harrison, A. (2010). *A Rapid View of Access to Care*. London: King's Fund.

British Medical Association (2016). *Safe Working in General Practice. One Approach to Controlling Workload and Dealing with the Resulting Overspill through a Locality Hub Model*. London: BMA.

British Medical Association (2017). General practice in the UK. https://www.bma.org.uk/-/media/files/pdfs/.../press%20briefings/general-practice.pdf (accessed January 12, 2019).

Carper, B. (1978). Fundamental patterns of knowing in nursing. *Advances in Nursing Science* 1 (1): 13–24.

Clay, H., Stern, R (2015). Making time in general practice. Freeing GP capacity by reducing bureaucracy and avoidable consultations, managing the interface with hospitals and exploring new ways of working. Primary Care Foundation. https://www.nhsalliance.org/making-time-in-general-practice (accessed January 12, 2019).

Department of Health (2000). The NHS plan. A plan for investment. A plan for reform. https://webarchive.nationalarchives.gov.uk/20110503161023/http://www.dh.gov.uk/prod_consum_dh/groups/dh_digitalassets/@dh/@en/documents/digitalasset/dh_4082154.pdf (accessed January 12, 2019).

Department of Health (2010). *Advanced level nursing: a position statement*. London: DH.

International Council of Nurses (2008). *The Scope of Practice, Standards and Competencies of the Advanced Practice Nurse*. Geneva: ICN.

Jakimovoc, M., Williams, D., and Stankiewicz, G. (2017). A systematic review of experiences of advanced practice nursing in general practice. *BMC Nursing* 16 (6): https://doi.org/10.1186/s12912-016-0198-7.

NHS Health Education England (2015). The handbook to the NHS constitution. https://assets.publishing.service.gov.uk/government/uploads/system/uploads/attachment_data/file/474450/NHS_Constitution_Handbook_v2.pdf (accessed January 12, 2019).

NHS Health Education England and Royal College of General Practitioners (2016). General Practice Forward View. https://www.england.nhs.uk/wp-content/uploads/2016/04/gpfv.pdf (accessed January 12, 2019).

Nursing and Midwifery Council (2005). Implementation of a framework for the standard of post registration nursing. Agendum 27.1 C/05/160 December. http://aape.org.uk/wp-content/uploads/2015/02/NMC-ANP-Dec051.doc (accessed January 12, 2019).

Ogden, J. (2001). Health psychology. In: *Health Studies. An Introduction* (ed. J. Naidoo and J. Wills), 69–100. Basingtoke: Palgrave.

Paniagua, H. (2011). Advanced nurse practitioners and GPs: what is the difference? *Practice Nursing* 22 (7): 383–388.

Radford, M. (2011). Power dynamics and professional expertise in the communication between specialist nurses and doctors in acute hospital settings. Unpublished PhD thesis, Birmingham City University, Birmingham

Royal College of General Practitioners (2013). *The 2022 GP. A Vision for General Practice in the Future NHS*. London: RCGP.

Royal College of General Practitioners (2015). *General Practice Advanced Nurse Practitioner Competencies*. London: RCGP.

Royal College of General Practitioners (2016). *The RGCP Curriculum: Professional and Clinical Modules*. London: RGCP.

Royal College of Nursing (2008). *Clinical Imaging Requests from Non-medically Qualified Professionals*. London: RCN.

Royal College of Nursing (2012). *Advanced Nurse Practitioners. An RCN Guide to the Advanced Nurse Practitioner Role, Competences and Programme Accreditation*. London: RCN.

PART 4

Developing Advanced Practitioners' Skills

Legal and Ethical Issues Related to Professional Practice

Nicola J Stock

Key Issues
- Ethical theories
- Mental capacity
- Consent
- Negligence
- Whistleblowing
- Improving care quality

LEARNING OBJECTIVES

By the end of this chapter you will be able to:

- Identify the key differences between virtue ethics, deontology, consequentialism, and principlism.
- Discuss the concepts of "mental capacity" and "deprivation of liberty safeguards."
- Explore the link between consent and autonomy.
- Describe the components of negligence and differentiate between negligence and misconduct in the context of a complaint.
- Discuss the "duty of candor" and the difference between whistleblowing and raising concerns.
- Explore how a transparent, respectful culture of excellence in care can be developed through ethical leadership, and how this can enable discussion related to difficult decisions.

Advanced Practice in Healthcare: Dynamic Developments in Nursing and Allied Health Professions,
Fourth Edition. Edited by Paula McGee and Chris Inman.
© 2019 John Wiley & Sons Ltd. Published 2019 by John Wiley & Sons Ltd.

13.1 Introduction

This chapter explores professional, legal, and ethical issues in the context of advanced professional practice. The aim of the chapter is not to provide an extensive discourse on jurisprudence or the philosophical origins of ethical theory (there are texts suggested at the end of the chapter that dedicate themselves to these endeavors), but to encourage readers to reflect on their daily practice from various perspectives, such as applying the Mental Capacity Act (MCA) 2005 and the duty of candor, and to consider how, as advanced practitioners, their knowledge and actions have a direct impact both on patient care and on their clinical colleagues. This focus on care is carried through the chapter to the latter sections, where we consider how incremental improvements in care quality can be introduced or facilitated by ensuring that legal obligations are met and by incorporating ethical principles into routine clinical practice.

The chapter begins by laying the groundwork on which later discussion is built. However, right from the start, the emphasis is not on grand theories but on everyday clinical practice, and this is reflected in the early introduction of a case study that will illustrate key theoretical points as they are raised throughout the chapter. It is based on Margaret, a 79-year-old retired civil servant, who is admitted to hospital after a fall. There is little that is unusual about Margaret and this is the point – that application of ethical theory and overt consideration of legal obligations should not be thought of as anything especially unusual, but simply another facet of clinical care.

13.2 Ethical Theories

It is not uncommon for a discussion on ethics in healthcare to begin with a note on the origins of the word and to advise that "ethics" is from the Greek *ethikos*, meaning "study of morals," or late Latin *ethicus, ethica,* and *ethicum,* meaning "relating to morals" or "the treating of moral questions as a science." It is perhaps due to this start point and the tendency toward a big-issues approach to ethics, emphasizing discussion on such subjects as abortion, euthanasia, human genetics, and the like, that ethics is seen as a subject divorced from everyday healthcare practice (Sellman 2011). If, however, the etymological roots of ethics are followed to their origin, instead of viewing ethics from an academic perspective or a treatise on the science of moral ideals, a viewpoint originating from *ēthos*, or "personal disposition," can be seen as equally valid and actually predates the more commonly applied definitions (Ayto 2005).

With this new starting point based more around the individual than on theoretical discourse, the question "Who should I be?" which is often subjugated to "What should I do?" becomes central to the study of ethics in healthcare. Consideration of "Who should I be?" goes much further in meeting the requirements of validation, safeguarding, and other professional obligations than routine adherence to a set of moral rules and principles that are at risk of being an afterthought or a side issue, rather than core components of care. With this in mind, the approach to healthcare ethics described here, whilst acknowledging philosophical underpinnings, is firmly rooted in everyday practice and is consistent with Sellman's (2011, p. 203) conclusion where he echoes Aristotle: "to know what to do, when, in what way and for what reason requires practical wisdom and not merely technical or intellectual capacities." As Shafer-Landau says (2012), it is a complicated skill, but one that requires the kind of "know-how" that comes from extensive training and experience rather than super-human intelligence.

13.2.1 Virtue Ethics, Deontology, and Consequentialism

Most, though not all, virtue ethics approaches have their roots in Ancient Greece, and in particular in Aristotle's *Nicomachean Ethics* (Aristotle 2009). Aristotle, and others such as Socrates and Plato, were known for lengthy discussions of character traits or "the virtues." At the heart of Aristotle's reasoning, though, was the notion of "phronesis" or practical wisdom. In Book VI of *Nicomachean Ethics*, Aristotle explores the soul. The soul, he says, is divided and includes a rational and an irrational part; the rational part, which includes practical wisdom, is further subdivided into a calculative part that deals with the practical matter of being human, a reasoning, contemplative, intellectual being that enables us, after proper deliberation, to make the right choices. The right moral choice, Aristotle argues, requires experience of particular situations and cannot be achieved through the mechanical application of general rules. This is consistent with Health Education England's (HEE) Advanced Clinical Practice (ACP) Framework (HEE 2017), which includes the need for experience in their definition of ACP, so, although Aristotle's work is well over 2000 years old, it is still relevant today. Let us consider this in the context of our case study.

CASE STUDY (i)

Margaret is a 79-year-old retired senior civil servant. She is a widow, her husband having died in his 50s from a myocardial infarction some 30 years ago. She lives alone in a park home with her West Highland terrier; her daughter lives a three-hour drive away, is married, and has two adult children.

Margaret's closest companion is a neighbour, Alan, himself a widower. She is a moderate to heavy smoker and consumes around 5 units of alcohol each day. She rarely cooks for herself, preferring to snack throughout the day, but she will have a meal in a café or restaurant if she is out.

Aristotle infers that, through a combination of training and direct acquaintance with practical situations, we develop an insight into life and the lives of others and have an "eye" for what is appropriate (Singer 1991); this extends to behavior. Codes of conduct, such as the Nursing and Midwifery Council's (NMC) Code (2015) and the Health and Care Professions Council's (HCPC) Standards of Conduct, Performance and Ethics (2016), require practitioners to treat people as individuals, so Margaret is treated as an individual and not labeled or subjected to discriminatory behavior because assumptions have been made based on how she lives. Aristotle would advise that through practical wisdom we not only know what is the right thing to do, i.e. to follow the rules and principles set in front of us, but how to do the right thing, at the right time, within a particular set of circumstances.

This is in stark contrast to Immanuel Kant, who believed that moral decisions were wholly a matter of following rules, rules that allow no exceptions and must be followed regardless of the circumstances or consequences. Kant's rules, or imperatives, are formulated in such a way that they will always apply; in other words, they are universal. It is not difficult to think of a few rules that could be universally applied, but Kant's system of moral reasoning, also referred to as a deontological theory, requires that all rules are universally applied, all of the time, and that one cannot justify the breach of a deontological principle simply by referring to the consequences. For example, if one takes the principle that it is wrong to lie, telling a lie on the grounds that the truth may hurt cannot be justified, and there is no such thing as a "little white lie." With its principle of adherence to the rules regardless of the consequences, deontology is sometimes referred to as nonconsequentialism.

Where a nonconsequentialist may answer the question "Do you like my new hairstyle?" with a negative, even though it may hurt the feelings of the questioner, a consequentialist will consider whether their answer will produce a good or a bad outcome, or what will produce the greater pleasure. At a first glance, it could appear that consequentialism is very nebulous and unpredictable: What is "good"? Good or bad for whom? Must every conceivable potential consequence be considered in our decision making? One of the most widely applied consequentialist theories that attempts to address this is utilitarianism, which holds that the best judgment is the one that produces the greatest human happiness. This highlights a major problem, in that a utilitarian argument can produce an outcome that feels instinctively wrong. For example, if a healthy person were kidnapped and killed so that their organs could be used to save the lives of five others, there would be five happy people instead of just one. Clearly, it would be wrong to try to justify such an action, and this has led to some consequentialists adopting a version of utilitarianism known as "rule utilitarianism," which suggests that we adopt a set of rules that will govern how we act and will, if followed correctly, produce the best outcome. It is not a huge leap here to find ourselves back at the question of "How do we know how to follow the rules correctly?" and to the criticism that ethical debate is of limited practical use when it comes to decision making. This may in turn explain, at least in part, the popularity of principlism in general, and Beauchamp and Childress' (2013) four principles in particular.

13.2.2 Principlism

Principlism, or the notion that we can base decisions on adherence to a set of ethical principles, is sometimes described as a middle-level approach between deontology and consequentialism. There have been many versions of principlism, spanning more than two centuries (Mallia 2013), but by far the most well known is the four-principle approach as described by Tom Beauchamp and James Childress (Beauchamp and Childress 2013). Their four principles – respect for autonomy, nonmaleficence, beneficence, and justice – have arguably been so widely adopted that those in the caring professions, or who conduct research on human subjects, consider that they "do ethics" by ticking off each of the principles. Introducing the four principles, Dudgeon (2015) states: "Ethics is nothing more than a system of principles or values which can help us in decision-making." Along with the "big-issues" approach, the oversimplification of Beauchamp and Childress' (2013) principles can also be seen as:

- Contributing to the continued treatment of ethics as a distinct subject rather than an integral part of care delivery.
- Rooted in "What should I do?" rather than "Who should I be?"

Whilst there is a place for the four-principle approach, and the intent here is not to dismiss principlism, the ethos of *ēthos* is not that we "do ethics," but that we are ethical in our practice. That returns us to practical wisdom and the adopted stance that choosing the best course of action cannot be reduced to an algorithm (Fowers 2003).

13.2.3 Practical Ethics and Practical Wisdom

Fowers (2003) argues that it is inconceivable that healthcare professionals can act ethically in the wide variety of situations in which they find themselves without the moral perception, and by implication practical wisdom, to recognize an issue as requiring ethical consideration in the first place. He argues in favor of careful deliberation and consultation with others and highlights Aristotle's perspective that, as advanced thinkers, we should move away from formal decision-making processes that will automatically guide us to the "right" answer. Significantly, in the context of the practical approach to ethics supported here, he recognizes that there is no need to abstract ethical issues from the rest of life, but we should instead see those issues in the context of the world inhabited by the individual patient or service user who is the subject of, and where able a contributor to, those deliberations.

Whilst there will be some ethical issues that require a multidisciplinary approach and possible lengthy discussion, the day-to-day issues that fall under the umbrella terms of healthcare law, ethics, and professionalism are not always matters for grand philosophical debate, but are problems that need to be addressed in a succinct and timely fashion in the clinical area. In the following sections, the issues of mental capacity, autonomy, consent, negligence, professional misconduct, management of complaints, whistleblowing, and clinical leadership are discussed with reference to our case study.

CASE STUDY (ii)

Margaret is admitted to an acute hospital ward late on Thursday with a fracture of her left humerus following a fall; she is right hand dominant. In addition to it being late and her living alone, there is some uncertainty over the reason for Margaret's fall. On Friday, she hasblood tests, an ECG and a comprehensive assessment of her medical condition,mental health, functional capacity and social circumstances, after which she is declared medically fit for discharge, but requiring support in the short term. An NHS Continuing Healthcare assessment is completed and late on Friday afternoon Margaret is advised that she is unlikely to be discharged before Monday. Margaret responds by saying that she does not want to stay in hospitalover the weekend. Her statement is first reviewed in the context of the MentalCapacity Act 2005.

13.3 The Mental Capacity Act

All providers of health and social care are required to have a good understanding of the MCA 2005 and the Deprivation of Liberty Safeguards (DoLS). Care Quality Commission (CQC) inspectors will expect staff to be able to discuss these during an inspection visit. The MCA was introduced to make new provision for persons who lack capacity. It established the Court of Protection and made provision in connection with the Convention on the International Protection of Adults (http://www.europarl.europa.eu), signed at The Hague on January 13, 2000, for the safeguarding of vulnerable adults. There are five key principles:

- Individuals are presumed to have capacity unless proven otherwise.
- All practical steps must be taken to support someone in decision making.
- A person is not to be treated as lacking capacity even though they make an unwise decision.
- An action taken on behalf of a person must be in their best interests.
- An act or decision must be the least restrictive of a person's individual rights and freedoms.

The MCA requires that all decision making must be time and decision specific and bans blanket decision making. In other words, just because a person lacks capacity in one area, such as finance or welfare, it does not automatically follow that they lack capacity to consent to treatment. Capacity to consent requires that a person can understand and retain information, weigh up the risks and benefits involved, and make a decision. Consent is valid if the patient has been given sufficient information, they have made their decision freely, and are able to communicate the decision. For example, a patient with early-stage dementia has a cut requiring treatment at a Minor Injuries Unit and a tetanus injection. Every effort should be made to communicate the pros and cons of the injection to enable him to make a decision. He may have Lasting Power of Attorney for property and finances, but this does not mean that he cannot make a decision about the injection. If he decides to refuse consent, provided that decision is a valid refusal of consent to treatment then, even though it may be considered an unwise decision, the emergency nurse practitioner or emergency care practitioner working in the department must respect his decision.

In our case study, Margaret is presumed to have capacity and there is no reason to think otherwise. She is perhaps considering an unwise decision, but her desire to go home may not be unwise in her view. The staff providing her care need to explore her reasoning, provide her with information relating to why it is considered better that she stays in hospital, and then support her decision making. In researching ethical issues surrounding discharge against medical advice, Machin (2015) found that there is still a very paternalistic and negative attitude toward patients who consider self-discharge that is in conflict with the notion of shared decision making in healthcare. Where an individual who lacks capacity is unable to make a decision, the decision must be made for them. The key principle under the MCA is that this must be in the patient's best interests.

The MCA allows for restraint and restriction, if it is considered to be in a person's best interests, such as physically preventing a person from self-harming or removing items from their possession that they may use to self-harm. Article 5 of the Human Rights Act (1998) states that everyone has the right to liberty and security of person and that no one is to be deprived of their liberty, except in defined circumstances and in accordance with an appropriate legal process. To provide this legal process, safeguards were introduced to provide protection to individuals where deprivation of liberty seems to be unavoidable.

13.4 Deprivation of Liberty Safeguards

DoLS were introduced in 2009 as an amendment to the MCA to protect some of the most vulnerable people in society. They are applicable only in England and Wales, to adults lacking capacity, and currently only apply to care homes and hospitals.

In other settings, such as in the community, DoLS authorizations are managed by the Court of Protection. DoLS do not apply to anyone detained under the Mental Health Act 2007. In a landmark legal case (*Cheshire West and Chester Council v P* [2014] UKSC 19), the Supreme Court clarified the meaning of "deprivation of liberty" with two important questions to be asked when determining whether a person is being deprived of their liberty:

- Is the person subject to continuous or complete supervision and control? *and*
- Is the person free to leave regardless of whether they want to or have attempted to?

If someone is under complete supervision and control and is not free to leave, then it is likely that they are deprived of their liberty. Examples of this may be the frequent use of sedating drugs or other medications to calm the person or to control behaviour; the use of bedrails, wheelchair straps, and some types of splint; or requiring a person to stay somewhere against their wishes. If the *managing authority* – that is, the staff in a care home or hospital – believes that they need to deprive someone of their liberty, they must request a standard authorization from a *supervisory body*, usually the local authority where the person is ordinarily resident. The supervisory body has up to 21 days in which to decide whether to grant a standard authorization, so a system of urgent authorization, which can be granted by the managing authority itself for up to seven days, is also in place. Once this occurs, the managing authority must also apply for a standard authorization and must have reasonable belief that this will be granted.

For example, Jim has learning difficulties and has been admitted to a community intermediate care unit for treatment of a leg ulcer, as he needs continuous supervision to deter him from removing his dressings and picking at his wound. The unit has a keypad entry and exit system on the doors and Jim has often tried to open the door. When unsuccessful, he climbs out of his window. The manager of the unit completes an urgent authorization for window locks to be fitted, as this will deprive Jim of his liberty to leave the unit. She also requests a standard authorization from the local authority.

The Law Commission has been reviewing the DoLS procedure in light of the Cheshire West judgment, which highlighted that the same standards apply to all, regardless of whether or not they have a disability. The Commission will streamline and extend the DoLS protections beyond care homes and hospitals into some community living facilities and patient transport. Currently, DoLS does not apply whilst a patient is in transit, even if it is acknowledged they may be deprived of their liberty once they reach their destination (DoLS Code of Practice [2.14]). The proposed Liberty Protection Safeguards (LPS) scheme would replace DoLS and provide a broader, less onerous system.

CASE STUDY (iii)

Margaret has agreed to stay in hospital over the weekend. However, on Sunday morning, the care assistant assigned to Margaret's bay reports that Margaret has declined to wash or shower, has no clean clothes, and will not wear hospital-supplied clothing. The registered nurse also notes that Margaret is not at her bedside when medications are being distributed. Margaret arrives with a blanket wrapped around her shoulders, carrying her cigarettes.

Before reading on, consider Exercise 13.1.

EXERCISE 13.1

There are five key principles of the MCA 2005. How do these relate to Margaret and the current situation?

Would it be appropriate to apply for DoLS authorization to prevent Margaret from leaving the ward to smoke?

How do the professional, legal, and ethical principles discussed so far relate to Margaret now? There is a risk that she will be treated negatively. What can an advanced practitioner, with enhanced knowledge, skills, and experience, do to avoid this?

13.5 Consent, Autonomy, and Advocacy

Mental capacity is closely linked to the twin issues of consent and autonomy. In the Court of Appeal in *R (on the application of Burke) v GMC* 2005, it was said that "where a competent patient makes it clear he does not wish to receive treatment which is, objectively, in his medical best interests, it is unlawful for doctors to administer that treatment. Personal autonomy, or the right of self-determination prevails" (para 30; see Table 13.1). So, if a patient wishes to withhold their consent, even if it is considered an unwise decision, it is unlawful to continue with that medical treatment, whether it is something that may appear trivial or

TABLE 13.1

Legal cases.

Bolam v Friern HMC [1957] 2 All ER 118
Maynard v West Midlands RHA [1985] 1 All ER 635
R (on the application of Burke) v GMC [2005] 3 FCR 169
R v Adomako [1994] 3 All ER 79
Roylance v GMC (no. 2) [2000] 1AC 311
S v St George's Healthcare Trust [1998] 3 All ER 673
Shakoor v Situ (trading as Eternal Health Co.) [2000] 4 All ER 181
Siddaway v Bethlem RHG [1985] 1 All ER 643
Stockdale v Nicholls [1993] 4 Med LR 190
All cases are freely available at the British and Irish Legal Information Institute, http://www.bailii.org

even in the event of life-saving surgery (*S v St George's* 1998; Table 13.1). For the advanced practitioner, being the patient's advocate in these circumstances is not simply a matter of recording that the patient has withheld their consent, but also establishing why.

It is important that all practitioners are confident that the patient has been provided with sufficient information to make their decision, which will vary from one patient to the next. Advocacy, says the NMC, requires impartiality, resilience, compassion, and emotional competence (NMC 2017). This suggests that autonomy, as well as being one of Beauchamp and Childress' (2013) "four principles," is again linked with the need for practical wisdom, as it in turn demands that the attributes of emotional maturity and emotional intelligence are well developed (Shafer-Landau 2012). These are demonstrated by returning to our case study, where the nurse needs to draw on the professional qualities described by the NMC to both act as Margaret's advocate and ensure accountability.

CASE STUDY (iv)

Margaret declines any paracetamol or codeine, stating that they are ineffective and that her pain is more muscular, and in her shoulder rather than at the fracture site. When the nurse attempts to discuss this further, Margaret responds angrily and says, "Stop treating me like a child or some old demented crone." A physiotherapist waiting to speak to the nurse mutters "shut up," loudly enough to be heard by two student nurses, who laugh.

Before reading on, consider Exercise 13.2.

this will have a negative impact not only on patient satisfaction and increased compliance with prescribed medication, but also on the team providing her care (Greenhalgh and Heath 2010). It can be seen here how one comment, whether defined as thoughtless, harmful, unprofessional, or misconduct, can have much wider implications than the immediate vicinity in which it is made.

Before reading on, undertake Exercise 13.3.

EXERCISE 13.2

How is Margaret's statement about her medication related to consent and autonomy?

For Margaret, the therapeutic relationship has broken down. There is evidence that

EXERCISE 13.3

Consider the exchange between the physiotherapist and student nurses. What impact might it have on Margaret, on the students, and on the nurse who witnesses the event? Who else might be affected?

13.6 Negligence

When a healthcare professional has harmed a patient through negligence, there are a number of potential legal consequences. First, though rarely, there may be a criminal prosecution, most likely for gross negligence manslaughter – as in *R v Adomako* [1994] 3 All ER 79 (Table 13.1), where an anesthetist failed to notice that oxygen tubing had become dislodged – but could also involve a charge of battery in the absence of consent. However, most cases will be brought as civil actions, with a claimant suing for damages. In either of these circumstances, there may also be professional disciplinary proceedings or action through the NHS complaints procedure (https://www.nhs.uk/nhsengland/complaints-and-feedback).

The test for criminal liability in gross negligence manslaughter was established in *R v Adomako* (1994) All ER 79 and requires the prosecution to prove, beyond reasonable doubt, that:

- The defendant owed the deceased victim a duty of care.
- The defendant breached their duty of care.
- The breach caused, or significantly contributed to, the death of the victim.
- The breach was so grossly negligent as to constitute a crime.

In common with medical negligence, once a duty of care has been established, a jury must consider the extent to which the defendant's conduct departed from the proper standard of that care. The test for this was first held in *Bolam v Friern HMC* [1957] 2 All ER 118, where it was stated that "a doctor is not guilty of negligence if he has acted in accordance with a practice accepted as proper by a responsible body of medical men skilled in that particular art" (Table 13.1). The test refers to doctors, but is applicable to all healthcare professionals, and has been widely cited in other cases and approved in the House of Lords, in *Maynard v West Midlands RHA* [1985] 1 All ER 635 and *Siddaway v Bethlem RHG* [1985] 1 All ER 643, for example (Table 13.1). In *Maynard*, the House of Lords held that a judge is not in a position to decide between conflicting expert medical opinions. So as long as there is a school of thought that endorses the care provided, the doctor (healthcare professional) will not be negligent, though this was qualified in *Bolitho v City & Hackney Health Authority* [1998] AC 232, where Lord Browne-Wilkinson added that the opinion had to have a logical basis and be defensible (Table 13.1). Further qualifications on the standard of care a professional is expected to exercise can be found in *Stockdale v Nicholls* [1993] 4 Med LR 190 and *Shakoor v Situ (trading as Eternal Health Co)* [2000] 4 All ER 181. These held that a general practitioner is to be assessed on the skills of general practice, a Chinese herbalist on traditional Chinese medicine.

It follows, then, that an advanced practitioner will be expected to practice in accordance with the skills of an advanced practitioner (Table 13.1). These were published by the Royal College of Nursing (RCN 2012) and further defined by Health Education England (HEE 2017).

The RCN (2012) raised the question of whether advanced nurse practitioners are more likely to be held liable for their actions than other nurses, and concluded that they were no more likely to be the subject of claims of negligence than other nurses, because their practice is underpinned by an educational program that enhances the ability to acknowledge limitations to competence and to set limits to their own practice. However, in 2016 the Medical Defence Union (MDU) reported that its nurse practitioner members were at an increased risk of claims and complaints. The MDU reported 25 medical negligence claims arising in 2015, with the commonest reason for cases being wrong or delayed diagnosis, followed by delayed referrals and prescribing errors. The MDU issued some sound advice, which echoes the Health and Care Professions Council's (HCPC 2016) and NMC's (2015) codes, that advanced practitioners keep their knowledge up to date, work within their level of competence, and, if there is any doubt about a diagnosis, seek advice or refer the patient on for further investigations or treatment. It also advised that, with roles such as running minor injury clinics, assessing and diagnosing patients, and prescribing medicines on the increase, practitioners are at an increased risk of being held individually accountable; and that, in line with the NMC requirement, having an appropriate indemnity arrangement in place is in the best interests of patients, clients, and registrants in the event of claims of professional negligence.

Not all claims and complaints will lead to a proven finding of negligence, even though the burden of proof in civil cases relating to professional cases is lower than that required for criminal charges or gross negligence manslaughter. Civil cases are decided on the balance of probabilities; or, rather, it is more likely true than not true that the basic elements of negligence – that is, duty of care, breach, causation, and harm – are proven. It may be, though, that even if a claim of negligence is unsuccessful, the practitioner will still face a professional disciplinary hearing and may be subject to sanctions by their regulatory body if their fitness to practice is found to be impaired due to lack of competence or misconduct. In *Roylance v GMC* (no 2) [2000] 1AC 311, misconduct is defined *as* "a word of general effect, involving some act or omission which falls short of what would be proper in the circumstances" (Table 13.1). The NMC and the Health Care Professions Tribunal Service Conduct and Competence Committees work in a very similar fashion and impose similar sanctions, which may result in a registrant being struck off or suspended, having practice conditions imposed, or receiving a caution. Practitioners registered with both regulatory bodies, for example a paramedic who is also a registered nurse, may receive sanctions from both bodies.

13.7 Handling Complaints

In England, complaints handling is governed by the NHS Health and Social Care Complaints (England) Regulations 2009, which cover all NHS healthcare provision, whether it is through NHS Trusts, independent organizations, voluntary bodies, or private companies providing care under arrangements with the NHS; there are separate arrangements for Scotland, Wales, and Northern Ireland. It does not cover complaints made by employees in relation to their work, nor does it include complaints made by one NHS body against another. All organizations are required to have a responsible person to oversee the complaints procedure, which must be publicized and accessible to all service users. Patients, or their representatives, can register a complaint locally, or can report the issue to the Parliamentary and Health Service Ombudsman. The vast majority of complaints are dealt with locally. Complainants are normally current or former patients, or their nominated representatives, and it is usual to expect patients over the age of 16, who have capacity, to complain for themselves. If a third party complains, it is necessary to ensure that they have the patient's authority and that confidentiality is not breached. Complaints may be verbal or written, but would normally be expected to be a formal statement of complaint, not a passing comment; a verbal complaint that can be dealt with in one working day does not need to be acknowledged in writing (MDU 2016). All other complaints, whether written or verbal, are deemed "official complaints," must be fully investigated, and must receive a written response within three working days. It is expected that all staff will have a good knowledge of local complaints procedures.

Before reading on, consider Exercise 13.4.

EXERCISE 13.4

With reference to the NMC Code and HCPC Code of Conduct, how should Margaret's remark about how she is being treated be responded to?

Consider the complaints policy in your area of work. Is it relevant to Margaret's comment?

13.8 Whistleblowing

Both the NMC and the HCPC impose a duty on their registrants to report any concerns that put people in their care or the public at risk. This is not just related to safety issues, but encompasses all aspects of care and treatment, and includes issues to do with individual attitudes, behavior, and prejudices and concerns over the organization as a whole, such as resources, staffing, or institutional prejudices.

It can be difficult for a registrant to know whether they need to make a complaint, are raising a concern, or are whistleblowing. These three terms are essentially about doing the same thing – speaking out – but the process to be followed, and the protections in law, will depend on the nature of the wrongdoing or harm. The common factor is that, unlike the service user complaints procedure, the concerns here are being reported by an employee or registered healthcare professional. For example, if an employee makes a protected disclosure in the public interest in relation to the mistreatment of patients, failure to comply with legal obligations, or the endangerment of the health and safety of any individual, that person is protected by the Employment Rights Act 1996 and must not be subjected to harassment, bullying, dismissal, or any other detrimental treatment. The Public Interest Disclosure Act 1998 was introduced to protect workers who raise genuine concerns in the public interest; it too protects against victimization and dismissal. Personal grievances, such as a complaint about pay or working conditions or relating to bullying, harassment, or discrimination, do not fall into "public interest disclosure" and as such are not covered by the same law. Grievances of this nature are dealt with through employers' complaints procedures.

The NHS has a whistleblowing helpline that offers free advice to all workers and employers in the NHS and social care organizations. If the concern is not resolved satisfactorily, it is then escalated to a prescribed body. This could be, for example, the CQC, NMC, HCPC, Healthcare Improvement Scotland, or the Healthcare Inspectorate Wales or, if appropriate, the Member of Parliament for the constituency where the concern originates (Department for Business, Energy & Industrial Strategy 2016). In relation to issues concerning the practice of individual registrants of a regulatory body, it would be appropriate to report concerns to that body. Here, for nurses and midwives, the NMC is quite clear, stating that "failure to report concerns may bring your fitness to practise into question and put your registration at risk" (NMC 2015b). The HCPC states that its registrants "must report any concerns about the safety or well-being of service users promptly and appropriately" and "must follow up concerns ... and, if necessary, escalate them" (HCPC 2016). This, they say, always comes before any professional or other loyalties.

In order to raise a concern, the NMC recommends that registrants seek advice from their professional body, from a trade union, or from Public Concern at Work (www.pcaw.org.uk), an independent whistleblowing charity that provides confidential advice to employees who have witnessed wrongdoing or malpractice and are uncertain how to proceed (NMC 2015b). If an employee is instructed to cover up a wrongdoing or harm, or told not to pursue a concern, the person giving that instruction is committing an offense; it will be a disciplinary, professional, or criminal offense, depending on the circumstances, and is contrary to the duty of candor, which requires that all NHS and non-NHS providers of services to NHS patients in the UK are open and transparent with service users about their care and treatment, including when these go wrong.

Before reading on, consider Exercise 13.5.

EXERCISE 13.5

In the case study, are there sufficient grounds for the registered nurse to raise a concern about the physiotherapist? If you consider there are, how might this be handled? Does the NMC's guidance on raising concerns *require* that the nurse report the incident?

13.9 Duty of Candor

Almost 50 years before the public inquiry into Mid-Staffordshire NHS Foundation Trust (Francis Report 2013), the book *Human Guinea Pigs: Experimentation on Man* (Pappworth 1967) uncovered and publicized the details of doctors carrying out unethical research involving human subjects. The catalyst for Pappworth's inquiry was said to be his concern that junior doctors whom he taught as postgraduate students felt they had little choice but to facilitate and participate in such research experiments for fear of ruining their careers. Pappworth's work precipitated a strengthening of research codes of conduct and the introduction of research ethics committees, but was definitely not the last time the twentieth century would see criticism of organizational cultures that failed patients.

The final report of the independent inquiry into care provided by Mid-Staffordshire NHS Foundation (Francis Report 2013) recommended that an obligation is placed on all healthcare professionals to be open and transparent when things go wrong and a service user has, or may have, suffered harm. The statutory duty of candor that arises from this requires not just the truthful answering of any questions or completion of statements, but, under Regulation 20 of the Health and Social Care Act 2008 (Regulated Activities) (Amendment) Regulations 2015, the notification and volunteering of information that may initiate an inquiry whenever a notifiable safety incident occurs. The Francis Report's recommendations and subsequent Regulation 20 were intended to put in place the systems and processes necessary to ensure that healthcare providers and the professionals working for them are accountable for the performance and quality of their services. One of the key challenges for healthcare providers is to nurture a culture of continuously improving care quality, within the context of limited resources.

13.10 Improving Care Quality

Care quality is almost synonymous with inspections, targets, and league tables, so it is important here to restate and emphasize Aristotle's practical wisdom: to know what to do, when, in what way, *and for what reason*. The true gauge of quality is not necessarily the standard of care when the inspectors call, though this does provide an insight, but the care provided when no one is looking. Professionalism leads to improved health outcomes through the realization of enabling environments (NMC 2017); and statutory obligations, regulations, and codes of practice tell us what we must do to mitigate against poor standards or errors; but working in an ethical workplace can teach us that striving to improve care quality is a good thing to do, an end in itself. An ethical workplace is one in which the leaders – and, by implication, this includes advanced practitioners – are committed, through role modeling, to preserving others' dignity and human rights, providing a safe environment for learners and others to raise concerns about workplace practices, and managing professionalism dilemmas with emotional sensitivity (Monrouxe and Rees 2017). Creating an ethical workplace can begin with a simple commitment to the preservation of dignity, as defined by regulation 10 of the Health and Social Care Act 2008 (Regulated Activities) Regulations 2014, and endorsed by the CQC. It includes making sure that people have privacy when they need and want it, treating them as equals, and providing any support they may need in order to be autonomous and independent. In this context, not only is physical dignity preserved, but difficult subjects can be raised and discussed with patients and those close to them, and with other members of the multidisciplinary team.

Before concluding this chapter, consider your answer to Exercise 13.6.

EXERCISE 13.6

Given that the creation of an ethical workplace can begin with role modeling a commitment to the preservation of dignity, how might an advanced practitioner demonstrate this in practice?

13.11 Conclusion

This chapter has explored professional, ethical, and legal issues related to advanced clinical practice not as ends in themselves, but as integral features of care delivery. The approach put forward is one that requires the advanced practitioner to have knowledge, skills, and experience and to apply those attributes wisely, whilst treating people as individuals and enabling increased involvement in decision making about planned care. All of these are features of an ethical workplace that actively seeks to continuously improve care quality by ensuring that all of the team involved in care delivery know, as appropriate to their role, what to do, when, in what way, and for what reason, and what they should do when things go wrong.

Key Questions

1. Codes of professional conduct for healthcare workers generally include a clause that urges their registrants to treat people as individuals. What are the implications of this for day-to-day practice?
2. This chapter focuses on practical wisdom and advances the idea that ethical decision making cannot be reduced to following an algorithm. Do you agree, or are there ethical decisions that can be made using algorithms?
3. Advanced practitioners work with a high degree of autonomy and are involved in complex decision making, sometimes forwarding innovative solutions to improve patient outcomes. Are advanced practitioners more vulnerable to charges of negligence as a result of deviating from accepted practice?

Glossary

Autonomy: the capacity to make deliberated or reasoned decisions for oneself and to act on the basis of such decisions.

Beneficence: the moral obligation to do good.

Care Quality Commission (CQC; www.cqc.org.uk): an independent body that monitors, inspects, and regulates health and social care services.

Consequentialism: moral theories maintaining that the result of actions (their outcome) is what matters most.

Deontology: theories of what is absolutely right or absolutely wrong according to rights and duties.

Duty of candor: a professional responsibility to be transparent and open when something goes wrong with treatment or care. Healthcare professionals must tell the patient what has happened, the possible outcomes, apologize, and offer whatever is needed to correct the situation (General Medical Council and Nursing and Midwifery Council 2017).

Duty of care: used to define when a professional (or organization) has assumed responsibility for patients or others.

Health and Care Professions Council (HCPC; http://www.hcpc-uk.co.uk): regulates 16 health and care professions in the UK, maintains a register of qualified individuals, sets standards, and approves training programs for those professions.

Justice: the moral obligation to be fair and treat others equally.

Medical Defence Union (www.themdu.com): provides indemnity for doctors, dentists, and other healthcare professionals.

Mental capacity: the ability to make decisions for and about oneself. In healthcare, exercising individual capacity may sometimes conflict with the need for protection from harm.

Misconduct: professional or personal action that provokes a disciplinary response.

Negligence: failure to provide care to the standard expected from similar colleagues, with similar training, skills, and experience.

Nonmaleficence: the moral obligation to avoid doing harm.

Nursing and Midwifery Council (www.nmc.org.uk): the professional regulator for nurses and midwives in the UK.

Parliamentary and Health Service Ombudsman (www.ombudsman.org.uk): makes final decisions about complaints that have not been resolved.

Practical wisdom: deliberation which gives equal weight to what one ought to do morally and what one can do in practice, which leads to a decision and effective action. Sound judgment is its key feature.

Principlism: an applied approach to ethics based on following a number of moral principles.

Royal College of Nursing (www.rcn.org.uk): a trade union and professional body for nurses, midwives, and healthcare assistants in the UK.

Whistleblowing: where a member of staff, such as a healthcare worker, draws the attention of external agencies to a problem in their institution, such as poor clinical standards or unprofessional practices.

References

Aristotle (2009). *The Nicomachean Ethics* (ed. W.D. Ross and L. Brown). Oxford: Oxford University Press.

Ayto, J. (2005). *Word Origins: The Hidden Histories of English Words from A to Z*, 2e. London: A. & C. Black.

Beauchamp, T.L. and Childress, J.F. (2013). *Principles of Biomedical Ethics*, 7e. Oxford: Oxford University Press.

Department for Business, Energy & Industrial Strategy (2016). Whistleblowing: list of prescribed people and bodies. https://bit.ly/1BtaAU3 (accessed July 23, 2017).

Dudgeon, J. (2015). Medical ethics made easy. https://bit.ly/2HHi5k9 (accessed August 28, 2017).

Fowers, B.J. (2003). Reason and human finitude: in praise of practical wisdom. *American Behavioural Scientist* 47 (4): 415–426.

Francis, R. (2013). Final Report of the Mid-Staffordshire NHS Foundation Trust Public Inquiry. http://webarchive.nationalarchives.gov.uk/20150407084231/http://www.midstaffspublicinquiry.com/report (accessed August 5, 2017).

General Medical Council and Nursing and Midwifery Council (2015). *Openness and Honesty When Things Go Wrong: The Professional Duty of Candour*. London: GMC and NMC.

Greenhalgh, T. and Heath, I. (2010). *Measuring Quality in the Therapeutic Relationship*. London: King's Fund https://bit.ly/2HjspQj (accessed January 6, 2018.

Health and Care Professions Council (2016). Standards of conduct, performance and ethics. https://bit.ly/1nLmyo5 (accessed August 17, 2017).

Health Education England (2017). Advanced clinical practice definition. https://hee.nhs.uk/our-work/advanced-clinical-practice (accessed August 20, 2017).

Machin, L. (2015). The ethical aspects of self discharge from hospital. https://bit.ly/2HIR146 (accessed January 5, 2018).

Mallia, P. (2013). *The Nature of the Doctor-Patient Relationship; Health Care Principles through the Phenomenology of Relationships with Patients*. Dordecht: Springer.

Medical Defence Union (2016). Medico-legal guide to the NHS complaints procedure. https://www.themdu.com/guidance-and-advice/guides/nhs-complaints (accessed August 6, 2017).

Monrouxe, L.V. and Rees, C.E. (2017). *Healthcare Professionalism: Improving Practice through Reflections on Workplace Dilemmas*. Chichester: Wiley Blackwell.

Nursing and Midwifery Council (2017). Enabling professionalism in nursing and midwifery practice. www.nmc.org.uk/standards/professionalism/read-report (accessed August 5, 2017).

Nursing and Midwifery Council (2015). The Code: professional standards of practice and behaviour for nurses and midwives. www.nmc.org.uk/standards/code (accessed August 17, 2017).

Nursing and Midwifery Council (2015b). Raising concerns: guidance for nurses and midwives. https://bit.ly/2vDkLL2 (accessed August 5, 2017).

Pappworth, M.H. (1967). *Human Guinea Pigs: Experimentation on Man*. Boston: Beacon Press.

Royal College of Nursing (2012). Advanced nurse practitioners – an RCN guide to advanced nursing practice, advanced nurse practitioners and programme accreditation. www.rcn.org.uk/professional-development/publications/pub-003207 (accessed August 6, 2017).

Sellman, D. (2011). *What Makes a Good Nurse: Why the Virtues Are Important for Nurses*. London: Jessica Kingsley.

Shafer-Landau, R. (2012). *The Fundamentals of Ethics*, 2e. Oxford: Oxford University Press.

Singer, P. (1991). *A Companion to Ethics*. Oxford: Blackwell.

CHAPTER 14

Advanced Practice in a Diverse Society

Paula McGee

Birmingham City University, Birmingham, UK

Key Issues
- Human rights
- Promoting equality
- Tackling discrimination
- Difficult conversations

LEARNING OBJECTIVES

By the end of this chapter you should be able to:

- Explain the key concepts of equality, diversity, discrimination, and harassment.
- Critically discuss the application of advanced competences in promoting equality in healthcare.
- Critically explore strategies for tackling inappropriate behavior.

14.1 Introduction

The term *diversity* is a very broad concept which refers to the differences between individuals and groups present in any society. These differences can provide new perspectives and connections, stimulate change, and create new economic opportunities, all of which contribute to the development of thriving communities, which in turn may improve quality of life. Healthcare services derive considerable benefit from diversity. For example, since its inception in 1948, the UK's National Health Service has depended quite heavily on recruitment from other nations. Recruiting offices were opened in many countries, including

Advanced Practice in Healthcare: Dynamic Developments in Nursing and Allied Health Professions,
Fourth Edition. Edited by Paula McGee and Chris Inman.

India in the early 1960s, where doctors were encouraged to come to the UK by the then Health Minister, Enoch Powell (Esmail 2007). The international recruitment of doctors, nurses, and other professionals has continued ever since creating a dynamic working environment based on a workforce that is drawn from many different countries and represents multiple cultures and languages. Nurses form a significant part of this workforce. The Royal College of Nursing (RCN 2017) reported that, of the 689 738 nurses on the Nursing and Midwifery Council's (NMC) register, 36 259 had been recruited from another country in the European Union (EU) and a further 67 683 from outside both the EU and the European Economic Area. These figures represent quite a substantial proportion of the nursing workforce that is providing patient care and contributing to the economy via taxation (RCN 2017). Overall, it is estimated that, in a workforce of 1.2 million, at least 139 000 members of staff originate from outside the UK, and that their absence could provoke a staffing crisis in some areas (House of Commons 2018).

However, the presence of differences and the changes they may bring mean that diversity can also be regarded as a threat, particularly by those who perceive themselves as having something to lose. In this context, the presence of differences such as in ethnicity, disability, sexuality, or economic status are perceived as undesirable, outside established social "norms." All societies and groups, large and small, establish norms, unwritten codes that determine behavior and are linked to culture, tradition, and shared identity, all of which provide a sense of belonging, a sense of "us" as opposed to others, "them" who are "not us." Social distinctions and judgments create a basis for opposition and resistance. Diversity may then become a focal point for those in more powerful social positions who have a strong tendency to consider themselves superior to others, to make negative value judgments about people, and even dehumanize them. It is in these situations that prejudice and discriminatory behavior arise and are enacted on a day-to-day basis as a way of reinforcing social hierarchies.

This chapter examines the notion of diversity in relation to both healthcare in general and, more specifically, advanced practice. It begins with a short discussion of human rights and health inequalities. It then progresses to examine ways of tackling discrimination and promoting equality with reference to UK legislation, the Public Sector Equality Duty, and the competences of advanced practitioners. The chapter closes with a case study which focuses on tackling a situation in which discrimination has taken place, and some guidelines for conducting conversations with individuals who have behaved in this way.

14.2 Human Rights

The idea of human rights is quite difficult to pin down. On a political level, human rights are enshrined in statements about how countries should treat the members of their populations. One such statement, the Universal Declaration of Human Rights (United Nations 1948), was developed by the victors of World War II and reflects the locus of political power in the West, the context of the atrocities and injustices committed by the Nazis, and the desire for protection against tyrannical state violence (Freeman 2011). For example, Article 1 of the Declaration states that "All human beings are born free and equal in dignity" (United Nations 1948) and are thus entitled to certain rights on an equal basis with everyone else. These include "life, liberty and security of person" (Article 3), equality in law (Article 6), freedom from slavery (Article 4) and from torture (Article 5), and "equal protection against any discrimination" (Article 7). The European Convention on Human Rights (1950) provides similar statements, adding that the "rights and freedoms set forth in this Convention shall be secured without discrimination on any ground such as sex, race, colour, language, religion, political or other opinion, national or social origin, association with a national minority, property, birth or other status" (Article 14). Member states of the European Union are required to sign the Convention, which is enforced through the European Court of Human Rights.

The human rights put forward in these documents are a political construct devised by humans to facilitate certain standards of behavior by governments and societies. In this context, they can be said to represent an attempt, albeit a flawed one, to address the questions of how human beings should live together in modern societies and in a globalized world. However, consideration of social and philosophical perspectives on human rights raises a number of issues. First, the Declaration and the Convention reflect the continued political power and Judeo-Christian-based values of Western nations, which may not be applicable in other societies. For example, religious freedom (Article 18) may not be regarded as a right in states which are effectively theocratic and view their beliefs as the only ones to be followed. Rights drawn up in societies based on different value systems might differ, and questions then arise as to whether it is possible for there to be agreement between such differing perspectives.

A second issue is whether all rights are absolute and equal, or whether some may actually be conditional on other factors. For example, "the right to liberty" (Article 3) raises questions about whether an individual's liberty can be curtailed or removed as a consequence of their behavior. If not, then the right to liberty may conflict with other rights such as Article 12, the "right to the protection of the law against such interference or attacks." Other rights may be dependent on local circumstances and seem more like aspirations. The right to "favourable conditions of work" (Article 23) may be impossible to achieve in very poor countries where unemployment is high and the regulation of workplaces is limited. In addition, some rights such as that to a "standard of living adequate for health and well-being" (Article 25) are vague, poorly defined, and, again, not universally achievable.

Further criticisms focus on whether human rights are legal rights or a special category of rights that each individual acquires simply by being human (Freeman 2011). If human rights are indeed a special category, then there is a need to establish how, why, and when these are conferred. The implication is that humans are a special species, separated from all others by these rights. In this argument, humans, their lives, and their experiences are intrinsically important and valuable; "humanism," or "gaining faith in humanity," marks an important change in the way humans view themselves (Hariri 2015, p. 259).

Perhaps "faith in humanity" (Hariri 2015, p. 279) will enable movement toward more peaceful and equitable ways of life in which everyone has a fair share. The Vienna Declaration certainly seemed like step in the right direction. It upheld the current statements about human rights, but moved the discourse on by including references to contemporary issues such as terrorism; it also set out a plan of action for signatories, which included the provision of healthcare services (Office of the United Nations High Commissioner for Human Rights 1993). Most importantly, the Declaration acknowledged that some social groups

TABLE **14.1**

The Millennium Development Goals.

Eradicate extreme poverty and hunger

Achieve universal primary education

Promote gender equality and empower women

Reduce child mortality

Improve maternal health

Combat HIV/AIDS, malaria, and other diseases

Ensure environmental sustainability

Develop a global partnership for development

Source: Data from United Nations (2015) The Millennium Development Goals Report 2015. Available http://www.un.org.

required special consideration and interventions: women and girls, minorities, indigenous peoples, refugees, and those living in poverty. In every society these are the groups which lack power and against whom prejudice and discrimination are commonly directed, with specific and potentially catastrophic results. The eight Millennium Development Goals were intended to address the inequalities experienced by these groups by 2015 (Table 14.1). Some improvements were made. For instance, extreme poverty and hunger declined, although they were still a major problem; more girl children were attending school, but the numbers still lagged behind those for boys (UN 2015a). However, inequality has deep roots that spread widely and success was only partial. In response, a new agenda for sustainable development was launched (UN 2015b). This set out a series of goals, more than twice the number of the Millennium Goals, but with similar aims, to be achieved by 2030. Whether this agenda will be successful remains to be seen.

Discussion about inequalities and human rights may seem a long way from the realities of daily clinical practice, but consideration of these rights links directly with the treatment and care of patients and how professionals should behave toward those who are ill and vulnerable. Health professionals are charged with obligations to provide treatment and care for all patients, irrespective of their individual differences. Each profession sets out the values to which it expects members to adhere and how professionals should behave toward patients and colleagues. For example, nurses and midwives are expected to "treat people as individuals and uphold their dignity … treat people with kindness, respect and compassion … avoid making assumptions and recognise diversity" (NMC 2015, p. 4). They must also treat "people fairly and without discrimination, bullying or harassment" (NMC 2015, p. 15). Similar statements can be found in other codes. Health professionals generally are expected to be aware of the ways in which their behavior may affect that of others and to act always "in non-discriminatory, non-oppressive ways" (Chartered Society of Physiotherapists 2011, p. 11), irrespective of the patient's illness and even if that person's "actions or lifestyle have contributed to their condition" (General Medical Council 2014, p. 19). As senior professionals with enhanced levels of competence, advanced practitioners have additional responsibilities in providing clinical and professional leadership. The NHS Constitution sets out the rights of patients with regards to access to healthcare on an equal basis for all, ensuring that no one is "excluded, discriminated against or left behind" (NHS Health Education England 2015, p. 5). However, it also makes clear that staff have rights too in terms of "healthy and safe working conditions and an environment free from harassment, bullying or violence" and the right "to be treated fairly, equally, and free from discrimination" (NHS Health Education England 2015, p. 12). Advanced practitioners therefore need to have an understanding of the multiple ways in which prejudice and discrimination can arise and the ability to take appropriate action.

They also require a sound understanding of the impact of inequalities on health. The Marmot Report (2010, p. 16) made clear that "Inequalities in health arise because of inequalities in society – in the conditions in which people are born, grow, live, work, and age. So close is the link between particular social and economic features of society and the distribution of health among the population, that the magnitude of health inequalities is a good marker of progress towards creating a fairer society." The report went on to note that, in poorer areas of England, people were likely to die earlier and have a higher risk of disabilities and long-term health problems than their wealthier counterparts. By 2016, the gap in life expectancy between men born into wealthier and poorer areas was nearly 10 years; the gap for women was 7.4 years (Office for National Statistics 2018). Advanced practitioners need to be knowledgeable about the inequalities and challenges faced by their patients and find innovative approaches that help them to cope. They also have responsibilities for guiding colleagues and others away from blaming people for what they are or for what they are not.

14.3 Tackling Discrimination

Equality is about treating people equally, irrespective of any particular characteristics they may or may not possess; no one should receive less favorable treatment because they are regarded as inferior to others. Such discrimination may be direct, targeting a particular individual or group, or indirect, occurring, for example, as a result of the culture or procedures in an organization. Exposure to discrimination perpetuates inequalities by reducing opportunities through denying access to education, employment, services, and other avenues that are open to others. Thus, discrimination limits freedom to develop and achieve; it curtails aspirations; and it discourages full participation in society. It also creates constant stress and anxiety because, even if discrimination does not actually occur in a particular situation, there is always the possibility that it might arise; this anticipation gives rise to an ever-present state of hyperarousal. Consequently, persistent physiological changes occur in which the fight-or-flight mechanism is activated, raising the heart rate and levels of cortisol, with negative long-term effects on health (Harrell et al. 2011; McGee 2016).

Promoting equality is about establishing a fairer society by actively promoting the rights of those who have been, and still are likely to be, exposed to discrimination and social exclusion. Promoting their rights is about improving their poorer life chances, so that each person has the same opportunities as everyone else to develop their potential. Bringing about societal change on this level requires huge investment and multiple avenues of development, one of which is legislation. In the UK, the Equality Act 2010 provides protection against discrimination with regard to nine characteristics (Table 14.2). It specifically

TABLE **14.2**

TABLE 14.2

Equality Act 2010: protected characteristics.

Age
Being or becoming a transsexual person
Being married or in a civil partnership
Being pregnant or having a child
Disability
Race
Religion
Sex
Sexual orientation

Source: UK Government Equalities Office. https://www.equalityhumanrights.com/en/equality-act

TABLE 14.3

Equality Act 2010: when protection against discrimination applies.

Protection against discrimination applies when someone is:
Seeking work or in employment
At school, college, or university
Accessing any public service such healthcare, the police, or the fire service.
Buying or renting goods or property
Joining or visiting a club or association
Related to, is a friend of, or has any other connection with a person who has a protected characteristic.

Source: Summarized from Discrimination: your rights. UK Government Equalities Office. https://www.gov.uk/discrimination-your-rights

prohibits discrimination with regard to particular settings such as public services (Table 14.3). This not only safeguards the individual who possesses a protected characteristic, but also anyone associated with them. Anyone who has made a complaint about discrimination is also protected (https://www.gov.uk/equality-act-2010-guidance).

Before reading on, undertake Exercise 14.1.

EXERCISE **14.1**

Read the three examples below. In your opinion, do these count as discrimination?

a. MJ is a receptionist. She is unable to walk very far and depends on a wheelchair for mobility. The building is due for demolition and the company is moving to the first floor in another building that is still under construction. The architect's plans could easily be adapted to include a lift, but the company rejects this idea because of cost and makes MJ redundant.

b. A magazine aimed mainly at young South Asian women is advertising for South Asian girls to model this season's bridal wear.

> **c.** AL and his daughter both work for the same organization. His daughter is on maternity leave and has received a letter terminating her employment. She believes that this is due to her pregnancy. She has instigated legal proceedings against the organization. Meanwhile, AL has applied for promotion, but recently overheard his manager telling someone that the application would not be successful because "that family are just trouble."

The Equality Act 2010 replaced earlier laws which focused on single issues: disability, sex, and race. It is complemented by other legislation, including the Age Discrimination Act 2004, the Race Relations Amendment Act 2000, and the Protection from Harassment Act 1997. This last Act made harassment a criminal offense, although what constitutes harassment is not defined. It depends on how the victim perceives the behavior; it is the repeated nature of certain behaviors that are often the most troublesome.

Before reading on, consider Exercise 14.2.

> **EXERCISE 14.2**
>
> Read the three examples below. In your opinion, do these count as harassment?
>
> **a.** A senior member of staff regularly makes derogatory remarks about the Traveler family that is parked near to where she lives. When she discovers that one of the nurses is from a Traveler background, she demands to know, every day, "When are your lot moving on?" and later, "I suppose you'll be off with them next."
> **b.** Teasing a colleague about their team losing the match on Saturday.
> **c.** Circulating texts about a colleague's sexual orientation as a gay man planning to marry his partner.

A second avenue for promoting equality and bringing about change is the Equality and Human Rights Commission (EHRC). This is a statutory regulatory body which is responsible for enforcing the Equality Act 2010, "safeguarding and enforcing the laws that protect people's rights to fairness, dignity and respect." It provides advice, guidance, and information for organizations, and if necessary uses "the courts and tribunals to secure binding, positive judgments that reinforce, strengthen or expand people's rights" (www.equalityhumanrights. com). EHRC investigations have included those into the harassment of people with disabilities, home-based care for older adults, and human trafficking in Scotland. The Commission is currently investigating a range of issues arising from the Grenfell Tower fire in 2017, in which over 70 people died. Among the many issues involved in this investigation are whether the management company's policies and practices discriminated against all or any of the tenants, the treatment of children who survived the fire, and potential breaches of the state's and local borough's responsibilities to provide safe social housing.

The breadth of this investigation alone reveals a number of important issues about the complex nature of inequality. The first is the concept of *intersectionality*. This is a situation in which different sources of power intersect and cannot be separated. They interlock, causing individuals to experience discrimination on multiple, overlapping grounds. For example, a woman may experience discrimination on the grounds of gender, pregnancy, race, and religion, all at the same time.

Second, the nine protected characteristics do not encompass all the individuals and groups who may be victims of discrimination. Inequality permeates so many aspects of daily life and may be so taken for granted that it is not always easy to discern. Recognizing the vulnerability of certain groups and protecting them through legislation is a step forward in promoting equality, but, with the passage of time, other inequalities and discriminatory behaviors will come to light. For example, in the UK, discrimination on the ground of caste is an emerging issue. Caste is a fundamental part of Hindu society. Dalits are people who do not belong in any of the four Hindu castes; in South Asia they experience high levels of discrimination and social exclusion. Caste systems also operate in other societies and, as people migrate, so do their value systems and discriminatory practices. Organizations such as the Dalit Solidarity Network UK (http://dsnuk.org) and Caste Watch UK (www.castewatchuk.org) monitor the incidence of caste discrimination and have lobbied for better recognition of this form of discrimination. A public consultation was conducted in 2017, resulting in a decision to rely on developing case law through the courts rather than legislate formally against this type of caste discrimination (Government Equalities Office 2018).

Finally, the EHRC's inquiry into the fire at Grenfell Tower highlights the responsibilities of public bodies such as local boroughs and councils, schools, and organizations such as the police and the National Health Service. The Public Sector Equality Duty, which became law in 2011, provides another approach to actively promoting equality. Public-sector organizations must take active steps to:

- "Eliminate unlawful discrimination, harassment and victimisation and other conduct prohibited by the Act.
- Advance equality of opportunity between people who share a protected characteristic and those who do not.
- Foster good relations between people who share a protected characteristic and those who do not." (Government Equalities Office 2011a, p. 3)

Inherent in the Public Sector Equality Duty is the requirement to treat people as having equal value and to provide them with equal opportunities that promote equity and fairness. Meeting these requirements may involve making some adjustments to policies and practices so that individuals with protected characteristics can function on a level with those without. In other words, the Public Sector Equality Duty is the antithesis of treating everyone the same.

In addition, public-sector organizations are required to publish three types of information. The first concerns members of staff who share a particular protected characteristic and who may be disadvantaged in some way by the organization's practices and procedures. Public-sector employers must report the action taken to meet the needs of staff with protected characteristics; treat them as having equal value; and ensure that they have equality of opportunity to enable them to do their work and participate fully in the life of the organization. The second type of information required concerns the organization's clients, policies, and procedures, and the steps taken to ensure equitable service provision. Finally, organizations are required to publish "measurable equality objectives which will help them to further the three aims of the Equality Duty" (Government Equalities Office 2011a, p. 6; 2011b). Compliance with the Public Sector Equality Duty requires a whole-organization approach, from board level to front-line staff; from strategic planning to dealing with clients, equality is everyone's business and responsibility (Government Equalities Office 2011b).

14.4 Advanced Practice Competences

As clinical and professional leaders, advanced practitioners hold positions of influence as role models for less experienced professionals and as experts in their field. Their actions can, therefore, have a profound effect on patient care and treatment, not only clinically but also in the ways in which people are treated. Care is care if it is based on respect and genuine concern for others. Caring requires paying attention to suffering and action to alleviate this (Papadopoulos 2018). Effective caring depends on communication between caregiver and recipient, to identify the cause of the suffering and establish a mutual trust-based understanding of how it may best be resolved for that person. In a diverse society, caring also includes recognition of individual differences and the ways in which those with protected characteristics may be disadvantaged. Advanced practitioners are well placed to provide leadership in caring for members of minority groups and in ensuring that they receive care on the same basis as everyone else.

14.4.1 Developing a Knowledge Base

A minority group is a social group whose members differ or are perceived to differ from those who hold power and who, as a result, experience low status, inequality, or discrimination. Thus, minority status is essentially about a power differential and not about numbers. In addition, whilst it is frequently used in connection with race and ethnicity, it has a much broader application. Women, for example, can be considered as a minority in circumstances in which they lack power, even though they usually make up half the population of any society. Minority groups include, but are not limited to, all those listed in the Equality Act 2010 (Table 14.2). Members of minorities are likely to experience inequality and discrimination, and so the first step in developing a knowledge base is to identify who they are and find appropriate ways of engaging with them. This can be challenging and requires patience. The best source of information is the people themselves, because it is through this that barriers are overcome; development of personal contacts transcends minority status, transforming it into "people I know."

Before reading on, consider Exercise 14.3.

> **EXERCISE 14.3**
>
> What information do you have about people with protected characteristics who the access the services in which you practice?
>
> How is this information shared with others?

Involvement in *direct care* to patients provides the advanced practitioner with opportunities for learning about their particular values, beliefs, challenges, and needs and how these can be addressed in the care setting. The advanced practitioner can also utilize *research skills* to facilitate information gathering from members of local communities, patient associations, and community groups. This can be helpful, but it is important to include a broad range of people, particularly among those not accustomed to being listened to or who have experienced abuse because of their differences. Making initial contacts cannot be rushed; it can sometimes take time to build relationships and trust. Identifying appropriate places to meet is important. These should be where people feel comfortable, so that they are relaxed and confident. There will have to be agreements about how discussions will take place, who will come, and for how long. Finally, whatever information is obtained needs to be regularly updated. Encouraging members of minorities to form or join patient advisory groups, for example to promote better care for transgender people, may provide channels for better long-term engagement by and with people with protected characteristics.

14.4.2 Making Changes

The most important consideration of all is that engaging directly with people who have protected characteristics creates hope and the prospect of change, which raises the issue about how the information gained will be shared and used. Too often the learning that occurs from caring for a patient with a protected characteristic is set aside when that person is discharged, so that, when another with similar differences requires care, everyone has to begin again. The advanced practitioner's role in "developing the self and others" is relevant here in enabling staff to share and embed knowledge (Department of Health 2010, p. 2). Storytelling can help in this, because "the oral tradition is effective in setting up salient memories. Stories are more memorable than lists of warnings that must be memorized out of context" (Benner et al. 1996 p. 208). In encouraging colleagues to share stories, the advanced practitioner can tap into rich resources that can be used as a basis for coaching and guiding.

Storytelling is a social activity. It enables the storyteller to make sense of events by explaining them and expressing feelings. It engages the listeners and in doing so it can facilitate reflection and help to make visible actions that might otherwise be overlooked (Holloway and Freshwater 2007). For example, caring for a patient following a stroke requires specific clinical interventions. Storytelling might also reveal that, prior to the stroke, the patient attended a gender identity clinic and was planning to undergo surgery for gender reassignment. This could lead into discussion about the care needs of this person with gender dysphoria and how these could be met in future.

14.4.3 Organizational Opportunities

Healthcare organizations have responsibilities under the Public Sector Equality Duty to take active steps to address inequalities. However, across a country, variations in readiness to meet these responsibilities vary. Advanced practitioners will have to make judgments about where their employing organization stands. At the most *basic level*, organizational activities will be purely reactive and focused on only satisfying the minimum requirements. Beyond this is the *project level*, where specific topics become the focus of attention for small groups. Examples might include siting ramps to improve physical access, creating prayer spaces, or improvements to catering. The associated publicity enhances the organization's image. Projects do not have to be expensive or require huge amounts of effort; small, incremental changes can make a lot of difference. Nevertheless, projects can also be risky. As with the previous level, there may be no real organizational commitment to change; only those charged with carrying out the projects have any involvement in equality issues.

Challenging the status quo in organizations in which in which equality and diversity are addressed at the basic or project levels will not be easy for advanced practitioners and they will need to operate strategically as leaders in order to bring about change. Three documents will be helpful. The first is the government objectives for the health service as a whole (Department of Health and Social Care 2018). This sets out what healthcare organizations are expected to achieve and how performance will be assessed. These objectives should be reflected in the second document, the corporate plan, in which an individual organization sets out its goals for a specific period and how these will be achieved. Scrutinizing the corporate plan can reveal opportunities for the advanced practitioner to package plans to address equality and diversity in ways that will contribute to achievement of the corporate plan (NHS England 2019). This means that the advanced practitioner needs to develop skills in identifying what people at the most senior levels see as priorities and communicating effectively in their terms. At the same time, the advanced practitioner will also need to present the same plans to middle managers and front-line staff in ways that reflect their priorities in getting through each day's work. The third document to include is the organization's most recent inspection report from the Care Quality Commission (CQC; www.cqc.org.uk). This will provide information about what is going well in the organization and any improvements required before the next inspection. Contributing to such improvements by addressing equality and diversity may provide additional avenues for the advanced practitioner to explore (Table 14.4).

Finally, at the *committed level,* the organization takes equality seriously. The strategic plan and mission statement incorporate equality issues; there is a commitment to change. Everyone, at all levels, from board level through every department to the front-line staff, receives mandatory training in addressing equality and diversity; these are now everyone's responsibility. The organization provides effective leadership in helping and supporting staff to bring about improvements through valuing and respecting people, recognizing inequalities, and developing strategies that enhance the capabilities of staff to provide equal care for everyone. The commitment of the organization is also evident in the allocation of budgets, in policies and procedures, and in the actions taken if those are breached.

TABLE 14.4

Questions to consider in promoting equality and tackling discrimination in your field of practice.

Are we clear about what needs to change and why?

How do we know this?

What do we have the power to do ourselves?

What sort of support do we need?

How can we gain this support from others/managers/board members to support us?

What do we need them to do?

How much will making a change cost and who will pay?

What steps will we take to introduce the change?

What is our measure for success?

Mr. J is 57, white, married with two children, and works in a bank. He was admitted to hospital with pneumonia and an acute exacerbation of asthma; the ward specializes in respiratory disease. As his condition is improving, his bed has been moved to a bay further down the ward, away from the area directly in front of the nurses' desk, so he is no longer directly observable all the time. He has a pleasant manner and enjoys company, therefore he welcomes the move as he is feeling slightly better and able to talk to other patients.

Nurse H qualified in Nigeria, where she was head nurse in a tuberculosis clinic. She relocated to the UK when she married her British husband and she is now a British citizen. Nurse H has worked as a Band 6 nurse in this particular ward for two years, and is currently studying for a qualification in managing chronic obstructive pulmonary disease.

Mr. J seems to get on well with all the staff, except Nurse H. Whenever she comes to carry out care activities, he speaks abruptly to her. On several occasions over the next two days, he tells her that he does not understand what she says and makes her repeat it several times. On leaving the bay, Nurse H sees him grin at the other patients and give a thumbs-up sign. When other staff attend to Mr. J, he behaves quite differently. He speaks to them politely and is cheerful, but on several occasions remarks that they are much better than Nurse H who, he says, is rough and rude. He is overheard telling the other patients that he "doesn't think black people should be in the country, that they are inferior and should go back to where they came from."

Before reading on, consider Exercise 14.4.

EXERCISE 14.4

As an advanced practitioner, what do you think may be happening here?

Later on the second day, the ward manager receives a complaint about Nurse H from the relatives of another patient in the bay, Mr. R. They allege that she has a bad attitude toward Mr. R and they do not want her to go near him again. The manager informs Nurse H that she has received a complaint about her.

Before reading on, undertake Exercise 14.5.

EXERCISE 14.5

How do you think Nurse H is feeling?

In your opinion, what should the ward manager do?

The manager asks each member of staff who has worked in the bay whether they have observed any problems, but does not tell them about the complaint. She then visits each patient in the bay and asks them whether they have heard or seen Nurse H display a bad attitude toward Mr. R. One of them tells the ward manager: "I was there all the time. She was very kind and gentle with Mr. R. He wasn't well this morning and she helped him and made sure he was alright before she left. There was no way she did anything wrong." Further conversations with patients reveals that it was Mr. J who told Mr. R's relatives about Nurse H and suggested they make a complaint. He was not present in the bay whilst she was caring for Mr. R. The ward manager discusses the outcome of her investigation with Mr. R's family and the complaint is dropped.

Before reading on, answer the questions in Exercise 14.6.

EXERCISE 14.6

As the advanced practitioner do you think that Nurse H has been treated fairly? Give reasons for your answer.

What interventions might you consider?

Black African nurses have reported experiencing racism from white patients and relatives, particularly older people. Examples included refusing to allow the nurses to care for them, ignoring them in favor of white staff, even if these were healthcare assistants, and generally regarding the black nurses as incompetent. The nurses have also encountered racism from ward managers: "they described how other nurses from overseas were allowed to perform certain procedures even when they were not competent, but Black African nurses were prevented from performing the same procedures even when they were competent." The nurses felt that their competence was overlooked, that managers did not trust them, that their prior experience did not count, and that if "they voiced this to their managers, they were labelled confrontational" (Likupe and Archibong 2013, p. 236). Archibong and Darr (2010) noted that nurse members of black and other minority ethnic groups were more likely to face disciplinary proceedings. When complaints arose, they also lacked support from informal networks, leading to feelings of isolation alongside fears about the possible outcomes. Those referred to the professional regulator are more likely than their white colleagues to face harsher outcomes (West and Nayar 2016).

The case study shows Nurse H in a similar position. She was told about the complaint, but was not given any information about it. She did not know what she had done. She was not offered any support or advice about what to do or who to speak to. She was not even informed that the complaint had been dropped. The case study also shows the insidious nature of prejudice and discrimination. Initially, Mr. J's behavior might be dismissed as a personality clash, but his comments to other nurses and patients indicated that it was more than this. His behavior escalated because it was unchecked; no one reported it and eventually Mr. J deliberately incited others to make a complaint against a black nurse.

The ward manager acted correctly in starting to investigate the complaint, but did not speak to Mr. J or record the matter. There was far more that she could and should have done, but she herself may have lacked confidence in approaching Mr. J. and worried that he might then complain about her. She might not have received training about how to deal with situations like this and might also have concerns about whether managers would support her actions. Mr. J would be discharged soon and so she may have felt that there was no need to pursue the matter.

Doing nothing, or not doing enough, in the face of difficult situations allows them to continue. However, taking action can also be challenging. A multimethod study of 1700 doctors and nurses showed that, whilst they had observed many examples of negative behavior such as broken rules, lack of respect, and incompetence, they did not report these incidents. It seems that people avoided action because (i) it was not their job; (ii) they thought reporting inappropriate behavior would not do any good; or (iii) they feared being criticized and made to feel that they were the ones at fault. In contrast, the small minority who did take action were able to bring about improvements. This is not to say that taking action was easy, but that it could be done (American Association of Critical Care Nurses 2005).

14.5 A Way Forward – Having That Difficult Conversation

Even in healthcare organizations that are committed to promoting equality for all staff and patients and take seriously their responsibilities toward those with protected characteristics, there is a need to ensure that staff:

- Have the confidence and capability to engage in difficult conversations with individuals who perpetrate inappropriate behavior.
- Are confident of the support of managers and the organization in reporting inappropriate behavior.

Advanced practitioners need to develop the skills required for difficult conversations, not only for dealing with equality issues, but also in tackling other situations in which individuals may not have acted appropriately, and in coaching and guiding staff like the ward manager. Advanced practitioners also need to know about sources of help and support for people who find themselves in professional difficulties; Nurse H, for example, should have been informed about the nature of the complaint and advised to contact her union representative.

Having a difficult conversation with someone about their behavior requires preparation. Witnessing bad behavior may provoke an immediate shocked or angry response, but try to lay aside the emotion and identify what actually happened: Who said or did what? How? And, if possible, why? Clarify also why you think this behavior is wrong. Consider as well where you can speak to the person concerned. This should be away from the immediate environment, other people, and interruptions. No one likes to be challenged in front of others and, if they are, then they will have a reason not to listen. Speak calmly and assertively when telling the person how you see the situation. Opening phrases such as "Are you alright?" "I don't really understand what happened out there," or "It seemed to me that you were [whatever the bad behavior was]" will be more helpful in starting the conversation than an aggressive or accusatory challenge. When you have explained how you see the situation and listened to the response, then you can move on to clearly stating what you want to see happen. However, stick to the matter in hand; avoid detours into previous events.

Consider the range of possible responses. There may be a reasonable explanation for the behavior, mitigating circumstances, or some other factors that you were unaware of which mean that simply asking someone not to repeat the behavior may not be enough. Recognize and acknowledge these responses, but try to avoid getting drawn into them. If necessary, these can be incorporated into what you want to see happen, but keep the focus on your main objective: that the person's behavior was not appropriate, why, and what needs to be done to put things right.

Be prepared for difficult responses: excuses, tears, and anger. Tears and excuses are easy ways to deflect your attention away from what has happened toward feeling sorry for the person concerned. Instead of the difficult conversation, you may find yourself mopping up tears and telling the person that there is no need to worry. Anger, shouting, and noise are also ways of deflecting your attention. They may lead into diatribes about how "You/they are always picking on me," and challenges such as "How dare you speak to me like this, you have no right?" or personal criticisms. Try not to respond with similar behavior or show that you feel threatened; stay calm. If the person storms out, let them go. Another difficult response is silence. There may be several reasons why the person does not respond. They may be feeling ashamed and not know what to say, or they may be afraid of what they think you may do as a result. Silence can be very uncomfortable. A minute can feel like a very long time. Nevertheless, give the person time to respond and if after that they still do not say anything, there is probably nothing more you can do (Sullivan and Garland 2013). Finally, when the conversation is over, make a record of the behavior, the conversation, and the outcome, and, if necessary, ensure that you have complied with organizational policies regarding reporting of inappropriate behavior.

14.6 Conclusion

Human rights are predicated on a value system in which all human beings are seem as having equal worth. Individual differences do not in any way alter an individual's status or the rights to which they are entitled as a person.

The recognition of these rights challenges established norms and associated prejudices, which form the basis for discrimination against particular social groups. Tackling discrimination, inequality, and social exclusion is important in creating fairer, more equal societies in which everyone can participate. Health professionals have a role to play in providing treatment and care for everyone in a nonjudgmental, nondiscriminatory manner, irrespective of any distinguishing characteristics. Whilst this is not always easy to achieve, as senior members of their respective professions, advanced practitioners can apply their skills to facilitate positive working environments.

Key Questions

1. How does inequality affect people's health and healthcare in your practice setting? What are the implications for you as an advanced practitioner?
2. As an advanced practitioner, how would you use your leadership, coaching and guiding, and direct care skills to facilitate the care of a patient who is:
   a. Learning disabled?
   b. Blind?
   c. Bisexual?

3. How would you ensure equal treatment for a colleague who is:
   a. Pregnant?
   b. Undergoing gender reassignment?
   c. Fasting for religious reasons?

Glossary

Discrimination: unequal and unjust treatment of others. Discrimination may be directed at an individual or social group because they are considered in some way inferior and/or undeserving. Discrimination may be carried out by individuals or members of a social group. It may also occur through the policies and procedures of an organization, which may disadvantage people with protected characteristics, even if the staff themselves do not behave in prejudiced or discriminatory ways. See MacPherson (1999).

European Economic Area (EEA; http://www.efta.int/eea): the area that allows free movement of people, goods, and services across the EU and with some non-member states.

European Union (EU; https://europa.eu/european-union): The political and economic union of states in Europe, which operates a single market for goods and services, and facilitates the free movement of people.

Millennium Development Goals 2000 (https://sustainabledevelopment.un.org): eight goals launched by the United Nations to improve the lives of the poorest people by 2015. These were then superseded by the Sustainable Development Goals, to be achieved by 2030.

National Health Service (NHS): launched in 1948, it provides healthcare services within the UK that are free to patients at the point of access and available to all. It is funded out of taxation.

NHS constitution (www.gov.uk): sets out the guiding principles of the NHS, including patients' rights and responsibilities.

Nursing and Midwifery Council (www.nmc.org.uk): the professional regulator for nurses and midwives in the UK.

Office of the United Nations High Commissioner for Human Rights (www.ohchr.org): an office within the United Nations that is responsible for monitoring, protecting, and upholding human rights.

Prejudice: negative ideas, beliefs, and feelings based on actual or perceived differences in others.

Royal College of Nursing (www.rcn.org.uk): a trade union and professional body for nurses, midwives, and healthcare assistants in the UK.

References

American Association of Critical Care Nurses (2005). Silence kills. The seven crucial conversations for health care. https://www.aacn.org/nursing-excellence/healthy-work-environments/~/media/aacn-website/nursing-excellence/healthy-work-environment/silencekills.pdf?la=en (accessed January 12, 2019).

Archibong, U., Darr, A. (2010). The involvement of black and minority ethnic staff in NHS disciplinary proceedings. A report of research carried out by the Centre for Inclusion and Diversity, University of Bradford on behalf of NHS Employers and NHS Institute for Innovation and Improvement. https://www.brad.ac.uk/research/media/CfID-Briefing-9-BME-disciplinaries.pdf (accessed January 12, 2019).

Benner, P., Tanner, C., and Chesla, C. (1996). *Expertise in Nursing Practice. Caring, Clinical Judgment and Ethics.* New York: Springer.

Chartered Society of Physiotherapists (2011). *Code of Members' Professional Values and Behaviour.* London: CSP.

Council of Europe (1950). *European Convention on Human Rights.* Strasbourg: Council of Europe.

Department of Health (2010). *Advanced-level Nursing: A Position Statement.* London: DH.

Department of Health and Social Care (2018). *The Government's Mandate to NHS England for 2018–19.* London: DHSC.

Esmail, A. (2007). Asian doctors in the NHS: service and betrayal. *British Journal of General Practice* 57 (543): 827–834.

Freeman, M. (2011). *Human Rights*, 2e. Cambridge: Polity Press.

General Medical Council (2014). *Code of Conduct for Council Members.* London: GMC.

Government Equalities Office (2011a). *Public Sector: Quick Start Guide to the Specific Duties.* London: Government Equalities Office.

Government Equalities Office (2011b). *Equality Act 2010: Specific Duties to Support the Equality Duty. What Do I Need to Know? A Quick Start Guide for Public Sector Organisations.* London: Government Equalities Office.

Government Equalities Office (2018). *Caste in Great Britain and Equality Law: A Public Consultation: Government Consultation Response.* London: Government Equalities Office.

Hariri, Y. (2015). *Homo Deus. A Brief History of Tomorrow.* London: Vintage.

Harrell, C.J.P., Burford, T., Cage, B. et al. (2011). Multiple pathways linking racism to health outcomes. *Du Bois Review* 8 (1): 143–157.

Holloway, I. and Freshwater, D. (2007). *Narrative Research in Nursing.* Chichester: Wiley.

House of Commons (2018). Research briefing. NHS staff from overseas: statistics. https://researchbriefings.parliament.uk/ResearchBriefing/Summary/CBP-7783 (accessed January 12, 2019).

Likupe, G. and Archibong, U. (2013). Black African nurses' experiences of equality, racism, and discrimination in the National Health Service. *Journal of Psychological Issues in Organizational Culture* 3 (S1): 227–246.

MacPherson, W. (1999). *The Stephen Lawrence Inquiry: Report of an Inquiry by Sir William MacPherson, Cm4262–1.* London: Home Office.

Marmot, M. (2010). *Fair Society, Healthy Lives. The Marmot Review. Strategic Review of Health Inequalities Post 2010.* London: Institute of Health Equity.

McGee, P. (2016). Race and ethnicity. In: *Sociology for Nurses*, 3e (ed. E. Denny, S. Earle and A. Hewison), 250–272. Cambridge: Polity Press.

NHS Health Education England (2015). The handbook to the NHS constitution. https://assets.publishing.service.gov.uk/government/uploads/system/uploads/attachment_data/file/474450/NHS_Constitution_Handbook_v2.pdf (accessed January 12, 2019).

Nursing and Midwifery Council (2015). *The Code. Professional Standards of Practice and Behaviour for Nurses and Midwives.* London: NMC.

Office for National Statistics (2018). Statistical bulletin. Health state life expectancies by national deprivation deciles, England and Wales: 2014 to 2016. https://www.ons.gov.uk/peoplepopulationandcommunity/healthandsocialcare/healthinequalities/bulletins/healthstatelifeexpectanciesbyindexofmultipledeprivationimd/englandandwales2014to2016 (accessed January 12, 2019).

Office of the United Nations High Commissioner for Human Rights (1993). Vienna declaration and programme of action. https://www.ohchr.org/en/professionalinterest/pages/vienna.aspx (accessed January 12, 2019).

Papadopoulos, I. (2018). *Culturally Competent Compassion. A Guide for Healthcare Students and Practitioners.* Abingdon: Routledge.

Royal College of Nursing (2017). *The UK Nursing Labour Market Review 2017.* London: RCN.

Sullivan, E. and Garland, G. (2013). *Practical Leadership and Management in Healthcare.* Harlow: Pearson.

United Nations (1948). Universal Declaration of Human Rights. http://www.un.org/en/universal-declaration-human-rights (accessed January 12, 2019).

United Nations (2015a). The Millennium Development Goals Report 2015. http://www.un.org/millenniumgoals/2015_MDG_Report/pdf/MDG%20 2015%20rev%20(July%201).pdf (accessed January 12, 2019).

United Nations (2015b). Transforming our world. The 2030 agenda for sustainable development. https://sustainabledevelopment.un.org/post2015/transformingourworld (accessed January 12, 2019).

West, E. and Nayar, S. (2016). *A Review of the Literature on the Experiences of Black, Minority and Internationally Recruited Nurses and Midwives in the UK Healthcare System.* London: NMC.

CHAPTER 15

Educational and Professional Influences on Advanced and Consultant Practitioners

Chris Inman

Birmingham City University, Birmingham, UK

Key Issues

- Master's-level education for advanced practitioners in the UK
- International collaboration in education for advanced practitioners
- The consultant practitioner role in the UK and Australia
- The interface between medicine and advanced and consultant roles

LEARNING OUTCOMES

By the end of this chapter you will be able to:

- Discuss the advantages of two approaches to Master's-level education for advanced practitioners.
- Explain the consultant role.
- Critically examine the interface between medicine and advanced and consultant roles.
- Discuss your own role in promoting health and preventing disease.

15.1 Introduction

This chapter commences with an overview of developments in the education of advanced practitioners in the UK, and outlines the key issues in current educational programs at Master's level. This is followed by an account of

Advanced Practice in Healthcare: Dynamic Developments in Nursing and Allied Health Professions,
Fourth Edition. Edited by Paula McGee and Chris Inman.
© 2019 John Wiley & Sons Ltd. Published 2019 by John Wiley & Sons Ltd.

international collaboration between universities in the Netherlands and one in the UK. Research carried out by a student who participated in this collaboration is used to demonstrate how the Master's-prepared advanced practitioner can pioneer new approaches to care and treatment that empower patients to take charge of their own health issues. The chapter then moves on to introduce the consultant practitioner role which has developed, in slightly different ways, in the UK and Australia. Both the advanced and consultant roles are then discussed with reference to social and socioeconomic factors that may influence their interface with medicine. The chapter concludes by returning to the case study in considering the role of the advanced practitioner in actively promoting health.

15.2 The Education of Advanced Practitioners in the UK

Master's courses in advanced nursing practice in the UK started to emerge in the 1990s in response to multiple factors, which included:

- Practitioner demand for Master's-level education.
- Increasing numbers of patients, particularly those with complex health needs.
- Changes in practice and pharmacological/technological advances in healthcare; shorter working hours for medical staff (DH 2003).
- Evolving National Health Service (NHS) policy (Foot et al. 2014; Gantz et al. 2012).

These courses were initially informed by developments in nursing in the USA and gradually evolved to meet the expectations of both national bodies and healthcare providers (Department of Health [DH] 1999a, b; United Kingdom Central Council for Nursing, Midwifery and Health Visiting [UKCC] 1990). Curricular and assessment methods were not constrained by regulation, hence they developed innovatively, but kept pace with changes in healthcare and regional demand. Courses began to admit allied health professionals (AHPs) alongside nurses, thus promoting interprofessional shared learning (DH 2002; Wenger-Trayner 2015). The only national body to retain a focus and represent advanced practice in education throughout its two decades of development is the Association of Advanced Practice Nursing Educators (AAPNE), which changed its name to the Association of Advanced Practice UK in order to accommodate AHP educators (AAPE UK 2017; AAPNE 2007).

Currently, nurses, AHPs, and pharmacists wishing to become advanced practitioners normally enroll on generic Master's courses, but lack of a standardized curriculum means that there continues to be considerable variation between courses. A small number of specialized courses is available, where NHS workforce demand exists; examples include emergency medicine, children, and neonatal care (Inman 2015). However, the possibility of more specialized courses is currently under consideration by Health Education England (HEE; NHS Health Education England 2017).

An additional development occurred, in 2006, with the introduction of independent and supplementary prescribing for nurses who had successfully completed a tightly structured prescribing course with five rigorous assessment methods (Nursing and Midwifery Council [NMC] 2006). In contrast to advanced practice, prescribing is regulated and approval to prescribe is recorded by the NMC (2006). By 2014, over 19 000 nurses had qualified as independent and supplementary prescribers and many more had limited rights, allowing them to prescribe specific items such as wound dressings (Royal College of Nursing [RCN] 2014). Some AHPs such as those in radiography and dietetics have also been granted prescribing rights within their spheres of expertise. The prescribing course is available for all advanced nurse practitioners (ANPs) and for AHPs whose field of practice is approved for prescribing.

Supervised clinical practice is a crucial element in Master's preparation. Student advanced practitioners are employed in clinical settings and are supervised by practice mentors. Mentors are normally practitioners in the student's field of practice and/or senior doctors (Inman 2009). Mentors support, assess, and document the student's progress in building on previous experience to develop advanced clinical skills and to complete a set of generic competences. As they come to understand the advanced practice role, mentors are able to promote the role in their organization, facilitate positive attitudes to advanced practice, and be instrumental in transforming service culture (Manley et al. 2009).

Before reading on, consider Exercise 15.1.

EXERCISE 15.1

What do you consider to be the advantages and disadvantages of:

- Generic advanced practice courses for nurses, AHPs, and pharmacists?
- Specialist advanced practice courses for nurses, AHPs, and pharmacists?

15.3 Collaboration with the Netherlands

In the UK, postgraduate education has served for over 20 years to strengthen knowledge, skills, competence, and confidence for advanced practitioners. Master's-level education has fostered higher-level clinical skills and critical thinking. The research produced by Master's graduates has generated an innovative approach in many services. Clinical career progression has been an added benefit for some (Jackson and O'Callaghan 2009).

Postgraduate education has also been exported through international collaboration between universities, a factor that is increasingly common (Wagner and Leydesdorff 2005). One example is collaboration between the Master's course at Birmingham City University (BCU) in the UK and several universities in the Netherlands, including Saxion and Fontys. This developed because the Dutch universities wished their courses to be mapped against a UK course, for the following reasons:

- One of BCU's professors also had a professorial role in one of the Dutch universities and was engaged in collaborative research. The professor spoke the language and was available to supervise Dutch Master's and doctoral students in their own country.
- The UK Master's dissertation required deeper methodological and epistemological analysis and allowed a larger and longer piece of practice-focused research that often built on the student's previous work.

- The Dutch students were self-selected, highly motivated advanced practice healthcare graduates who wanted to complete further practice-focused research and needed academic support to write and publish it in English.
- International collaboration and shared teaching between universities were highly valued and viewed positively in the higher education system.

The research carried out by some of the Dutch students enabled them to develop some highly innovative work; as a result, several graduates collaborated with government ministers and initiated changes in healthcare which were rolled out nationally. The case study presented here is an example of research completed by Connie, a successful Dutch student who wrote and was supervised in English.

CASE STUDY

After completing the Dutch Advanced Nurse Practitioners course, a general practitioner (GP) and I collaborated in setting up a social medical healthcare program for people who were homeless. This brought together the GP, an NP, statutory health services, and health insurance to remove the barriers to social and medical care for people who were homeless, regardless of whether or not they had health and social care cover. In 2009, I completed a research study on reproductive and contraceptive healthcare for female street sex workers who were addicted to drugs. The aim was to gather information about the women's reproductive history, attitudes, opinions, and motives for using or rejecting contraceptives. The results showed that the reasons were complex, highly personal, and originated from the women's backgrounds and experiences.

Before reading on, complete Exercise 15.2.

EXERCISE 15.2

Identify three advanced practice characteristics that underpinned Connie's role and provide your own working definition of each one.

How might you apply these competences in your own practice setting?

It became evident that vulnerable persons with complex and multifaceted problems and unwanted pregnancies tended to have poor pregnancy outcomes. They also had difficulties in child rearing, with the result that often youth welfare was, or needed to become, involved. The definition of vulnerability varied and was complex. For some women it was clear that their

pregnancy was unwanted and unplanned, and the question had to be asked why the repeated unwanted pregnancies occurred. Unplanned and unwanted pregnancies can be an ethical, extensive, and complex problem and therefore an important issue in public health. It seemed that these problems might need another approach. Increasing understanding of the problems could help provide solutions that could contribute to preventing unwanted pregnancies.

I embarked on an additional Master's research project at BCU. This qualitative project was designed to explore the effectiveness of a pilot program offering birth control to vulnerable women who did not regularly use contraception, and for whom a pregnancy was not desirable. Since it was not a homogeneous group, solutions to the questions and needs of these women could only be found at an individual level with individualized care planning. This meant that healthcare workers had to invest in establishing personal relationships in order to determine what triggered the related behavior and attitudes. Once the mix of factors and motivations was identified, I could offer a tailored approach. If I had neglected these individual factors, resources could be wasted and service usage continue to fail.

Before reading on, undertake Exercise 15.3.

EXERCISE 15.3

Identify the advanced practice competences that underpinned Connie's role in this pilot program.

Reflecting on one episode of care in your own sphere of practice, which competences are involved and why?

The program is now implemented in three cities in the Netherlands. The results showed that over 80% of the women are motivated to postpone pregnancy by voluntarily choosing adequate contraception. The suggestion is that the program is transferable and consistent.

15.4 Consultant Practitioners

Aside from the UK and Australia, few countries identify consultant practitioner roles, although a small number of appointments were reported in Hong Kong which were aimed at rectifying service problems (Lee et al. 2013). In Australia, the consultant practitioner role is confined to nursing (Giles et al. 2014, 2018). Clinical nurse consultants (CNCs) are classified as senior to advanced practitioners (Cashin et al. 2015). Regulation is managed by the Australian Health Practitioner Regulation Agency, although it is said to be based on subjective criteria (Leidel 2013). Despite the CNC role being established since the 1980s, Baldwin (2013) suggests that the role in Australia is still inadequately defined. There are no AHP consultant practitioners.

In the UK, consultant nurse, midwife, and AHP practitioners were introduced as part of the health service reforms introduced by the Labour government which came to power in 1997 (DH 1999a, 2000). These reforms encouraged experienced practitioners to enhance their roles and levels of responsibility (DH 2008; Inman and McGee 2009). Consultant practitioners were envisaged as clinical leaders who would link expert care with the strategic development of services. Master's or doctoral preparation was essential, and would incorporate clinical practice, research, education, and leadership (Dewing and Reid 2003). The grading of consultant posts was to be higher than those for advanced practitioners and the consultant role itself was not clearly defined (Dyson et al. 2014). These two factors contributed to wide variations in conditions of employment, substantial salary differences, and discontent (Booth et al. 2006; Coster et al. 2006). Dyson et al. (2014) and Jasper (2006 p. 2) both suggest that this caused consultants to expend their energy "fighting the system," rather than immersing themselves in role-development activities. Retaining the consultant practitioner role in the UK continues to generate debate (Inman 2017). In Australia, there are three performance grades at 1, 2, and 3 for CNCs and some differences in the domains of practice, which include clinical service and consultancy, clinical service planning, and management, as well as research and education (Cashin et al. 2015; Fry et al. 2012).

In the UK, the DH (1999a) initially saw the consultant role as having a strong clinical focus, with 50% of the time being spent in practice settings. Alongside this were three other areas to be included: professional leadership and consultancy; education, training, and development; and practice/service development linked to research and evaluation. These relate to at least six substantial areas of practice, which were all supposed to interact with one another. For example, expert practice would be based on knowledge of research evidence, leadership skills, and interaction with patients and/or other staff, which would involve education. Woodward et al. (2006) and Cashin et al. (2015) emphasized how, for the consultant role to be successful, it was essential to integrate the key roles of research, education, practice and system support, and leadership, and not only focus on the clinical domain.

A number of studies have reported positive perceptions of the clinical impact of the consultant role, but these reports are predominantly based on self-evaluation, which limits their credibility (Booth et al. 2006; Fairley and Closs 2006; Osbourne 2001; McKenna 2006; McSherry et al. 2007; Woodward et al. 2006). Other evaluations based on service audit results suggest that consultant practitioners were perceived to improve services (Coster et al. 2006; Humphreys et al. 2007). Studies in Australia indicate that CNCs work in a range of specialties, including stoma therapy, diabetes, infection control, pediatrics, and in community outreach work (Currey et al. 2011; Gregorowski et al. 2012; Walters 1996). Health service consumers appear to have supported the development of a CNC role which integrated physical health assessments into mental health services, but cautioned against an excessively medical approach to care (Happell et al. 2016). In the mental health field, Giles et al. (2018) reported CNCs engaging in collaborative and interprofessional working.

Before reading on, think about Exercise 15.4.

> **EXERCISE 15.4**
>
> To what extent and why are consultant and advanced practitioner roles needed in your field of practice?

15.5 Consultant Roles and Research

Doctoral studies have become the preferred level of educational preparation to enable consultant practitioners to focus their research on issues in depth and increase their impact on services (Inman 2009). Research opportunities allow consultant practitioners to facilitate the development of person-centered, individualized services (Manley and Titchen 2016). Inman (2009) argued that the credibility of the consultant role is influenced by the practitioner's knowledge of research methodologies and collaboration with research communities (Inman 2009). Motivation also plays a part via the satisfaction gained from increasing professional knowledge and the opportunities afforded by doctoral research in terms of developments in status, role, career, and patient care (Ormrod 2003). The synergy of personal and professional interests corresponds with Bryant's (2004, p. 33) statement that "doctoral study becomes increasingly connected with professional development in many social sciences." This reinforces the need for high levels of cognitive activity in successfully functioning to interconnect the complex concepts and practice needed for the consultant role. Figure 15.1 highlights the strength of the motivation, because intrinsic and extrinsic influences are present which, when combined, assist in maintaining momentum in research.

However, doctoral studies take time and many remain works in progress, which means that, in the UK, consultant practitioners often hold postgraduate degrees at a lower level. A similar situation was reported in Australia, where Cashin et al. (2015) found that, of the 37 CNCs who participated, only one achieved a PhD; 49% held a Master's degree, others held lower postgraduate awards, and six had an undergraduate degree or less. Those without at least a Master's degree have been found to struggle with the role (Woodward et al. 2006). These findings indicate that even the minimal educational level of a Master's degree is achieved by fewer than 50% of consultant practitioners. This

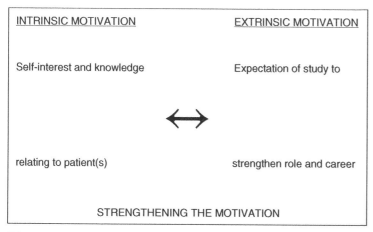

FIGURE 15.1 Potential to strengthen motivation for study. *Source:* Inman 2009.

situation may in part explain why the number of consultant practitioners in the UK failed to reach targets, because too few practitioners had the educational, academic, and clinical requirements (Manley and Titchen 2016). Scott (2013) states that 130 consultant practitioners were in post by 2001 and 1139 by 2012, when new appointments slowed. Anxiety was voiced in 2013 in several RCN newsletters about the future of the consultant practitioner role. Some regions in the UK ceased to have any in post, which threatened clinical career opportunities for expert clinical nurses and skill loss to patient services (Scott 2013). An additional factor is that many consultant practitioners have found it difficult to protect their primary research time, because service evaluations and medical research were prioritized (Dyson et al. 2014).

15.6 The Interface between Medicine and Advanced and Consultant Practitioners

Foucault (1984) suggested that medical professionals possess high professional status and power in relation to both the health agendas of governments and within healthcare organizations. The creation of clinical careers for non-medical health professionals such as advanced and consultant practitioners has blurred the interface with medicine, but the extent of the change is debatable (Jackson and O'Callaghan 2009). Where advanced and consultant practitioners currently fit in terms of status or position in relation to medicine reflects an evolving situation in which power may gradually be redistributed (Trowler et al. 2012).

The concept of academic tribes provides one way of analyzing the interface between medicine and the new advanced and consultant practitioner roles in relation to the culture, strength, coherence, and internalization of authority achieved by different disciplines (Becher and Trowler 2001). This concept is particularly apt in relation to the medical profession as a distinct discipline with a discrete body of knowledge, a clearly defined function, and a single professional regulator. However, it is debatable whether advanced and consultant practitioners can claim to be one tribe. Their roles are associated with quite diverse bodies of knowledge, their functions vary considerably both between and within different professional groups, and, as an overall group, they are subject to more than one professional regulator. Thus, advanced and consultant practitioners form a set of disparate groups, which may limit their status.

Various social and socioeconomic factors reinforce the position and functions of health professions. These include the influence of social background, type and level of education, and many other factors. The family backgrounds of nurses are more variable than those of doctors, with nurses tending to originate from a mixture of middle-, lower middle-class, or working-class backgrounds, which influences academic achievement and socioeconomic status (Marmot et al. 2010). In contrast, most AHPs fall somewhere between doctors and nurses in terms of socioeconomic background and educational achievement. Thus, there is an implicit inequality between members of different health professions.

The level of professional education is a second factor in considering inequality. In the UK, initial nurse education was below degree level until 2013 (RCN 2018). In academic terms, this placed it below the level of initial education for many AHPs. The entry requirement for both nursing and AHP courses was below that required for medical school. This situation in no way reflects the ability of individual nurses and AHPs, but it demonstrates how, from the outset, professional preparation contributes to the creation of a hierarchy of health professions, with medicine at its peak. However, modern academic development for advanced and consultant practitioners may challenge this hierarchy and change the professional status of new and emergent clinical roles as they interface with medicine.

The hierarchy of health professions may also be perpetuated by public perceptions of different professional roles and ways of working. AHPs provide consultations or episodes of care lasting a limited time, which is comparable with the practice of some consultant doctors. Many nurses provide periods of care normally lasting for between 7 and 12 hours at a time and have the opportunity to work in partnership with patients, developing rapport. Both professional groups may seem closer, more accessible to patients. Patients themselves may not always understand the differences between these two groups of practitioners, let alone those between them and advanced and consultant practitioners. In addition, patients may expect to be treated by doctors and not realize that advanced and consultant practitioners may be equally well qualified (Inman 2009). It may be suggested that in some instances, advanced and consultant practitioners who have studied at PhD level may actually be better qualified in their field of practice than some doctors, but, as one consultant practitioner stated, "a nursing PhD is inferior" to a doctor's (Inman 2009, p. 63). In other words, no matter what academic qualification consultant practitioners achieve, the status gap between them and medical practitioners persists.

15.7 The Advanced Practitioner's Role – Enhancing the Impact on Care

The final section of this chapter focuses on one aspect of the current nursing strategy in England: health and well-being (NHS England 2014, 2016a). This emphasizes the importance of taking every opportunity to tackle major public health issues such as obesity, smoking, and alcohol consumption. Advanced practitioners are well placed to engage in the prevention of illness and disease, both through their direct clinical practice and patient education, and indirectly through service development and leadership. The drive to prevent people from becoming ill rather than directing every effort to treating them when they are ill reflects the salutogenic approach developed by Antonovsky (1996). This addresses the prevention of illness in preference to, rather than instead of, treating it after it has occurred. Thus, the salutogenic approach can help to prevent or at least reduce harm, improve the quality of people's lives, and reduce the economic, social, and psychological burden of disease (Mittelmark et al. 2017).

To return to the case study, it is evident that Connie applied a salutogenic approach in three classic stages, adapted from Downie et al. (1996):

- *Primary stage:* responding to a perceived need to help women avoid unwanted pregnancies by initially setting up a multiprofessional service. However, it became clear that this was not enough.
- *Secondary or early action stage:* developing a pilot program specifically designed to help women avoid pregnancies.
- *Tertiary stage:* caring, treating, and supporting women who have contracted a sexually transmitted disease, helping them avoid further infections if possible, and managing long-term health problems such as human immunodeficiency virus (HIV).

Developing such a service requires an appraisal of structural factors affecting care, such as staffing and the siting of services; process factors, which focus on the technical, clinical, interpersonal, administrative, and organizational systems required; and anticipated outcomes (Donabedian 2005). Inherent in this approach to prevention is the need for empowerment not only of patients to enable them to exercise control over their own lives, but also of advanced practitioners to enable them to take the lead in promoting health (Foot et al. 2014).

15.8 Conclusion

This chapter has provided information regarding the education and development of Master's courses for advanced practitioners in the UK. It has introduced the concept of consultant practitioners in the UK and Australia. It has examined the importance of study at doctoral level and the contribution that this affords to patient care. Despite considerable progress in the development of advanced and consultant practitioner roles, the interface with medicine still needs to be addressed. Finally, consideration was given to the advanced practitioner's role in tackling major current challenges to health, and the way in which innovative services may help to improve the well-being of service users and the level of control they have over their lives. Such initiatives may support government policy identified earlier, including NHS Sustainability and Transformation Plans (NHS England 2016b) and Integrated Care Systems (Ham 2018).

Acknowledgment

The case study was contributed by Connie Rijlaarsdam, Nurse Specialist, MANP, MSc, Program Manager, Nu NIet Zwanger, NHS Utrecht, The Netherlands. The program started in Tilburg, followed by Rotterdam and Nijmegen. The Dutch government then decided that it should be implemented all over the country. Connie is the Program Manager for this national scheme.

Key Questions

1. With reference to your own Master's dissertation, how do your findings inform your practice? What factors affected your ability to implement your findings and why?

2. How might you use the salutogenic approach to promote health for your patients?

3. Is it necessary to have a clinical career structure beyond advanced practice for nurses and AHPs? If you think it is, what shape should this take?

Glossary

Association of Advanced Practice Nursing Educators (AAPNE; http://aape.org.uk): a national network linking universities that provide courses for aspiring advanced practitioners.

Health and Care Professions Council (http://www.hcpc-uk.co.uk): regulates 16 health and care professions in the UK, maintains a register of qualified individuals, sets standards, and approves training programs for those professions.

Health Education England (https://hee.nhs.uk): the education-funding branch of the NHS in England that determines the resources to be invested annually for all health professionals, including advanced clinical practice, courses, and sponsorships.

NHS England (https://www.england.nhs.uk): leads the NHS for England. Following devolution, Scotland, Wales, and Northern Ireland have their own organizations.

Nursing and Midwifery Council (www.nmc.org. uk): the UK-wide regulatory body for nursing, midwifery, and health visiting. Nursing has four first qualification levels for adults, children, mental health, and learning disabilities. The NMC also sets standards for prescribing courses as approved by government, and adds the qualification to registered practitioners' existing qualification on the register. It does not currently regulate advanced practice/advanced clinical practice or consultant practice.

Royal College of Nursing (www.rcn.org.uk): a trade union and professional body for nurses, midwives, and healthcare assistants in the UK.

References

Antonovsky, A. (1996). The salutogenic model as a theory to guide health promotion. *Health Promotion International* 11 (1): 11–18.

Association of Advanced Nursing Practice Educators (AANPE) (2007). History and development. http://aape.org.uk/about (accessed January 12, 2019).

Association of Advanced Practice Educators UK (AAPE UK) (2017). Governance Committee minutes items. http://aape.org.uk/governance (accessed January 12, 2019).

Baldwin, R. (2013). The role and function of Clinical Nurse Consultants, an Australian advanced practice role: a descriptive exploratory cohort study. *International Journal of Nursing Studies* 50: 326–334.

Becher, T. and Trowler, P. (2001). *Academic Tribes and Territories: Intellectual Enquiry and the Culture of Disciplines*, 2e. Buckingham: Society for Research into Higher Education and OU Press.

Booth, J., Hutchinson, C., Beech, C., and Robertson, K. (2006). New nursing roles: the experience of Scotland's consultant nurse/midwives. *Journal of Nursing Management* 14 (2): 83–89.

Bryant, M. (2004). *The Portable Dissertation Advisor*. Thousand Oaks, CA: Corwin Press.

Cashin, A., Stasa, H., Gullick, J. et al. (2015). Clarifying Clinical Nurse Consultant work in Australia: a phenomenological study. *Collegian* 22 (4): 405–412.

Coster, S., Redfern, S., Wilson-Barnett, J. et al. (2006). Impact of the role of nurse, midwife and health visitor consultant. *Journal of Advanced Nursing* 55 (3): 352–363.

Currey, J., Considine, J., and Kwaw, D. (2011). Clinical nurse research consultant: a clinical and academic role to advanced practice and the discipline of nursing. *Journal of Advanced Nursing* 67 (9): 2275–2283.

Department of Health (1999a). *Making a Difference: Strengthening the Nursing, Midwifery and Health Visiting Contribution to Health and Healthcare.* London: DH.

Department of Health (1999b). Nurse, Midwife, and Health Visitor Consultant: Establishing Posts and Making Appointments. HS Circular 1999/217. Leeds: NHSE

Department of Health (2000). *The NHS Plan. A Plan for Investment. A Plan for Reform.* Wetherby: Stationery Office.

Department of Health (2002). *Liberating the Talents: Helping Primary Care Trusts and Nurses to Deliver the NHS Plan.* London: Stationery Office.

Department of Health (2003). *Protecting Staff, Delivering Services. Implementing the European Working Time Directives for Doctors in Training.* Health Service Circular 2003/001. London: DH.

Department of Health (2008). *High Quality Care for All: NHS Next Stage Review Final Report.* London: Stationery Office.

Dewing, J. and Reid, B. (2003). A model for clinical practice within the consultant nurse role. *Nursing Times* 99 (9): 30–32.

Donabedian, A. (2005). Evaluating the quality of medical care. *Millbank Quarterly* 83 (4): 691–729. First published 1966.

Downie, R., Tannahill, C., and Tannahill, A. (1996). *Health Promotion: Models and Values*, 2e. Oxford: Oxford University Press.

Dyson, S., Taynor, M., Liu, L., and Mehta, N. (2014). *Scoping the Role of the Nurse Consultant.* London: Middlesex University.

Fairley, D. and Closs, S. (2006). Evaluation of a nurse consultant's clinical activities and the search for patient outcomes in critical care. *Journal of Clinical Nursing* 15 (9): 1106–1114.

Foot, C., Gilburt, H., Dunn, H. et al. (2014). *People in Control of their Own Health and Care: The State of Involvement.* London: King's Fund.

Foucault, M. (1984). The subject and power. In: *Power Critical Concepts* (ed. J. Scott), 218–233. London: Routledge.

Fry, M., Duffield, C., Baldwin, R. et al. (2012). Development of a tool to describe the role of the clinical nurse consultant in Australia. *Journal of Clinical Nursing* 22: 11–12.

Gantz, N., Sherman, R., Jasper, M. et al. (2012). Global nurse leader perspectives on health systems and workforce challenges. *Journal of Nursing Management* 20 (4): 433–443.

Giles, M., Parker, V., and Conway, J.M.R. (2014). Recognising the differences in the nurse consultant role. *Journal of BMC Nursing* 13 (30): https://doi.org/10.1186/1472-6955-13-30.

Giles, M., Parker, V., Conway, J., and Mitchell, R. (2018). Knowing how to get things done: nurse consultants as clinical leaders. *Journal of Clinical Nursing* 27: 1981–1993.

Gregorowski, A., Brennan, E., Chapman, S. et al. (2012). An action research study to explore the nature of the nurse consultant role in the care of children and young people. *Journal of Clinical Nursing* 22 (1–2): 201–210.

Happell, B., Weart, S.B., Platania-Phung, C. et al. (2016). Embedding a physical health nurse consultant within mental health services: consumer' perspectives. *International Journal of Mental Health Nursing* 25 (4): 377–384.

Ham, C. (2018). Making sense of integrated care systems, integrated care partnerships and accountable care organisations in the NHS in England. The King's Fund https://www.kingsfund.org.uk/publications/making-sense-integrated-care-systems (accessed 9 May, 2019).

Humphreys, A., Johnson, S., Richardson, J. et al. (2007). A systematic review and meta analysis: evaluating the effectiveness of nurse, midwife and AHP consultants. *Journal of Clinical Nursing* 16 (10): 1792–1808.

Inman, C.E. (2009). Doctoral study for a new healthcare practitioner group: Exploring the motivations, experiences and practices of non-medical consultants pursuing PhD study. Unpublished doctoral thesis, King's College London.

Inman, C. (2015). Standardising education for advanced practice: survey of advanced practice programmes in the UK. Paper presented at the UK Association of Advanced Practice Educators UK Conference, Bournemouth, March 5, 2015.

Inman, C. (2017). Advanced practice: is the structure of advanced practice in transition? Paper presented at the Nursing Education and Professional Development: The Global Perspective conference, Royal College of Nursing, Cardiff, March 21, 2017.

Inman, C.E. and McGee, P. (2009). The careers of advanced practitioners. In: *Advanced Practice in Nursing and the Allied Health Professions* (ed. P. McGee), 210–226. Oxford: Wiley Blackwell.

Jackson, J.F.L. and O'Callaghan, E.M. (2009). What do we know about glass ceiling effects? A taxonomy and critical review to inform higher education research. *Research in Higher Education* 50 (5): 460–482.

Jasper, M. (2006). Editorial. Consultant nurses and midwives – are you making a difference? *Journal of Nursing Management* 14 (2): 81–82.

Lee, D.T.F., Kai, C.C., Carmen, W.H. et al. (2013). The impact on patient health outcomes of introducing nurse consultants: a historically matched controlled study. *BMC Health Services Research* 13: 431.

Leidel, S. (2013). Australia could do so much more with its nurse practitioners. *The Conversation* Nov. 21: https://theconversation.com/australia-could-do-so-much-more-with-its-nurse-practitioners-17693.

Manley, K. and Titchen, A. (2016). Facilitation skills: the catalyst for increased effectiveness in consultant practice and clinical systems leadership. *Educational Action Research* 25 (2): 256–279.

Manley, K., Titchen, A., and Hardy, S. (2009). Work-based learning in the context of contemporary health care education and practice: a concept analysis. *Practice Development in Health Care* 8 (2): 87–127.

Marmot, M., Goldblatt, P., and Allen, J. (2010). *Fair Society Healthy Lives (The Marmot Review)*. London: Institute of Health Equity.

McKenna, H. (2006). The introduction of innovative nursing and midwifery roles. *Journal of Advanced Nursing* 56 (5): 553–562.

McSherry, R., Mudd, D., and Campbell, S. (2007). Evaluating the perceived role of the nurse consultant through the lived experience of healthcare professionals. *Journal of Clinical Nursing* 16: 2066–2080.

Mittelmark, M., Sagy, S., Eriksson, M. et al. (2017). *The Handbook of Salutogenesis*. New York: Springer International.

NHS England (2014). The Five Year Forward View. https://www.england.nhs.uk/wp-content/uploads/2014/10/5yfv-web.pdf (accessed January 12, 2019).

NHS England (2016a) Leading change. Adding value. A framework for nursing, midwifery and care staff. https://www.england.nhs.uk/wp-content/uploads/2016/05/nursing-framework.pdf (accessed January 12, 2019).

NHS England (2016b). Sustainability and Transformation Plan. https://www.england.nhs.uk/wp-content/uploads/2016/02/stp-footprints-march-2016.pdf (accessed January 12, 2019).

NHS Health Education England (2017). *Multiprofessional Framework for Advanced Clinical Practice in England*. London: NHS https://www.hee.nhs.uk/sites/default/files/documents/Multi-professional%20framework%20for%20advanced%20clinical%20practice%20in%20England.pdf (accessed January 20, 2019.

Nursing and Midwifery Council (2006). *Standards of Proficiency for Nurse and Midwife Prescribers*. London: NMC.

Ormrod, J.E. (2003). *Education Psychology: Developing Learning*, 4e. London: Merrill Prentice Hall.

Osbourne, A. (2001). What does it take to be a consultant midwife? *British Journal of Midwifery* 9 (4): 218.

Royal College of Nursing (2014). *RCN fact sheet on nurse prescribing in the UK*. London: RCN.

Royal College of Nursing (2018). Become a nurse. https://www.rcn.org.uk/professional-development/become-a-nurse (accessed January 12, 2019).

Scott, G. (2013). Editorial: it would be a shame if this career option is lost. *Nursing Standard* 28 (8): 3.

Trowler, P., Saunders, M., and Bamber, V. (2012). *Tribes and Territories in the 21st Century*. London: Routledge Taylor & Francis.

United Kingdom Central Council for Nursing, Midwifery and Health Visiting (UKCC) (1990). *The Report of the Post Registration Education and Practice Project*. London: UKCC.

Wagner, C. and Leydesdorff, L. (2005). Network structure, self-organization, and the growth of international collaboration in science. *Research Policy* 34: 1608–1618.

Walters, A.J. (1996). Being a clinical nurse consultant: a hermeneutic phenomenological reflection. *International Journal of Nursing Practice* 2: 2–10.

Wenger-Trayner E Wenger-Trayner B (2015). Introduction to communities of practice. http://wenger-trayner.com/introduction-to-communities-of-practice (accessed January 12, 2019).

Woodward, V., Webb, C., and Prowse, M. (2006). Nurse consultants: organizational influences on role achievement. *Journal of Clinical Nursing* 15 (3): 272–280.

CHAPTER 16

Assessment of Advanced Practice

Chris Inman

Birmingham City University, Birmingham, UK

Key Issues

- Subjects and assessments included in UK advanced practice courses
- Clinical assessment and OSCE in universities and in practice
- Nonclinical assessments of advanced practice
- End-point assessment plan of apprentices for Master's courses

LEARNING OUTCOMES

By the end of this chapter you will be able to:

- Identify the focus of subjects learned as part of advanced health assessment.
- Explain the types of situations and stations to expect in an OSCE assessment.
- Critically discuss the strengths and limits of three clinical assessment methods.
- Critically debate the issues around who can assess advanced practitioners.

16.1 Introduction

A survey of advanced practice (AP)/advanced clinical practice (ACP) Master's courses delivered in nine universities in different countries and regions across Great Britain identified that eight included delivering and assessing clinical skill modules, mainly during the first, postgraduate certificate stage of the course. More theoretical subjects tended to be delivered and assessed during

Advanced Practice in Healthcare: Dynamic Developments in Nursing and Allied Health Professions,
Fourth Edition. Edited by Paula McGee and Chris Inman.
© 2019 John Wiley & Sons Ltd. Published 2019 by John Wiley & Sons Ltd.

> TABLE **16.1**
>
> ## Postgraduate certificate clinical subjects identified in a survey of nine universities.
>
> | Module titles and/or subject areas | No. of courses |
> |---|---|
> | Advanced Health Assessments/Skills for Clinical Practice | 7 |
> | Clinical Decision Making/Diagnostic Skills | 4 |
> | Pathophysiology | 3 |
> | History Taking | 1 |
> | Population Assessment | 1 |

the second postgraduate diploma stage, and research-type projects were mainly addressed in the third and final Master's stage (Inman 2015). Assessment in this context refers to examination of clinical skills, knowledge, and behaviors needed to address AP, as well as the critical thinking needed to meet Master's-level academic standards and quality for the Quality Assurance Agency for Higher Education (QAA 2009; Skills for Health 2018). Astin and Antinio (2012, p. 2) critiqued *assessment,* suggesting it was a tradition focused on student activity that supports accountability, but cautioning that it may "be seriously lacking with regard to student learning." Therefore, it may be useful to maintain a questioning perspective when considering the assessment methods referred to in this chapter.

Clinical modules taught and assessed in AP university courses were mainly at postgraduate certificate level and were required to enable advanced practitioners to safely carry out complete episodes of care with patients. Carney's (2018) qualitative survey suggested that in some circumstances in primary care, patients preferred consulting an advanced practitioner to a general practitioner, because they could be seen on the same day, be provided with a prescription if required, and often received clearer information. The 2015 survey of courses identified various module titles that represented advanced health assessment (AHA), including differential diagnosis/critical decision making and pathophysiology (see Table 16.1).

Table 16.1 suggests that at the time of the survey, considerable differences in emphasis were placed on the input of AHA modules. Whilst seven of the nine courses included AHA teaching, less than half, only four, indicated clearly assessment of critical thinking skills for clinical decision making, which is crucial for the AP role at Master's level. Even fewer, only three, stated pathophysiology, knowledge of which was needed at an advanced level to underpin clinical decision making for diagnosis and planning care. History taking was only identified as a separate entity in one course, as was population study of public health, health promotion, and epidemiology. This suggests variation in the content of clinical skill teaching when comparing the nine courses in the survey.

Before reading on, consider Exercise 16.1.

> EXERCISE **16.1**
>
> Suggest two types of examination of clinical assessment skills to test the ability of students to perform at advanced level.

Advanced health assessment for AP/ACP of necessity also depended on who was teaching the subject matter and the effectiveness of the learning. The survey did not request this information, but information from committee members of the Association of Advanced Practice Educators UK identifies that AP lecturers were teaching the courses, with some universities also employing medical doctors in support. Committee discussions have also suggested that course leaders may in the future need to be qualified advanced practitioners, which is not currently a requirement.

The main concern with learning noted for students enrolling for AP courses initially tended to be on different aspects of advanced clinical skills, with the assessment of these tending to overshadow other core subjects and skills. Clinical skills in the UK are taught and formally assessed in university and practice by Objective Structured Clinical Examinations (OSCE) and other methods, including a portfolio of practice. More theoretical subjects require written and presentation methods of assessment.

The survey of AP courses identified that five of the nine university courses prioritized clinically related teaching, and especially physical examination, to the extent that some omitted modules addressing other core subjects (Inman 2015). The three other core, more theoretical AP pillars of research, leadership, and education provide essential knowledge, reinforcing the effectiveness of the fourth, clinical, which is central to AHA and AP. The impact and adequacy of care may be diminished if these complementary subjects are not integrated into practice for the critical thinking required for AHA and differential diagnosis.

Assessment of the more theoretical pillars of advanced practice in the curriculum, although addressed lightly, is not omitted from this chapter. Their relevance is fundamental to developing holistically caring practitioners' understanding of social issues, the links between maintaining health and healthcare treatment, and differences in the causes of ill-health and the social "causes of the causes" of ill-health, including low income, limited education, and living in a deprived environment (Marmot and Allen 2014). These theoretical pillars include research knowledge and appraisal skills, to ensure ethically that care is underpinned by the strongest evidence available. Leadership knowledge is also essential for advanced practitioners/advanced clinical practitioners for them to act as role models and mentors for others, as well as strategically for service design. Education includes coaching and guiding, which may be required for patients and other clinicians, and for optimizing opportunities for health education. All of these knowledge areas underpin critical thinking for the clinical aspects of AHA.

16.2 Stages and Subject Areas of Advanced Practice Master's Courses in the UK

Postgraduate advanced practitioners and advanced clinical practitioners in the UK can adopt the AP title, providing their employer agrees, even if they have not completed a full Master's degree. In the absence of regulation, qualification recognition tends to be directed to Master's-level study, a description which is imprecise and has an impact on whether AP can be one *level of practice*. Master's

> **TABLE 16.2**
>
> **Assessment methods for university-delivered clinically related modules and teaching.**
>
> | Assessment methods | No. of courses |
> |---|---|
> | OSCE and viva | 2 |
> | OSCE and poster | 1 |
> | OCSE | 1 |
> | Case study | 1 |
> | Exam | 3 (including 1 with poster) |

in Advanced Practice–type courses in the UK mostly follow three stages, identified in the UK higher education postgraduate QAA (2009) model: postgraduate certificate, postgraduate diploma, and full Master's degree.

People with any of these three different awards and employer approval are all entitled to call themselves an advanced practitioner or an advanced clinical practitioner. The postgraduate certificate accounts for one-third of a full Master's award; the postgraduate diploma accounts for two-thirds; and the Master's degree is the final award. Since a full Master's degree is not required to enable clinicians to be called an advanced practitioner, uncertainty is created regarding their breadth and depth of knowledge, which may be less extensive than clinicians who complete a full award. The university-based assessment methods for the postgraduate certificate in AP tend to be more practice focused, whereas assessments for later modules are more theoretical or involve studying for a prescribing award (see Table 16.2).

Objective Clinical Structured Examinations (OCSE) have become an accepted method of assessment of clinical skills in most universities, and in the survey these were used in various combinations: in one university with a viva, in another with a poster presentation. They were claimed to be **O**bjective – each student was provided with an identical written brief and "actor" in the same situation. They were **S**tructured, with identical patient prompts, examination timing, and examiners' marking criteria (Feathers et al. 2012). Mock **C**linical settings were created for the **E**xamination. Roberts et al. (2006) claim that this is a valid and reliable method involving the testing of specific skills at a sequence of examination stations or points. It supports students' ability to "assimilate and apply theoretical knowledge to practice" (Henderson et al. 2013, p. 1459). Five of the seven courses teaching AHA included OSCE for assessments. Only three universities taught pathophysiology, assessing it by examination, one with a viva relating physiology to the OSCE, and one required pathophysiology to be included in a case study poster presentation. Only one university was assessing clinical skills by case study, whereas in the past more courses tended to include what can be a valuable assessment, where extensive research evidence and refined analysis are required to meet broad patient-focused learning outcomes. However, the case study has gradually been replaced by OSCEs in most courses, although the evidence base for OSCE being a more valid and reliable assessment is limited and preferred assessment can change over time.

16.3 Advanced Health Assessments and OSCEs in Universities in the UK

Advanced health assessments normally require university teaching by experienced advanced practitioners, and possibly also by medical practitioners, to provide knowledge, skills, and understanding, including the following aspects:

- Identifying what the patient is presenting with, date of birth, sex, and name.
- History taking in a structured, logical manner from the patient or carer, which, by following appropriate cues, may suggest the possible differential diagnoses – unless immediate life-saving action is required.
- Physical examination skills, as well as critical thinking to ensure the most appropriate system is examined relating to the information provided in the history taking, leading to possible differential diagnoses. For example (i) decision making regarding respiratory or cardiovascular systems; (ii) justifying the system chosen. If the patient reports extensive or generalized symptoms, examining two systems or a head-to-toe assessment may be required.
- Knowledge of the pathophysiology influences underpinning the presenting condition to inform critical thinking.
- Clinical decision making relating information accrued, diagnostic hypothesis, options available, investigations, and potential management – an action plan with identification of red flags (Feathers et al. 2012, p. xii).
- Discussion in partnership with patient and/or carer regarding options and preferred choices.
- Documentation of information in patient case records – if required, investigation requests and referrals completed.

University-based assessments may include OSCEs, vivas, poster presentations followed by questions and answers, or case study essays. However, due to time constraints and overburden of assessment, fewer areas may be assessed. Ideally assessments include all areas identified in the list provided, but these do not necessarily represent separate examination stations. For example, students may read a written outline of the patient's presentation and background information, allowing a set time of 5 minutes; OSCE stations may follow with an actor for history taking – 15 minutes; physical examination – 15 minutes; documentation/record keeping – 15 minutes; then related physiology viva – 10 minutes. That takes at least one hour for each student. These timings are suggested as typical, as this detail of OSCEs was not identified in the 2015 survey, although further exploration of OSCEs for advanced practitioners is planned. The survey suggested a tendency for module leaders to focus assessment for ACP students on the essential novel aspects of physical examination, since AP students may consider themselves already to be competent in other areas, e.g. history taking.

Informal conversations with AAPE UK module leaders, experience in my own and other universities as an external examiner observing OSCEs, plus the survey data suggest considerable variation in the number and types of OSCE stations, in the focus of the examination, and in the number of items and grading of the marking criteria (Inman 2015). For example, only one of the nine universities was assessing history taking, despite advanced practitioners needing a more probing style of open questions than may normally have been required as a registered nurse or allied health professional (AHP), who were likely to use electronic proformas designed for their own specialty for history taking.

Established medical texts highlight that for accuracy of diagnosis, history taking needs to allow for the patient to tell their story, the development of rapport, the practitioner asking relevant open-ended questions, listening and responding, noting nonverbal cues from the patient, and providing positive nonverbal cues so that information can be accrued and accurately interpreted (Talley and O'Connor 2014). The focus and outcome of physical examination can be compromised by inadequate history taking. Good history taking can enable patients to report symptoms prior to physical signs becoming manifest, and therefore in some patients may be a more essential source of information than physical examination, e.g. persistent headaches in central nervous system disorders with raised intracranial pressure.

In the survey, most of the university-based OSCEs normally involved assessing AP students' clinically related knowledge on one occasion during the postgraduate certificate stage of the course. Advanced practice course leaders, nurses, and AHPs became aware of the increasing use of OSCEs via knowledge circulating through networks including the Association of Advanced Practice Educators UK and the external examiner systems. External examiners are part of the QAA quality system that requires university course members from a different university that delivers a similar course to examine, observe, and comment on the assessment methods and the standard of examiners' grading and feedback for students. This facilitates the dissemination and sharing of knowledge of OSCEs throughout the higher education system.

OSCEs were developed in universities for AP/ACP students, possibly without fully appreciating the amount of time and people required to arrange them or the equipment or facilities needed. In terms of lecturer planning and preparation, the time required is extensive. During the OSCE, two examiners normally assess each station, a lecturer and a senior practitioner, and marking and feedback are time consuming, often involving reviewing and analyzing audio and video recordings. These resource-heavy assessments involve a smaller number of stations than those prepared for doctors and, in all but one AP/ACP course in the survey, OSCEs appeared to take place on only one occasion during the university course.

In comparison, OSCEs have been used for decades with medical students and are considered an essential component of assessment for doctors, which possibly influenced their adoption for advanced practice. Talley and O'Connor (2014) and Feathers et al. (2012) identify that the frequency and method of assessment in medicine differ from AP, as doctors may be assessed annually and their final examination can involve up to 19 OSCE stations, whereas for AP four or five stations seem more common. Each station is focused around a patient-centered scenario and students carry out assessment and examination of the patient, normally with two senior examiners observing, who may at the end ask related, rigorous questions in the form of a viva. The actor patient seems not always to be consulted for their views, which is an aspect of assessment that might be included.

OSCEs have been standardized for all students, reducing "examiner variation," and testing knowledge, attitude, and skill (Aronowitz et al. 2017, p. 121). To summarize, they are expensive to prepare, design, and manage in terms of staff: examiners and "actors" for each station, and an overall manager on the day to ensure students are in the right room at the right time and coping with the stress. They also require extensive specialized facilities, equipment, rooms, and recording equipment, so that external examiners can view them or in case a student disputes their results. Medical schools have established the resources required and have extensive budgets. Universities delivering AP courses with adjacent medical schools may as a privilege be able to negotiate use of specialist facilities, providing they fit examination dates around the needs of medical students. Less affluent universities may have less ideal facilities in which to examine students.

Actors can be an additional expense and were bought in for assessment in some universities. However, actors need briefing to ensure consistency of performance. For example, a young male advanced clinical practitioner was interviewing a young male patient who was a professional actor, and both were noted to respond by tending to develop a laddish cultural rapport. Nonprofessional actors such as outside lecturers and undergraduate nursing or medical students have been found to perform with at least as much consistency and effectiveness as professional actors. If they are students of a different year group or discipline, e.g. a paramedic student, they may consider involvement with and observation of the learning experience itself to be a form of remuneration, together with meal vouchers, book tokens, or university printing credit.

Before reading on, undertake Exercise 16.2.

EXERCISE 16.2

Which OSCE stations would you consider essential to ensure advanced practitioners could practice safely?

If you were planning OSCEs for AHA, which physical examination skills stations would you decide were essential for assessments to ensure safe advanced practitioners?

Who do you think would be suitably qualified people to assess and judge students' clinical skills and critical thinking?

Despite the substantial resources required, teaching and assessment of AHA have become an essential requirement for AP, and the use of OSCEs for assessment has snowballed. At the data collection time for the survey in 2015, they were used by five or 55% of the nine courses responding. It is likely that now, more if not all AP courses will be teaching AHA and using OSCEs but costs are high and fashions can change. A few AP courses may remain that focus more on one or more of the nonclinical pillars, e.g. leadership or research, and different methods of assessment may be used. Further research is required to ascertain current trends and practices.

16.4 OSCEs – Recent Published Research

Whilst most universities are assessing AP students using OSCEs, evidence of the benefits is scant. Kurz et al. (2009) and Aronowitz et al. (2017) explored the effect of OSCEs on AP students, and Henderson et al. (2013) and Nulty et al. (2011) examined the effect of guidelines and frameworks for implementing

OSCEs for non-medical students. Little tangible evidence was identified, although Kurz et al. (2009) attempted statistical analysis of data from small numbers (n=37) in a blinded, quasi-experimental study of AP students in the USA assessed by OSCE. Higher scores were reported for the advanced practitioners' intervention group when compared with the control group as assessed by teachers, blinded preceptors, and students' self-evaluation. Students reported they were generally more satisfied with course aspects when OSCEs were used with trained individuals called standardized patients (SPs), who simulated patient symptoms and gave feedback to students on the precision and comprehensiveness of the health assessment. The control group were said to be assessed by traditional methods, but these were not fully explained.

Aronowitz et al. (2017) also adopted the use of SPs, and proposed that OSCEs contributed to AP education, suggesting that high face validity existed. They emphasized that by using SPs, a safe learning environment was created, to assist in learning associated with increasing understanding and autonomy when practicing with complex patients. These authors further extended the OSCE learning experience by developing scenarios associated with health promotion and ethical issues, such as may arise if one partner of a married couple becomes human immunodeficiency virus (HIV) positive from undisclosed, extramarital relationships, and management of contact tracing required healthcare professionals to inform the marriage partner.

Henderson et al. (2013) trialed the OSCE guidelines produced by Nulty et al. (2011) and considered they required a structure, so developed a framework for their implementation. This involved four Os:

- Opportunity – focusing on commonly occurring consultation to learn the knowledge and skills required. Students sometimes tend to focus on rare cases that they were unlikely to encounter again.
- Organization – practicing and learning the skills to ensure a structured and systematic approach to patient assessments.
- Oversight – using a generic, comprehensive marking guide to improve reliability and avoid omission.
- Outcomes – developing the knowledge, understanding, attitude, and skills to deliver effective care in a setting that is safe for the patient and practitioner. Ensuring support and feedback were provided at an appropriate time to enable continuing reflection.

The strengths and limits of OSCEs in different settings can be identified. University-based OSCEs have the advantage of all students, whatever their discipline or practice setting, being assessed under the same conditions and by the same team of assessors. Some limitations include the artificial setting and that assessors may not belong to that specialty. Consequently, AP students must also be assessed for their own specialty and normal practice setting by mentors, who can include an experienced practitioner of their discipline and senior medical practitioners. At present, standardized practice documents are not required in the UK and each university devises its own practice portfolio, which includes competence criteria; some also have frameworks and requirements for practice-based OSCEs with real patients. Standardised ePortfolios are currently being planned in England for Advanced Clinical Practice. First impressions suggest practice based OSCEs should be a more valid process than in university. However, limitations still exist, because the mentor/assessor may be a longstanding colleague of the AP student with commitments to provide support. Therefore, rigor may be compromised in practice-based assessments.

Sam reflected on the uncertainty she felt about being assessed by OSCE for knowledge, attitude, and skills in history taking. She had worked for the past five years as a practice nurse in an inner-city general practice, and the time seemed right to take the challenge of completing the MSc ACP and becoming a nurse practitioner. The university module lead advanced practitioner was excellent, demonstrating, teaching, and giving vivid examples from practice, as was the doctor who assisted with teaching. Sam recollected that the practice sessions in clinical skills rooms with other students could at times be brilliant, depending who was in the group of three or four students turn taking around a bed as patient, ACP student, examiner checking the mark sheet, and prompter to correct if some aspect was omitted.

Parking and traffic seemed more stressful than normal on the day of the OSCE and her son Henry, aged 5, was being difficult and did not want to stay at school, which was stressful, so Sam was preoccupied when she entered the OSCE rooms corridor. The history-taking OSCE station had not caused as much concern as the prospect of the physical examination station, because she had performed history taking as a registered practitioner for the last eight years, although the tutors stressed the ways in which it was different for an advanced clinical practitioner. As required, Sam had prepared for the OSCE assessments, focusing on cardiovascular, respiratory, central nervous system, musculoskeletal, and mental health assessments. Three of these stations would be assessed, but Sam did not know which ones in advance, so she had prepared for them all.

A sheet was provided with brief information saying the patient (actor) was Jane, a 45-year-old woman, a single parent with three school-aged children, who had not attended the practice recently, but had been made redundant two months earlier when the department store where she had worked full time had gone into liquidation. Prior to commencing, Sam considered the marking criteria and their structure, and was aware through teaching sessions of the need to take a coherent history from the patient systematically and logically. Sam began in a professional manner to identify the patient's name and age, and to gain consent for the examination. When she engaged fully and observed closely to hear about the problem, she became alarmed, as Jane was clearly distraught, barely in control of her distress, with tissues in her hands being rolled and torn, and staring at the ground.

Sam gently asked: "How can I help you today?"

Jane glanced up, looking hopeless. When probed, she provided a little information on the distressing situation.

Sam then asked if Jane ever had suicidal thoughts, as that immediately seemed important. The patient nodded.

Even when asking so early in the consultation, awareness dawned on Sam that this was not the systematic approach that required other life factors to be explored first, to try to gain information and to develop rapport. Sam tried to revert to the structure she had been taught that asked about low mood, sleep pattern, engaging with others, interests, diet, and weight in a measured manner, but all the time she was preoccupied by knowing suicidal thoughts were present.

At the end of the history taking, she made an urgent referral to the mental health department. Nevertheless, Sam realized not only that she had deviated from the required structure, but that she had omitted requests for basic information, including allergies and recreational drugs.

Before reading on, consider Exercise 16.3.

EXERCISE 16.3

State two reasons why this could be a useful assessment for advanced practice students. Also consider whether this assessment may create any difficulties for students.

16.5 Practice Assessments and Requirements for a Portfolio of Evidence

Inman's (2015) survey revealed that all nine universities assessed practice. There was a wide range of types and numbers of assessments used, with some universities identifying as few as four main methods, ranging to the most excessive document requiring seventeen methods of assessment. These could include assessment of defined competence skills, reflections, OSCEs, other assessments of real patients in clinical practice, and sign-off statements by the main mentors. Mentors were also often assessors, and included medical practitioners and senior practitioners belonging to the students' discipline.

An almost unbelievable degree of diversity was displayed across the nine university practice documents, with 30 different assessment methods identified in the survey (see Table 16.3).

Whilst it is acknowledged that some of the methods identified may overlap and be similar, this also suggests that some standardization may be required. If students are being allowed protected learning time, adequately mentored, and supported in practice, they should be gaining a wide range of experience, knowledge, and skills. They need to prepare for their future by developing their own job descriptions and personal development plans, and some appeared to be being encouraged in this by having to undertake a strengths, weaknesses, opportunities, and threats (SWOT) analysis of themselves and their organization. This also suggests a need for some degree of consistency to improve the clarity and possibly the reliability and validity of the practice learning experience and of assessments, so that managers employing advanced practitioners have a clear idea of the learning and assessment they have undergone in acquiring the abilities that enable them to be called advanced practitioners.

Before reading on, consider Exercise 16.4.

EXERCISE 16.4

If you were invited to join a policy steering group to help design an electronic practice portfolio (ePortfolio) of eight assessment methods to be carried out in practice, what would you include?

Which do you think would be the most useful for assuring that an advanced clinical practitioner had the knowledge, understanding, appropriate attitude, and skills to provide advanced care and practice safely?

The many methods identified to demonstrate AP possibly lead to a requirement for further detailed information about practice portfolio assessment. It is more

---

TABLE 16.3

Assessment methods for practice.

Job description

Curriculum vitae and review

Visual Aural Read/write Kinesthetic (VARK) learning styles questionnaire

Attainment of competences

Personal development plan

Strengths, weaknesses, opportunities, and threats (SWOT) analysis

Contextual statements

Progress review reflections

Two case studies

Critical incident analyses

Expert competence statements

Witness statements

Three consultations (with patients)

Specialist training reflections

Visits

Practice-based OSCEs in year one (and year two for one university)

Assessments in practice

Action plan and review

Learning log

Specified number of reflections

Teaching sessions attended

Masterclasses attended

Clinical sessions attended

40 assessed cases in 2 years

Assessed cases (number not specified)

Self-assessment

Practice log of all other activity

Bespoke skills (for specialty)

Direct observed procedure skills (DOPS)

OSCE for clinical photography.

---

likely that a clear rationale is needed to determine the most accurate learning and assessment methods for advanced practitioners, and to ensure some equity across courses. For example, the rationale for 40 assessed cases, even over two years, needs justification. Some of the assessment methods used were adopted from medical practice, e.g. direct observed procedure skills (DOPS), and were clearly not designed for advanced practitioners, thus their reliability and validity could be questioned. Others were well established and accepted by tradition and more generally used in other educational settings, e.g. SWOT analysis and personal development plans. When several assessment methods are used, it may be described as triangulation or multiple method assessment. The variety and volume of assessment in different universities make it impossible to compare them for quality and outcome.

16.6 The Second and Third Stages of Assessment for a Master's Degree

Assessment methods for the theoretical modules, which were mainly in the postgraduate diploma, second stage of courses, conformed more closely to those conventionally associated with Master's-level study. They included universities teaching and assessing:

- **Research** in four courses, providing 15–30 credits. This was assessed in writing, requiring either a research proposal, a literature review, or a mini-lab examination.
- **Leadership** in three courses, providing 15–20 credits. This was assessed in writing, and in one with a viva.
- **AP** professional/critical/contemporary issues were taught in three courses, providing 15–20 credits. All were assessed by a 3000-word essay.
- **Independent and supplementary prescribing**. The remainder of the academic credits for the postgraduate diploma were provided by students completing independent and supplementary prescribing. This could be studied at degree or Master's level, and required the individual practitioner's regulatory body assessments strategy to be met, which often involved several assessment methods, including examinations, OSCEs, practice competences, professional reflections, and presentations.
- **Optional modules**. Practitioners who did or could not complete prescribing could select optional modules.

The Master's award was completed by a dissertation or management project for eight of the universities in the survey. One university with additional academic as well as clinical requirements in the practice portfolio of evidence encompassed the Master's credit within the portfolio.

16.7 End-point Assessment – Master's-degree Apprenticeship

The majority of this chapter has focused on information from a 2015 survey of UK AP courses. This final section relates to the assessment of the new Master's degree ACP apprenticeship, launched in September 2018 (Maclaine 2018; Skills for Health [SfH] 2018). The qualification has a heavily bureaucratic structure (Maclaine 2018). The end-point assessment for these apprenticeships will be briefly outlined, because it generated extensive debate among policy makers, clinically based experts and advanced practitioners, and academically based advanced practitioners. Discussions revolved around what to include in the assessment and who was qualified to assess Master's apprenticeship students for the final 20 credits of assessment that make up the 180 UK credits needed for a full Master's degree. Who could assess advanced practitioners' skill set was a particularly controversial issue in the early days for this new professional group.

Eraut (1994) considered similar issues, questioning whether anyone has the skill set to validly assess others:

- To perform assessments for innovative roles – with AHPs and nurses, few may have the knowledge and skill of people not only in specialist disciplines, but in subspecialties.
- When services are being changed, redesigned, and delivered by practitioners in roles that have not previously existed.
- For services in new settings, when few or no practitioners are employed with similar skills in comparable settings, who can assess whether skills and care will be optimal. Even if a few rare practitioners existed in distant locations, they were frequently such a scarce resource in high demand that they might have little opportunity to disseminate deep knowledge of their skills or assess others for similar abilities.

During the past two decades, the absence of advanced practitioner assessors specific to the individual has frequently led to medical practitioners being significantly involved in assessing the clinical skills of advanced practitioners. Whilst there may be overlap in some aspects of the roles in some settings, they can never be identical when student and assessor belong to different professions. The original intention for AP was for experienced health professionals employed in a particular area of practice to work at a higher level within their own profession, strictly avoiding any impression of being mini doctors. However, AP in the UK has tended in some settings to become synonymous with the ability to perform clinical examination skills, thus further blurring boundaries between advanced practitioners and medical practitioners.

The end-point assessment plan (EPAP) for apprenticeship is therefore worthy of comment, because it does not include OSCEs. The EPAP requires 50% weighting for the ACP element of the final assessment, to focus on three 1500-word case studies students have compiled. An open-book examination of these cases requires eight examination questions set by an EPA organization to be answered over two hours. The other 50% assesses the advanced clinical, education, clinical leadership, and research pillars of AP, and is based on a 35-minute presentation of a 1500-word clinical practice change report (SfH 2018, p. 9).

The examining panel for both elements will need to include a "representative employer organization and an independent external examiner" (SfH 2018, p. 10). Without knowledge of the assessments for the previous 180 credits achieved by the Master's in Advanced Clinical Practice, judgment cannot be made regarding the omission of OSCEs. Given the trend in the last decade toward OSCEs, it is however noteworthy that they were not considered necessary for the final part of the award. Furthermore, the patients' views of the advanced practitioner's ability to assess seem to be neglected, since a lay representative appears to have been omitted.

16.8 Conclusion

Issues around the assessment and examination of AP are likely to continue to generate debate, discussion, and change. In rapidly changing societies and with increasing consumer demand, the requirements of healthcare systems and budgets are likely to lead to further refinement, and possibly to more valid and reliable assessments of AP in the future. Higher education and the health service have demonstrated the ability to adapt to increases in numbers of disciplinary groups and specialties. The EPAP suggests that assessment of students' knowledge, skills, and behavior is likely to continue to evolve dynamically.

Key Questions

1. To what extent are OSCEs a valid and reliable method of assessment for advanced practice?

2. In your opinion, do advanced practice curricula include the most important subjects with regard to meeting current and future healthcare needs?

3. What are the potential advantages and disadvantages of apprenticeships for advanced practitioners?

Glossary

External examiner system: requires academic staff from one university to examine the quality mechanisms of a different university delivering similar courses. It involves examiners discussing and approving assessment methods, and viewing samples of students' work to ensure that standards, grading, and feedback for students are at the appropriate level for the award. External examiners also have opportunities to meet students, view assessments, and attend examination awards to ensure quality standards are maintained. This quality system is monitored by the QAA, which sets standards for degrees and provides guidelines and subject benchmarking statements. Universities are responsible for monitoring and auditing the external examiner system to test whether it is working in practice. It remains one of the key areas for institutional audit and review.

Master's degree structure in the UK: (i) postgraduate certificate – most courses assign the teaching and assessing of AHA-related modules to this stage, providing 60 Master's credit points; (ii) postgraduate diploma – leadership, research, and prescribing may be taught at the second stage, with a value of 60 further credit points, 120 in total; (iii) the Master's part – most courses require research dissertation work to be completed for the final 60 credit points awarded, totaling 180 credits for the full Master's award.

Quality Assurance Agency for Higher Education (QAA): an independent body funded by UK colleges, universities, and government departments. It states: "We safeguard standards and improve the quality of UK higher education wherever it is delivered around the world. We check that students get the higher education they are entitled to expect." Its function includes reviewing courses through benchmarking the provision against a quality code. The QAA advises the Privy Council of the UK on whether an organization can award degrees and call itself a university.

References

Aronowitz, T., Aronowitz, S., Mardin-Small, J., and BoRam (2017). Using objective structured clinical examination (OSCE) as education in advanced practice registered nursing education. *Journal of Professional Nurse* 33 (2): 119–125.

Astin, A. and Antinio, A. (2012). *Assessment for Excellence*. Plymouth: Rowman and Littlefield.

Carney H (2018). Patient satisfaction with consulting an Advanced Nurse Practitioner instead of a General Practitioner for a minor illness: a mixed methods survey. Unpublished Master's dissertation, Birmingham City University.

Eraut, M. (1994). *Developing Professional Knowledge and Competence*. London: Falmer Press.

Feathers, A., Lillis, A., Joy, and Lumley, J. (2012). *OSCE Stations for Medical Finals. Book 2*. Norwich: Carnegie Books.

Henderson, A., Nulty, D., Mitchell, M. et al. (2013). An implementation framework for using OSCEs in nursing curricula. *Nurse Education Today* 33 (12): 1459.

Inman C (2015). Standardising education for advanced practice: survey of advanced practice programmes in the UK. Association of Advanced Practice Educators UK Conference, Bournemouth, March 5.

Kurz, J., Mahoney, K., Martin-Plank, L., and Lidicker, J. (2009). Objective structured clinical examination and advanced practice nursing students. *Journal of Professional Nursing* 25 (3): 186–191.

Maclaine K (2018). Advanced clinical practitioner apprenticeships in England: a new module to consider. PowerPoint presentation. London South Bank University. http://www.npapn2018.com/wp-content/uploads/2018/09/59-Advanced-clinical-practitioner-apprenticeships-in-England-a-new-model-to-consider.pdf (accessed January 13, 2019).

Marmot, M. and Allen, J. (2014). Social determinants of health equity. *American Journal of Public Health* 104 (54): 5517–5519. https://ajph.aphapublications.org/doi/full/10.2105/AJPH.2014.302200.

Nulty, D., Mitchell, M., Jeffrey, C. et al. (2011). Best practice guidelines for use on OSCEs: maximising value for students learning. *Nurse Education Today* 31.

Quality Assurance Agency for Higher Education (2009). *Handbook for Instructional Audit.* Mansfield: QAA.

Roberts, C., Newbie, D., Jolly, B. et al. (2006). Assuring the quality of high-stakes undergraduate assessments of clinical competence. *Medical Teacher* 28 (6): 535–543. https://www.tandfonline.com/doi/full/10.1080/01421590600711187.

Skills for Health (2018). *End Point Assessment Plan Integrated Degree Apprenticeship for Advanced Clinical Practitioner at Level 7.* London: SfH https://haso.skillsforhealth.org.uk/wp-content/uploads/2017/04/2017.11.14-Advanced-Clinical-Practice-Apprenticeship-Standard-Final.pdf (accessed January 13, 2019.

Talley, N. and O'Connor, S. (2014). *Clinical Examination: A systematic Guide to Physical Diagnosis.* London: Churchill Livingstone.

CHAPTER 17

Leadership in Advanced Practice

Paula McGee

Birmingham City University, Birmingham, UK

Key Issues
- The nature of leadership
- Attributes of the leader
- Types of leadership

LEARNING OUTCOMES

By the end of this chapter you will be able to:

- Critically discuss the positive attributes of leaders and the pitfalls to be avoided in leadership roles.
- Explain three levels of leadership in healthcare organizations.
- Critically discuss the nature of clinical, professional, and organizational leaders with reference to your own sphere of practice.
- Explain the difference between leadership and management.

17.1 Introduction

Advanced practice has developed in the context of rapid changes in the provision and delivery of healthcare. Longer lifespans, technological advances, and aging populations are among the many factors that have challenged health service providers, raised public expectations, and increased costs. Any change can be unsettling for those who have to deal with the demands and anxiety it

Advanced Practice in Healthcare: Dynamic Developments in Nursing and Allied Health Professions,
Fourth Edition. Edited by Paula McGee and Chris Inman.
© 2019 John Wiley & Sons Ltd. Published 2019 by John Wiley & Sons Ltd.

creates, but the complex nature of healthcare and health service provision can place considerable pressure on practitioners, leaving them struggling to cope. It is in this context of change and high pressures that advanced practice has emerged, offering opportunities to experienced and appropriately prepared practitioners to apply their expertise as leaders.

Leadership is regarded as one of the core competences of advanced practice by policy makers and theorists alike. In UK policy, "leadership and collaborative practice" is one of the four main features of advanced practice, and the current strategy for nursing focuses strongly on the importance of leadership (Department of Health 2010, p. 2; NHS England 2016). The Nursing and Midwifery Council (NMC 2005) places a similar emphasis on leadership, and the Royal College of Nursing (RCN) regards it as a means of both introducing and managing change, and also as an essential element in credentialing advanced practitioners (NMC 2005; Royal College of Nursing 2018a, b). Theorists such as Hamric (2014) place leadership among the core competences of advanced practice. Leadership is an essential component in health service reforms, in clinical practice, in "professional organisations, within health care systems and in health policymaking areas" (Tracy and Hanson 2014, p. 268).

This chapter begins by examining the nature of leadership as an interpersonal activity that requires specific attributes, talent, and a burning desire to improve on the deficiencies of the status quo. Leadership is distinguished from management, before the chapter moves on to address clinical, professional, and organizational leadership and the different levels at which these may be utilized in healthcare organizations. A case study is used to illustrate how these three forms of leadership can be applied by advanced practitioners.

17.2 The Nature of Leadership

Leadership is a relational activity requiring at least two people and concerns the nature of the interactions between them. To lead is to cause someone else to follow, to influence them, to show them a way forward. Thus, leadership is a role that an individual adopts and one that requires the application of specific skills which encourage feelings of trust in others. Leadership also does not take place in isolation from other roles. No one is or can be a leader without, at the same time, also engaging in multiple roles: leader and therapist, parent, son, or daughter. Thus, although the literature about advanced practice separates the various competences involved, in the daily realities of practice they are performed simultaneously and interact with one another. A single therapeutic encounter with a patient may involve a combination of leadership with direct care or coaching, or with several competences at once: ethical decision making, leadership, collaboration, and clinical practice. Finally, leadership is a relational activity in that it is focused on a goal and how it may be achieved. Showing others a way forward provides a sense of direction for achieving the task and a sense of value; the task matters, it is worthwhile (Shaw 2007).

Before reading on, consider Exercise 17.1.

EXERCISE **17.1**

Who are the leaders you admire? Give reasons.

17.3 Attributes of the Leader

Leaders are restless people, "constantly challenging themselves to think of new ways to do things and are never content with doing something the conventional way if a better way is possible" (Tracy and Hanson 2014; Pilbeam and Wallis 2018, p. 45). Leaders make things happen. They have goals and set themselves tasks that they want to achieve. They are enthusiastic about these goals and tasks and their excitement is often contagious. Enthusiasm is a useful trait, but it is not enough to make someone a leader. The first most important attribute of a leader is integrity: being honest, being brave, and doing what is right irrespective of the consequences (Pilbeam and Wallis 2018). Honesty with oneself and in dealings with others is of "critical importance" because "it creates and maintains trust. Mutual trust between the leader and the led is absolutely vital: lose that and you have lost everything. Moreover, it is very hard to re-establish" (Adair 2018, p. 98). Honesty is the antithesis of corruption. The word "corruption" comes from the Latin *rumpere*, meaning "to break" and *com* meaning "with." Corruption is, therefore, a breaking of trust by using one's position or contacts for personal advantage. It may occur as a result of individual or group actions or decisions at any level in society or organizations. Leaders need to be aware of and guard against the subtle ways in which dishonesty and corruption may infiltrate their own activities.

However, corruption is not the same as political acumen. Leaders need a sound understanding of the impact of relevant health policies on both their particular work setting and on the healthcare organization as a whole. The *policy-competent* leader is able to apply this understanding by contextualizing innovation and change in ways that match the organization's priorities (Hewison 2009). Leaders understand what the healthcare organization is expected to do in order to meet policy demands, the organizational culture, how systems work and why, how funding is allocated and why, and they use this understanding to achieve their goals. Similarly, leaders need to develop a wide sphere of influence across the healthcare organization. This means forming supportive and collaborative alliances at varying levels, from immediate colleagues to those in senior positions, contributing to the formation of policies and protocols through active participation in committees and maintaining a visible presence. Outside the organization, active participation in professional and patient organizations may provide additional influence at local, regional, or national level. Politically astute advanced practitioners are well equipped with skills to act with integrity in using systems and alliances to their advantage in achieving their goals (Tracy and Hanson 2014).

Before reading on, undertake Exercise 17.2.

> **EXERCISE 17.2**
>
> To what extent do you think you are policy competent? How well do you understand current health policies and how these affect the healthcare organization in which you work?

Interpersonal competence is an essential attribute of a leader. The leader is responsible for communicating the goal or task to be achieved, sharing the criteria for success, and showing the way forward in terms of how these may be achieved. Good communication skills are required to convey clearly this message and the opportunities that it affords everyone concerned. The skilled leader recognizes and values people and seeks to actively incorporate them and their skills into the way forward. In using interpersonal skills in this way, the leader enables others to develop and achieve and, at the same time, avoids one of the major pitfalls of leadership, the "queen bee syndrome" (Tracy and Hanson 2014, p. 291). *Queen bees* accrue and hoard power to themselves, promoting their own interests and image even if this gets in the way of the work to be done; they do not allow anyone else to make decisions or use their initiative, and they feel threatened by anyone who challenges them. They use people for their own ends and employ criticism rather than praise to secure their position and keep others in their place. Queen bees are dishonest with themselves in thinking that they can do everything, that only their expertise and point of view matter. Eventually, queen bees can become the problem rather than the solution to achieving the goals and tasks required. Leaders who are self-aware will take a different path, "sharing opportunities, knowledge and expertise and acknowledging the contributions of others" (Tracy and Hanson 2014, p. 291). These leaders share power. They value people as ends in themselves and demonstrate faith in them by encouraging, mentoring, perhaps even pushing them, all of which can help to instill confidence and provide the freedom that enables others to achieve in their own right.

Before reading on, think about Exercise 17.3.

EXERCISE 17.3

As an advanced practitioner, what networks and working relationships have you developed? To what extent do these benefit (i) members of these networks and relationships, (ii) you? Give examples.

The leader's interpersonal skills convey authenticity, genuine interest in, and concern for others. Leaders are visible and involved. They connect, across the organization, with diverse individuals and groups, listening to and acting on their concerns and ideas, encouraging their efforts, clarifying and confirming the task, sorting out problems, and evaluating progress. They convey warmth (Adair 2018). They build teams, negotiate positions and access to resources, and make sure these are delivered. The enactment of these social skills caries an emotional charge; it connects with people at a deep level that creates a bond with the leader. In this context, those who are led will not be afraid to challenge if they think the leader is mistaken; the leader is not afraid to admit an error and vice versa. However, if those who are led feel that the leader is not really interested in them, is just using them as a means to an end, then the emotional bond will not develop and they are less likely to speak up if things go wrong.

Finally, the leader requires sufficient theoretical and practical knowledge about the field of practice, the task to be achieved, and the day-to-day work involved. The leader is capable and unafraid to join in when necessary and perform whatever jobs need doing at that moment, even, and perhaps especially, the unpopular ones. This does not mean that the leader has to be an expert in everything, but willingness to share the work demonstrates credibility and sets an example that others will follow. It also helps the leader to identify problem areas that might otherwise not be recognized. However, joining in the work cannot be the main focus of the leader's activities. It is the leader's responsibility to ensure that the goal is reached and that tasks are accomplished.

The attributes of integrity, interpersonal skills, knowledge, and credibility represent a mixture of innate ability, training, and experience. The leader must have an aptitude, a talent for the role, which can be enhanced by training and experience, although these are not enough. It is the synergy between aptitude, training, and experience that seems to be the key factor in forming the attributes that leaders require (Adair (2018). This synergy can be fostered through regular "thinking in action", bringing together the attributes of the leader, the task to be achieved, and knowledge of the people involved in a critical appraisal of a particular situation. Inherent in this is acknowledgment of failures, by oneself, by others, or in the achievement of the task, and an honest examination of the reasons they occurred. It is through "thinking in action" that the leader is able to grow and develop (Benner et al. 2011, p. 10; Adair 2018; Pilbeam and Wallis 2018).

17.4 Leadership and Management

Leaders do not necessarily hold the most senior positions within an organization and their power base may not always be rooted in the management or the organizational hierarchy. Indeed, the leader may sometimes be at odds with those levels. Shaw (2007, p. 28) makes clear that leadership is distinguishable from management: "Management is a process that focuses on maintaining systems to produce goods and services efficiently." Thus, whilst leaders provide a sense of direction, inspire others, and generally make things happen, managers are behind them making sure that finance is managed, staff are paid, employment procedures are followed, legal requirements are met, and computer systems work. Managers control budgets and spending has to be accounted for. Managers also control other functions such as ordering supplies and staff deployment. Managers therefore are part of the power structures in the organization and have their own spheres of influence. Consequently, there may be occasions when leaders find it useful to incorporate management into their role in innovation, managing change, and team development (RCN 2018a).

Before reading on, consider Exercise 17.4.

> **EXERCISE 17.4**
>
> How do you see yourself as a leader? What opportunities for leadership are available to you?

17.5 Leadership in Advanced Practice

The importance attached to leadership in advanced practice has arisen because the "presence and/or absence of effective leaders in health care can have a stark consequence on the quality and outcomes of care. The delivery of safe, quality, and compassionate health care and services is dependent on having effective leaders at the frontline" (McSherry and Pearce 2016, p. 11). In the UK, a number of reports have documented, in graphic detail, what happens when leadership is absent or incompetent: patients are neglected and ill-treated, sometimes with fatal consequences (see, for example, Francis 2010; Kirkup 2015). Health professionals directly involved in treating and caring for patients need leaders to ensure that standards, quality, and consistency are maintained and, where possible, improved. Leadership is crucial in ensuring patient safety and dignity, as well as in navigating the intricacies of health service reforms. The most recent reform of the National Health Service was introduced by the Health and Social Care Act 2012, which placed considerable responsibility on health professionals with regard to implementing the policies set out in the Five Year Forward View. This included measures to tackle major public health issues such as obesity and smoking, more engagement with local communities, changes in service commissioning, and reducing healthcare costs (NHS England 2014), which are also a major part of the most recent NHS Plan (NHS England 2019). Thus, the provision of healthcare services is far from simple. It requires the synchrony of multiple systems and large numbers of people to establish pathways through which treatment and care are delivered; leaders need to understand not only how these work, but also how to access and use them for maximum patient benefit (Swanwick and McKimm 2011).

In large, complex organizations such as those responsible for healthcare, leadership is essential, and it can broadly be divided into three levels. *Team leaders* are responsible for a small number of people and a specific function, for example community-based physiotherapy. *Operational leaders* are responsible for a section of the organization, for example surgical wards and operating theaters. *Strategic leaders* are responsible for the whole organization (Adair 2018). These three types of leadership provide advanced practitioners with opportunities to influence others and show the way toward the achievement of specific goals and tasks in three domains.

17.5.1 Clinical Leadership

The clinical leadership competence framework (NHS Leadership Academy 2011, p. 7) is based on five important elements of leadership: "demonstrating personal qualities" such as self-awareness and integrity; "working with others," for example through collaborative practice; "managing"; "improving services"; and "setting direction," in terms of managing and evaluating change. The framework is based on "shared leadership" and applies to all health professionals, at every stage of their careers, with regard to their share "of responsibility for the success of the organization and its services," irrespective of their position or status (NHS Leadership Academy 2011, p. 6). The notion of shared responsibility among employees is important in any organization; achieving success does require a commitment to the organization's goals and purpose. However, shared responsibility as an employee may not be the same as leadership in every context. Exactly how individuals emerge as clinical leaders is not particularly clear. In some instances, individuals may be appointed to leadership roles, but this may not make them leaders (Adair 2018). Clinical leaders in medicine are recognized as such by others because they are experts in a particular field. They are seen as "approachable, effective communicators and empowered" and able "to see improvements to services or … to address limitations" (McSherry and Pearce 2016, p. 13).

Moreover, these leaders uphold clinical governance standards. They motivate and are considerate of others, have integrity, and engage in critical thinking. It is to be hoped that the same may be said of advanced practitioners as clinical leaders.

The advanced practitioner's clinical expertise is based on a broad repertoire of technical and clinical experience, knowledge, and skills, accompanied by interpersonal competence, all of which has been acquired through practice in a wide range of settings and with diverse patient populations. This background enables the advanced practitioner to fulfill a range of activities focused on the provision of treatment and care for patients and their families, particularly those with multiple or challenging needs that require interventions from diverse professionals. For example, a patient with chronic obstructive pulmonary disease may receive treatment and care from doctors, nurses, physiotherapists, dieticians, and psychologists, who may never come together. There is no coherent and shared picture of the patient's health and progress; the patient is left feeling adrift between differing opinions and advice. In these circumstances, the advanced practitioner, as clinical leader, is able to act as a lynchpin on behalf of the patient by liaising with the other professionals and developing and coordinating a multidisciplinary team. Engagement in patient care as a clinical leader may also include the actual performance of care and treatment, for example in crisis intervention, in teaching through example, or in role modeling. These episodes are useful in maintaining clinical credibility and in reinforcing membership of the clinical team, but they are not the sole focus of the advanced practitioner's role in clinical leadership.

As clinical leaders, advanced practitioners are both present and future orientated; they look ahead to possible outcomes and seek to shape these through transformational processes. Engagement in practice provides clinical leaders with opportunities as team leaders to identify where change or innovation is needed, to supervise its introduction, and to evaluate its effects (RCN 2018a). Studies of the leadership role of advanced practitioners show that they are able to use their interpersonal skills, knowledge, and experience to build networks as either team or operational leaders. They create teams, support and encourage individuals to join them, and use mentoring skills to help them to achieve (Elliott et al. 2013). Unfortunately, and despite all this, advanced practitioners are not always recognized for what they do, or for the contribution that they make to patient care. Lack of clarity about their role, lack of administrative help, work overload, and lack of encouragement and support all contribute to this situation and need to be addressed in setting up future advanced practice roles (Higgins et al. 2014; Elliott 2017).

17.5.2 Professional Leadership

Developing their spheres of influence requires leaders to step outside their immediate workplace setting and be proactive in building networks across their organization and beyond, which provide the leader with opportunities to engage in indirect care activities (Koetters 1989; Table 17.1). These activities require the leader to apply clinical, technical, and interpersonal competence for the benefit of patients, but in a broader, multidisciplinary environment. Within the healthcare organization, this indirect care may include developing clinical procedure manuals, or promoting evidence-based practice. Leaders have to consider the cost, feasibility, and impact on all parts of the organization's clinical environment, as well as factors such as the geography of a hospital site or, in the community, the opening hours of the local pharmacy. Team or operational leadership in a professional context requires the advanced practitioner to draw on a wealth of experience and work collaboratively with colleagues to bring about innovation and change. However, this participation in the wider life of the healthcare organization can only be realized if the advanced practitioner makes the effort to be proactive in networking. Active participation in the healthcare organization includes attending meetings regularly. Simply having one's name on the list of members of a committee will not achieve anything; it may look superficially impressive on a CV, but that impression may be quickly dispelled by a few questions about the exact nature of one's contribution (Table 17.1).

Outside the healthcare organization, professional leadership activities focus on a wider stage at local, regional, or national level (Table 17.2). Engagement with patient associations and community groups provides opportunities for the leader to develop initiatives that show people how to improve their health and manage minor illnesses through self-care. Active participation in special interest groups or the work of a professional body enables the leader to develop a broader network and share expertise and concerns. Research, conference presentations, and publications enable the leader to influence others further afield.

Educational activities can also be seen as a form of indirect care. As professional leaders, advanced practitioners share their expertise to help improve patients' quality of life and to help colleagues deliver high-quality care in line with current knowledge. Teaching, coaching, and guiding challenge the advanced practitioner to develop both an understanding of how people learn and a broad repertoire of strategies to facilitate different approaches to learning. Interpersonal competence is particularly important, because learning involves change, moving from what is already known and understood to the incorporation of something new.

TABLE 17.1

Professional leadership: indirect care activities within the healthcare organization.

Providing education for groups of patients with specific conditions
Collaborating on the development of clinical procedure manuals, protocols, and policies
Participating in service evaluations and clinical audits
Acting as a source of advice for patients and staff based outside the leader's workplace setting
Promoting evidence-based practice
Coaching and guiding staff
Participating in or leading research
Teaching and assessing students
Providing staff support
Participation in multidisciplinary committees
Promoting cultural competence

TABLE 17.2

Professional leadership: indirect care activities outside the healthcare organization.

Collaboration with local community groups to promote health

Partnerships with patient associations

Research

Participation service commissioning

Participation in the work of a professional body

Presentations at conferences

Publications

Teaching

Finally, professional leadership also offers opportunities for advanced practitioners to promote cultural competence at team, operational and strategic levels. Culture is "a set of guidelines (both explicit and implicit) that individuals inherit as members of a particular society and that tell them how to view the world, how to experience it emotionally and how to behave in it in relation to other people, to supernatural forces or gods" (Helman 2007, p. 2). In a diverse society, culture is an important consideration in healthcare. It influences how people experience and respond to illness, treatment, and care, how they conceptualize health, and what they believe will enhance it. Everyone is born into a culture and this is usually linked to ethnic origins. However, throughout life individuals may also become part of social cultures, developed, for example, around particular characteristics or memberships. As an example, an individual with hearing impairment may belong to social organizations for people with similar differences that create their own culture. Cultural competence is a continuous process through which the practitioner develops expertise in providing "effective health care, taking into account people's cultural beliefs" (Papadopoulos 2006, p. 11). Achieving cultural competence depends on effort, self-awareness, commitment, and leadership; it also requires compassion. Thus, culturally competent, compassionate care is that in which the professional:

- Responds to the suffering of others with a commitment to relieve this within a culturally appropriate framework.
- Acknowledges their own feelings when encountering the suffering of others (Papadopoulos 2018).

17.5.3 Organizational Leadership

Operational and strategic levels of leadership require health policy competence and a thorough understanding of the goals, values, culture, and functions of the organization as a whole. The strategic leader combines these factors to create a shared vision of what the organization can achieve, by what means, over what period of time, and to what degree of success. In other words, the strategic leader sets out the path that the organization will follow and makes it happen;

works across the organization ensuring targets are met and that performance is high; identifies problems; and motivates, encourages, listens to, and praises people for their efforts. The strategic leader builds teams of operational leaders who are responsible for achieving particular aspects of this vision; they, in turn, devolve some of this responsibility to team leaders. Thus, at each level, people have the opportunity to develop as leaders; the strategic leader grows future leaders, including their own replacement. Strategic leaders are also engaged outside the organization promoting good relations with the local community, forming alliances, and participating in relevant regional and national bodies (Tracy and Hanson 2014; Adair 2018). Thus, strategic leaders require the same skills as any other advanced practitioner, but use them in a different context, both within and outside the organization.

Advanced practitioners wishing to become strategic leaders have to adapt their thinking to be able to function at this level. The first step is to engage in a dialog with the self. Negative voices in our inner dialog can easily prevent us from taking the first steps in becoming a leader, and may still be there to undermine us even when we hold a senior position. They tell us only what we cannot do and challenging them requires bravery, first in developing a positive mindset and second in taking action (Table 17.3). Confidence comes with rather than before taking action. Katie Piper's (2011) advice throughout her autobiography is to "fake it till you make it": act as if you feel confident and people will believe that you are. Given time, so will you.

TABLE 17.3

Eight habits for strategic leadership.

Be proactive	See what can be changed and make it happen Be brave
Focus on the end point	Be clear about what you want to achieve and the criteria for success
Prioritize	Manage your time and energy Plan a series of steps rather than trying to do everything at once
Negotiate	Try to see situations from other points of view Identify how others and you can benefit
Communicate	Respect people and listen to them rather than think about what you want to say to them Ensure that they understand what you are trying to achieve, what you would like them to do, and what they can gain from taking part
Synergize	Bring people and ideas together Recognize, create, and provide new opportunities
Make time for yourself	Be aware of your limitations Share responsibility Take time out and rest Grow your own replacements
Inspire people	Show warmth and kindness Leave them feeling better rather than worse Encourage and support people, and help them to achieve

Source: Summarized from Covey (2004, 2006).

A young man lies curled up in a hospital bed, clutching his abdomen. He is crying, in a lot of pain, and asking for analgesia. Several family members are with him. They are very upset and they are asking the nurse in charge to help him. The staff nurse is shouting loudly at the young man, telling him that he cannot have anything for another two hours and to stop making a noise.

The advanced practitioner approaches the nurse in charge to ask about the situation and is told what the problem is. The man was admitted, about two hours ago, in sickle cell crisis with a temperature of 38.8 °C. The nurse says: "Oh, he's got sickle cell and he just wants more pethidine. He's just an addict, you know. That's the only reason they come in."

Before reading on, think about Exercise 17.5.

With reference to clinical, professional, and strategic leadership, what is your first priority here?

This is an emergency situation in which the first priority is patient safety and care. Thus, the advanced practitioner initiates a care and treatment plan based on the patient's four main problems: distress, sickle cell crisis, high body temperature, and abdominal pain. As clinical leader, the advanced practitioner works collaboratively with the nurse and medical staff to resolve the situation and ensure core clinical standards are met. What is important at this point is to focus on the patient and not the nurse's behavior. A friendly, pleasant, but firm manner is more likely than criticism to encourage the nurse to work with the advanced practitioner (Table 17.4).

Before reading on, consider Exercise 17.6.

How would you address the professional leadership issues in this situation?

Nurses, and midwives have a duty of candor in treating and caring for patients (National Health Service Executive 2015). This duty has

TABLE 17.4

Clinical leadership issues: what the advanced practitioner ensures.

Managing distress	The patient and their family receive high-quality, compassionate care and are fully informed of what is happening. They are treated with respect and every effort is made to resolve their distress.
Acute painful crisis	The patient has received strong analgesia within 30 minutes of arrival in hospital. Their pain, pain relief, and vital signs are continuously monitored and recorded in line with hospital protocols. Patient-controlled analgesia is provided if other methods of pain relief are not successful. The hematologist has been notified of the patient's arrival.
Management of the febrile patient	The patient's high temperature of 38.8 °C is fully investigated: chest X-ray. Blood and other relevant cultures are undertaken. Antibiotic treatment is commenced alongside other care interventions to lower body temperature.
Abdominal pain	A differential diagnosis clarifies the cause of the pain, which may be due to the complications of sickle cell or to other conditions. Liver function tests are performed. A care and treatment plan is developed.
Complications of sickle cell disease	The presence of other complications of sickle cell disease are noted and included in the care and treatment plan.

Source: Based on Sickle Cell Society (2018). See also National Institute for Health and Care Excellence (2016).

three dimensions. First, when something has gone wrong, patients and families are entitled to receive a clear, open, and honest explanation as quickly as possible after the event has occurred. This explanation must be accompanied by an apology and a second explanation of what, if anything, can be done to rectify the situation and prevent its recurrence in future. All of this must be commensurate with what patients and families want to know and in a way that is meaningful and memorable. This first responsibility is complemented by transparency, in which errors and near misses are reported honestly, and openness, in which professionals feel able to raise concerns without risking reprisals (National Health Service Executive 2015; McSherry and Pearce 2016; NMC 2018).

In the situation described here, several things have gone wrong. Sickle cell is one of a group of inherited diseases that occur in people originating from African Caribbean, African, Eastern Mediterranean, and some Asian backgrounds. Abnormally shaped cells cause bouts of intense pain as they block blood vessels. Anemia, infection, and complications affecting major organs and other parts of the body also occur. Thus, sickle cell affects people of color and, unfortunately, not all health professionals are well informed about this disease. The advanced practitioner needs to recognize that not only were the young man's immediate care and treatment needs not met and the nurse was rude and uncaring, but also that ignorance, racism, and discrimination may well have contributed to this neglect. This situation requires the leader to engage in a series of difficult conversations with the patient, the family, and the staff nurse (Sullivan and Garland 2013; Chapter 14 in this volume). The advanced practitioner will have to be open and honest with the patient and his family, apologize, and rectify, as quickly as possible, the lack of care and treatment provided earlier. A separate conversation will have to take place with the nurse to make clear that her behavior is not acceptable. Finally, the advanced practitioner should also discuss the situation with the ward manager to facilitate a way forward in the provision of culturally compassionate care.

The advanced practitioner should consider the implication of the young man's experience in terms of the organization as a whole. This might begin by reviewing the organization's priorities and goals in terms of how these can be linked with the care and safety of people of color. Thus, a new possibility is envisioned and the strategic leader begins to open up new horizons and the routes by which they may be achieved.

17.6 Conclusion

Leadership is an important element of advanced practice. It requires integrity, competence, and a high level of people-orientated skills. Leaders value people, are interested in them, pay attention to them, and set them in motion, enabling them to become more than they themselves previously anticipated. In the complexity of modern healthcare, leaders who understand how things work, why, and how, and can help patients and colleagues navigate paths to success, are invaluable.

Key Questions

1. Select one aspect of your field of practice that requires change. What would you like to see in place instead and why? How would you present your argument to (i) your colleagues; (ii) patients; (iii) your manager; (iv) the organization's board?

2. Identify a situation in which you, as a leader, were not successful. What did you learn from this experience? To what extent did it help you?

3. Where do you see yourself in five years' time? How do you plan to get there?

Glossary

Clinical leadership: patient-focused activity by practitioners engaged in the provision of care and treatment, aimed at promoting the consistent provision of high-quality care and preventing or finding solutions to difficulties.

Organizational leadership: providing strategic direction for the whole or part of an organization.

Professional leadership: practitioner-focused activity by practitioners engaged in developing members of their profession or the profession as a whole at local, regional, national, and international levels.

Racism: unjust treatment of others because they are deemed inferior on the grounds of skin color or some other distinguishing characteristic.

References

Adair, J. (2018). *Lessons in Leadership. The 12 Key Concepts.* London: Bloomsbury Business.

Benner, P., Kryiadis, P.H., and Stannard, D. (2011). *Clinical Wisdom and Interventions in Acute and Critical Care,* 2e. New York: Springer.

Covey, S. (2004). *The 7 Habits of Highly Effective People: Powerful Lessons in Personal Change.* London: Simon and Schuster UK.

Covey, S. (2006). *The 8th Habit. From Effectiveness to Greatness.* London: Simon and Schuster UK.

Department of Health (2010). *Advanced Level Nursing: A Position Statement.* London: DH.

Elliott, N. (2017). Building leadership capacity in advanced nurse practitioners – the role of organisational management. *Journal of Nursing Management* 25: 77–81.

Elliott, N., Higgins, A., Begley, C. et al. (2013). The identification of clinical and professional leadership activities of advanced practitioners: findings from the Specialist Clinical and Advanced Practitioner Evaluation study in Ireland. *Journal of Advanced Nursing* 69 (5): 1037–1050.

Francis, R. (2010). *Independent Inquiry into Care Provided by Mid Staffordshire NHS Foundation Trust January 2005 – March 2009.* London: Stationery Office.

Hamric, A. (2014). A definition of advanced practice nursing. In: *Advanced Nursing Practice: An Integrative Approach,* 5e (ed. A. Hamric, C. Hanson, M. Tracy and E. O'Grady), 67–85. St. Louis: W.B. Saunders.

Helman, C. (2007). *Culture, Health and Illness,* 5e. London: Hodder Arnold.

Hewison, A. (2009). UK health policy and health service reform. In: *Advanced Practice in Nursing and the Allied Health Professions,* 3e (ed. P. McGee), 15–28. Oxford: Wiley-Blackwell.

Higgins, A., Begley, C., Lalor, J. et al. (eds.) (2014). Factors influencing advanced practitioners' ability to enact leadership: a case study within Irish healthcare. *Journal of Nursing Management* 22: 894–905.

Kirkup, B. (2015). *The Report of the Morecambe Bay Investigation.* London: Stationery Office.

Koetters, T. (1989). Clinical practice and direct patient care. In: *The Clinical Nurse Specialist in Theory and Practice,* 5e (ed. A. Hamric and J. Spross), 107–123. Philadelphia: W.B. Saunders.

McSherry, R. and Pearce, P. (2016). What are the effective ways to translate clinical leadership into health care quality improvement. *Journal of Healthcare Leadership* 8: 11–17.

National Health Service Executive (2015). New "duty of candour" guidance published for NHS staff. http://www.nationalhealthexecutive.com/Health-Care-News/new-duty-of-candour-guidance-published-for-nhs-staff (accessed January 13, 2019).

National Institute for Health and Care Excellence (2016). Sickle cell disease. https://cks.nice.org.uk/sickle-cell-disease (accessed January 13, 2019).

NHS England (2014). The Five Year Forward Review. https://www.england.nhs.uk/wp-content/uploads/2014/10/5yfv-web.pdf (accessed January 13, 2019).

NHS England (2016). Leading change. Adding value. A framework for nursing, midwifery and care staff. https://www.england.nhs.uk/wp-content/uploads/2016/05/nursing-framework.pdf (accessed January 13, 2019).

NHS England (2019). The NHS Long Term Plan. https://www.england.nhs.uk/long-term-plan (accessed January 20, 2019).

NHS Leadership Academy (2011). *Clinical Leadership Competency Framework.* Coventry: NHS Institute for Innovation and Improvement.

Nursing and Midwifery Council (2005). Implementation of a framework for the standard of post registration nursing. Agendum 27.1 C/05/160 December. http://aape.org.uk/wp-content/uploads/2015/02/NMC-ANP-Dec051.doc (accessed January 13, 2019).

Nursing and Midwifery Council (2018). The professional duty of candour. https://www.nmc.org.uk/standards/

guidance/the-professional-duty-of-candour (accessed January 13, 2019).

Papadopoulos, I. (2006). The Papadopoulos, Tilki and Taylor model of developing cultural competence. In: *Transcultural Health and Social Care: Development of Culturally Competent Practitioners* (ed. I. Papadopoulos), 7–24. Edinburgh: Churchill Livingstone.

Papadopoulos, I. (2018). *Culturally Competent Compassion. A Guide for Healthcare Students and Practitioners.* Abingdon: Routledge.

Pilbeam, D. and Wallis, G. (2018). *Leadership iD.* Harlow: Pearson Education.

Piper, K. (2011). *Beautiful.* Abingdon: Ebury Press.

Royal College of Nursing (2018a). *Advanced Level Nursing Practice: Introduction.* London: RCN.

Royal College of Nursing (2018b). *RCN Credentialing for Advanced Level Nursing Practice. Handbook for Applicants.* London: RCN.

Shaw, S. (2007). *Nursing Leadership.* Oxford: Blackwell.

Sickle Cell Society (2018). *Standards for the Clinical Care of Adults with Sickle Cell Disease in the UK.* London: Sickle Cell Society.

Sullivan, E. and Garland, G. (2013). *Practical Leadership and Management in Healthcare.* Harlow: Pearson.

Swanwick, T. and McKimm, J. (2011). What is clinical leadership...and why is it important? *Journal of Healthcare Leadership* 8: 22–26.

Tracy, M. and Hanson, C. (2014). Leadership. In: *Advanced Practice Nursing: An Integrative Approach,* 5e (ed. A. Hamric, C. Hanson, M. Tracy and E. O'Grady), 266–298. St Louis: Elsevier Saunders.

CHAPTER 18

Research Competence in Advanced Practice

Paula McGee

Birmingham City University, Birmingham, UK

Key Issues
- Critical appraisal of research findings
- Evidence-based practice
- Application of research skills in direct patient care
- Publication of research results

LEARNING OUTCOMES
By the end of this chapter you will be able to:
- Explain the factors to consider in assessing the quality of research.
- Critically discuss the use of social media in research.
- Explain the importance of impact with regard to research.
- Plan a research paper.

18.1 Introduction

Advanced practitioners are highly competent clinical practitioners and leaders, who pioneer innovations and who use their skills to engage in a range of activities to improve patient care, their healthcare organization's ability to provide appropriate services, and their respective professions as a whole. They understand the structures and processes through which healthcare organizations function and how to get something done. National and international links provide useful insights into the world outside the organization and enable advanced practitioners to ensure that innovations reflect current policy, practice, and research. Achieving all this requires advanced practitioners to approach practice from a critical standpoint, evaluating what is going well and identifying

Advanced Practice in Healthcare: Dynamic Developments in Nursing and Allied Health Professions,
Fourth Edition. Edited by Paula McGee and Chris Inman.
© 2019 John Wiley & Sons Ltd. Published 2019 by John Wiley & Sons Ltd.

what should be changed. It is their responsibility to ensure that practice in the workplace is based on the best available evidence and to systematically investigate those aspects of care that give cause for concern. This type of indirect care activity requires research skills that enable the advanced practitioner to assess and generate new evidence and, where appropriate, apply this to patient care.

This chapter presents three short discussions about advanced practitioners and research activities. First is a discussion about research competence, which is an essential prerequisite for both advanced practice and evidence-based practice (EBP). This discussion focuses on three levels of research activity: critical appraisal skills and tools, EBP, and conducting original research. The second discussion focuses on research activities in relation to direct patient care. This is the core, the essence of advanced practice, and provides many opportunities for practitioners to use their research skills for the benefit of patient care and treatment at national, local, and individual patient levels. Continued research into direct practice is essential to explore gaps in current knowledge, improve access to treatment and care on an equal basis for everyone, and assess the impact of health policies. Particular features of this discussion are the impact of new technologies in managing health and in conducting research. The third discussion focuses on the publication of research outcomes, how to set about this, and the issues to be aware of. It is presented as a case study through a series of questions that are intended to help all readers, but particularly those planning to write their first research paper. The final section of the chapter presents an agenda for research to which advanced practitioners can apply their skills.

18.2 Research Competence in Advanced Practice

Advanced practitioners are expected to "critically engage in research activity, adhering to good research practice guidance, so that evidence based strategies are developed and applied to enhance quality, safety, productivity and value for money" (NHS Health Education England 2017, p. 10). To achieve this, they must demonstrate ability in the application of research skills in order to evaluate practice, identify and investigate gaps in knowledge, and share their findings through conference presentations and publications (NHS Health Education England 2015; Royal College of Nursing 2018; Table 18.1). Thus, competence in research activities is considered an essential feature of the capabilities of advanced practitioners, that is to say the "extent to which individuals can adapt to change, generate new knowledge and continue to improve their performance" (NHS Health Education England 2017, p. 20). The concept of capabilities reflects the gradual development of advanced practitioners and their need for continuing professional education that enables them to enhance their expertise in research activities. These activities are divided here into three broad groups based on the work of DePalma (2009) and Gray (2014) as a basis for further discussion.

18.2.1 Critical Appraisal Tools

Advanced practitioners need to draw on a wide range of evidence from both within their own and other professional fields. They need to be adept at

TABLE 18.1

Ten key research skills for advanced practice.

Identification of questions for research

Use of research resources

Understanding of quantitative and qualitative research methods

Critical review of research studies and synthesis of findings

Application of relevant research findings in practice

Application of skills in auditing and evaluating practice

Planning and conduct of research investigations

Dissemination of research findings and their impact on patient care

Development of research governance systems

Development of local, regional, and national networks

Source: Summarized from NHS Health Education England (2017), Royal College of Nursing (2018).

TABLE 18.2

CASP critical appraisal guides.

Randomized controlled trials

Qualitative research studies

Quantitative research studies

Systematic reviews

Diagnostic test studies

Case control studies

Economic evaluations

Clinical prediction tool studies

Cohort studies

Source: Summarized from the Critical Appraisal Skills Programme (CASP; https://casp-uk.net).

critically appraising research reports and deciding whether and to what extent the evidence they provide will help their patients. The Critical Appraisal Skills Programme (CASP; https://casp-uk.net) provides a series of free guides to help practitioners evaluate different types of research. Each guide consists of a series of questions to facilitate decision making about the conduct of the study, the credibility of the findings, and the extent to which these may be helpful to the individual practitioner (Table 18.2). The Preferred Reporting Items for Systematic Reviews and Meta-Analyses (PRISMA) tools provide similar guidance for both evaluating and presenting these types of research (http://www.prisma-statement.org). Appraisal tools help to adopt a systematic approach to the examination of research reports. It is best to begin with tools that are straightforward and easy to use, and then progress to more complex approaches later on. What matters is identifying the best-quality evidence.

Before reading on, undertake Exercise 18.1.

EXERCISE 18.1

Review a research paper using a CASP guide and the PRISMA tool. Which was most help to you and why?

However, the sheer volume of evidence that is published every week makes it difficult to keep abreast of every development, and it is easy to feel overwhelmed by the amount of reading involved. This requires skill in developing clear questions and keywords to guide searching for information about specific issues; setting aside regular time periods for reading; having a reliable filing system; making brief notes that summarize the key points; and attending journal clubs and discussion with others are among the many strategies that can help (Poorman 2016).

Before reading on, consider Exercise 18.2.

EXERCISE 18.2

What strategies do you use to review research papers?

Which strategies really help you to manage and keep track of your reading?

18.2.2 Evidence-based Practice

Current ideas about using evidence to inform practice bring together a range of factors for consideration in relation to a patient's circumstances. In medicine, EBP has been defined as "the conscientious, explicit, and judicious use of current best evidence in making decisions about the care of individual patients. The practice of evidence based medicine means integrating individual clinical expertise with the best available external clinical evidence from systematic research" (Sackett et al. 1996, p. 71). In this definition, expertise and experience alone are not enough; they can deteriorate over time, become out of date, and encourage rigidity in thinking. Expertise needs the challenges posed by evidence which provides new knowledge, new techniques, and new perspectives. Similarly, evidence alone is not enough. It informs, but it "can never replace, individual clinical expertise" (Sackett et al. 1996, p. 71). This concept of evidence-based medicine gradually expanded to all health professions. EBP now brings together the practitioner and current evidence, but decisions about implementation depend on the advanced practitioner's professional judgment and expertise. Factors such as cost, resources, and the working environment must also be taken into account. Even the layout of the building in which the advanced practitioner works can have an impact on the feasibility of applying new evidence. Finally, new evidence may be sound but inappropriate in relation to the patient's condition, the side effects experienced, or their personal preferences. Thus, EBP is now seen as bringing together the evidence, resources, and clinical and environmental factors to be judged by the advanced practitioner in relation to the patient's state of health and preferences. McMaster University provides a range of further information and resources which are freely accessible at https://hslmcmaster.libguides.com.

TABLE 18.3
A hierarchy of evidence.
Summaries of evidence
Evaluations of meta-analyses
Meta-analyses
Systematic reviews
Randomized controlled trials
Studies published with expert reviews
Peer-reviewed single studies
Single studies
Opinion, editorials
Source: Summarized from Ingham-Broomfield (2011).

The fact that it was ever deemed necessary in the first place to make statements about the nature of EBP reflected and continues to reflect marked variations in healthcare practice and standards of patient care. Evidence is crucial to their provision, but not all of it is the same quality. To be useful, evidence must be relevant, valid, reliable, ethical, and robust. Advanced practitioners therefore need to be aware of how evidence is graded. Table 18.3 presents a simple hierarchy in which opinion is the least reliable and meta-analysis the best. Various versions of this hierarchy are available and can be helpful in distinguishing levels of research. However, they do not assist in determining quality. Using design to determine the place of a study in the hierarchy does not necessarily mean that the research is robust. The rigor employed in systematic reviews and meta-analyses may be flawed or obscure important findings (Murad et al. 2016). Certain types of research, particularly quantitative studies, may be privileged over others. The methods used to determine validity and reliability may not be useful in assessing qualitative studies. Thus, while hierarchies of evidence may provide some help in determining the quality of evidence, they are not the only way of doing so. The systematic summaries of evidence based on the Grading of Recommendations, Assessment, Development and Evaluations (GRADE) framework (https://gdt.gradepro.org/app/handbook/handbook.html) are now the preferred approach used in medicine. In addition, the *BMJ*'s free EBM pages (https://bestpractice.bmj.com) and McMaster University's guides and tutorials (https://hslmcmaster.libguides.com) provide further resources.

Discussion about the grading of evidence is heavily dominated by medical research and quantitative methodologies: large-scale surveys, pharmaceutical trials, the testing of medical devices. This is entirely appropriate, but it is not necessarily helpful in relation to other types of research. With regard to advanced practice, there is a large and ongoing body of research which investigates the advanced practice role, examining the scope of practice, work activities, role development, stakeholders' views and experiences, and evaluations of the impact of new roles. Most of this research reflects single, peer-reviewed studies that have contributed to the understanding and development of advanced roles. However, they also tend to employ qualitative methodologies and be based on small samples or, in some cases individual practitioners. There are far fewer systematic reviews or meta-analyses. Consequently, research about

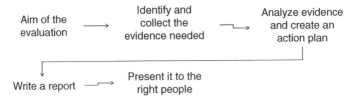

FIGURE 18.1 Key steps in evaluation.

advanced practice and the advanced practitioner's role may be perceived as at the low to mid-range level in current hierarchies (Table 18.3). This may create challenges for advanced practitioners in trying to gain support for the introduction of new evidence.

Finally, engaging in EBP enables advanced practitioners to evaluate current practice and lead the introduction of change based on the best relevant, valid, reliable, ethical, and robust evidence available (Gray 2014; NHS Health Education England 2015; Figure 18.1). In doing so, the advanced practitioner uses:

- Research skills in leading a team to critically evaluate current practice, identifying what needs to change and why, and appraise new evidence.
- Interpersonal skills and collaborative networking to generate support for change across the organization and develop new protocols to inform practice.
- Direct practice and coaching and guiding skills to facilitate the incorporation of new evidence into practice. Thus, research skills are integrated with other advanced competences as a basis for improving practice.

18.2.3 **Conducting Original Research**

The preparation of advanced practitioners usually requires them to conduct a small-scale research project as the basis for a dissertation. This enables them to demonstrate a sound grasp of the application of at least one methodology and experience of review by a research ethics committee or internal review board (IRB) and research regulation, for example by the Health Research Authority (https://www.hra.nhs.uk). A small scale project is usually linked to some aspect of the individual's practice and may enhance clinical knowledge or contribute to the introduction of change. However, it does not prepare them sufficiently for future research activities as members of collaborative research teams or, when more experienced, as project leaders. For example, NHS Health Education England 2017, p. 10) states that advanced practitioners should be able to engage in "seeking out and applying for research funding" and "develop and implement robust research governance systems," but as yet there is no formal system through which the expertise required may be gained. Lack of higher-level research skills, confidence, time, and supervision may all militate against the involvement of advanced practitioners in research.

18.3 Direct Patient Care

The NHS Constitution makes clear that everyone has a responsibility to look after their own health and take appropriate steps to protect themselves from ill-health (NHS Health Education England 2015). Accepting and exercising this responsibility require patients to be able and motivated to take charge of their own health and professionals to relinquish the idea that they always know what is best. Accepting responsibility involves changes in behavior. For patients, it may include adopting new behaviors that reduce the health risks posed by obesity, smoking, substance abuse, and lack of exercise. It may also include some reappraisal of attitudes, for example toward screening and immunization in order to avoid preventable disease (McGee 2013, 2015). For professionals, it may include new ways of enabling people to adopt such behaviors. The problem here is that "involving people [in their own health] is not one 'thing', and there is not a single lever that policy-makers, service designers and citizens can pull to make it happen. Rather, there is a range of approaches, with different philosophies, histories, perspectives and terminologies. At worst this can lead to confusion and paralysis, with decision-makers unsure what to make of the exhortations to 'engage', 'involve', 'share decisions', 'empower', 'personalize' and so forth" (Foot et al. 2014, p. 6).

Their close involvement with patients and families means that advanced practitioners are well placed to address the issues highlighted here in relation to national, local, group, and individual needs. At national level, there are a number of organizations that involve patients, families, and carers in aspects of healthcare. These include Involve (www.invo.org.uk), which promotes the inclusion of patients and the public in all aspects of the conduct of research; ethical review of research studies includes consideration of their involvement. Involve provides advanced practitioners with access to patient and public opinions from across the country. Patients and the public are also members of national committees. However, it cannot be assumed that patients and the public automatically know about the design and conduct of research, how the health service functions, or the role of the various bodies and professions involved. They need training, resources, and support if they are to make meaningful contributions. Similarly, professionals have to learn how to work effectively with patients and the public. NHS England (https://www.england. nhs.uk/participation) provides information and resources to support patients and the public and statutory guidance for commissioners, together with a range of good-practice examples.

The advanced practitioner's research skills are important in working collaboratively with local commissioners, professionals, and patient stakeholders to determine where change is needed and develop strategies for change. Research skills can be used in collaborative working with diverse local groups and communities to gain insights into their health needs and develop tailored, culturally competent interventions. Fostering networks between local organizations can lead to small-scale interventions that can make a positive difference to people's health. For example, a local authority and an NHS Community Trust developed a pilot project to examine the perceived health benefits of free access to exercise facilities for people in an economically deprived area over a period of six months. Evaluation showed that there was a marked increase in the use of the facilities, and participants reported improvements in their health with regard to general fitness, weight loss, stress reduction, and fewer visits to their general practitioner. The scheme was later extended to other similar areas (Rabiee et al. 2014). This example demonstrates not only the research itself, but also the *impact* of the results. Impact refers to making a difference, bringing about improvements, and, in the case of funded projects, demonstrating value for money (Economic and Social Research Council 2018; Vitae 2018). Impact may be professional, academic, social, or economic, but it must be supported by verification. This means that researchers have to look beyond their own results. For example, verification of the impact of Gym for Free might include confirmation from the local authority and NHS Community Trust about the decisions made to extend the scheme, further evidence of the effect of this on people's health or social issues such as loneliness, or influence on the development of an aspect of health policy. Thus, in planning studies, research teams need to consider the potential impact of their work, the type of evidence required to verify this, and how and when they will be able to collect this.

At an individual level, the advanced practitioner has many opportunities to promote health as part of direct care. The Five Year Forward View prioritized "hard-hitting national action on obesity, smoking, alcohol and other major health risks" (NHS England 2014, p. 4). One approach to this is the *Making Every Contact Count* program (www.makingeverycontactcount.co.uk), which is also emphasized in the most recent NHS Plan. This requires national and local organizations and professionals at every level to take advantage of any and every opportunity to provide practical help and advice to patients, relatives, carers, and the public at large about the actions they can take to improve their health. Advanced practitioners can contribute to this through their direct care activities by identifying individuals at risk and by investigating local factors that hinder or prevent access to health information and services. Members of socially marginalized and of black and minority ethnic groups do not always receive health-related information. For example, the high incidence of Type 2 diabetes among people of South Asian origin is well established (Hanif et al. 2014). It is attributed to changes in diet and other lifestyle factors. However, in the UK there is a significant number of people of South Asian origin who have difficulties speaking and/or reading English. In this context, a *Making Every Contact Count* moment during patient care could mean providing a timely intervention by suggesting that any relatives present could help them and the patient avoid the onset of Type 2 diabetes (Ali et al. undated). Research skills enable the advanced practitioner to evaluate the effectiveness of *Making Every Contact Count* interventions to determine which are most effective (Exercise 18.3).

EXERCISE 18.3

To what extent are you able to *Make Every Contact Count* in your dealings with patients? Give examples.

Direct care activities also provide opportunities for advanced practitioners to use research skills in developing resources for patients with specific conditions, or those whose lifestyles place them at risk of injury or particular health problems. Inherent in tackling these issues is the use of online resources and social media. The use of apps, FaceTime, WhatsApp, and other media is useful in forming groups, promoting self-help, and collecting data for research. Among the advantages of these tools are ease of use, general acceptability, and low costs. However, these online resources need good designers, and regular updating and refreshing; static pages, an out-of-date appearance, or difficulty in obtaining access may all deter rather than encourage use. The ubiquity of social media means that it is now a taken-for-granted part of everyday life. It has changed notions about privacy; people may reveal more about themselves or post material that they would be less inclined to reveal in face-to-face

> **TABLE 18.4**
>
> **Questions to ask about the use of social and other online media to collect data.**
>
> What data do I want to collect?
>
> Is this the best medium to collect data and, if so, why?
>
> Have I read the terms and conditions and the privacy policies for this media? What impact might these have on my data collection?
>
> Who will have access to the data?
>
> Who will own the data that I collect?
>
> How may they use the data?
>
> How long will they keep the data for?
>
> When and how will they destroy the data? How will I know they have been destroyed?

settings. Protection, management, and sharing of data, particularly personal and sensitive information, form an important issue (Table 18.4). The Data Protection Act 2018 sets standards for all aspects of data protection in the UK, and the General Data Protection Regulations 2016 do the same in relation to the processing and transfer of data within the European Union. The Information Commissioner's Office's (https://ico.org.uk) Data Protection Self-assessment Toolkit provides guidance that researchers can use to manage data appropriately and further information about compliance with the law with reference to health and social care. In addition, the use of social media to make contact with hard-to-reach groups such as male sex workers may require clear protocols to protect practitioners (Hains and McGee 2006). Thus, engaging in research activities that involve the development and/or use of online facilities requires organizational support. Employers have a responsibility to make sure that they understand what innovation and research involve and to take appropriate steps to ensure compliance with legal requirements and other regulatory issues, rather than just leaving the individual practitioner to cope alone.

Before reading on, think about Exercise 18.4.

> **EXERCISE 18.4**
>
> To what extent are online resources and social media helpful in your field of practice?

18.4 Publication of Research Results

The first purpose of research is discovery. It is through systematic investigations that professionals find out what works and what does not, how patients experience treatment and care, what needs changing or improving and why, and what effect innovations have on people's health. However, discovery has little or no significance if it is not shared and, unfortunately, sharing does not seem to be a routine outcome of research. There are many unpublished research studies, including dissertations and theses that are moldering, forgotten, on people's shelves, having contributed little to knowledge about health because no one knows about them. Publishing research in professional and academic journals allows others to learn and to draw on the knowledge gained so that they do not have to repeat the same work. Even negative findings should be shared, because it is important to know if something does not work. Publishing enables students to learn. It contributes to national or even global communities of professional discourse on specific topics. In this context, publishing helps to raise the profile of advanced practice researchers, to widen their sphere of influence, to expand their professional networks, and to create opportunities for collaborative research. Publishing certain types of research, for example about patient satisfaction, may also help to raise the profile of the organization concerned and encourage colleagues. Finally, health professionals seeking to advance their careers will find that publishing their research, especially in high-ranking journals, will enhance their CV. Universities assessed on the quality of their research, such as the UK's Research Excellence Framework, also look to staff to generate publications.

A second aspect of sharing the outcomes of research is respect for participants who provided access to their bodies, experiences, and lives because they believed that the research in which they took part might help others. Failure to inform participants about the outcomes of a project suggests a lack of respect for their efforts, that they have simply been used as means to an end. Researchers have a duty to tell participants about their discoveries in meaningful terms and using appropriate media (Table 18.5).

TABLE 18.5

Strategies for informing participants about the outcomes of a research project.

Include in the initial consent process written consent from participants wishing to be notified of the results.

Invite participants to a feedback session to present results in nontechnical language. Provide refreshments.

Develop a short written summary in plain language. Use post, email, or a website, providing that participants have given permission for contact.

Develop a good-quality recording of the short summary for participants who cannot read.

Request a short interview on local and/or national radio.

Present findings at patient association conferences.

Write a short article for a patient association newsletter or magazine.

Preparing to publish research results requires careful planning. This case study is presented as a series of exercises to help you prepare a research paper for publication. It also explains some wider issues that you may encounter in getting your paper published.

WHAT DO YOU WANT TO WRITE ABOUT?

In planning to write your research paper, you will need to consider how best to focus on the most important aspects of your research. A large-scale project such as a PhD thesis could be divided into a series of papers based on specific areas such as the literature, methodology, findings, or impact. Alternatively, you may want to write an overview of the whole project. What is important here is clarity about what you want to tell people. Exercises 18.5 and 18.6 are two ways to help you.

EXERCISE 18.5

Take a blank sheet of paper and place your research topic in the center.

In no more than five minutes, brainstorm all the aspects of your research. Figure 18.2 represents the many different strands that might be present in a large project about Type 2 diabetes.

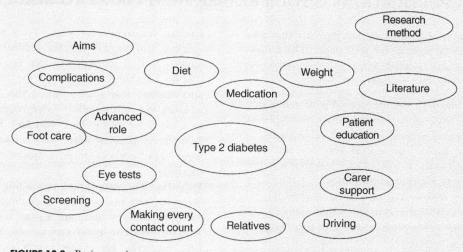

FIGURE 18.2   Brainstorming.

Next, prioritize each one.

Take another sheet of paper and place your research topic in the center, and insert around it all the points you think are most important.

Repeat this exercise until you have only the most important points on the paper. Figure 18.3 represents a more focused approach to one aspect. Arrange the points in logical order starting with the aim of the project.

EXERCISE 18.6

Most journals set word limits between 2000 and 5000 words. A 2000-word paper will have to include an introduction, a brief overview of the literature, the aims, method and sample, the findings, a discussion, and references. Roughly how many words would you use in each section?

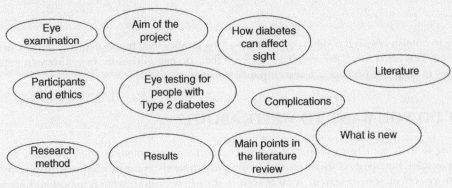

FIGURE 18.3 Repeat brainstorming.

WHO DO YOU WANT TO READ YOUR PAPER?

The most successful presenters on radio and television know their audiences very well. Some speak to "my listener," imagining only one; others to "our viewers." Audiences differ. Some want entertainment, others information or debate, and so it is with readers. Clarifying who you want to read your paper will help you decide what you want to tell them and the level of detail or explanation required.

WHAT PUBLICATIONS IS YOUR READER MOST LIKELY TO READ?

Review a sample of academic journals that you think may be suitable for your paper. The following points are intended to help you choose the one that best suits your research:

- Readership, who the journal is intended for.
- The type of papers published, the types of research, and the academic level required.
- The topics covered. If you are not sure whether the subject of your research matches a journal's, contact the editor.
- Peer review. A good journal should have a peer review system in which papers are appraised by professionals with knowledge of the subject area.
- Presentation, the layout of the pages, use of illustrations, tables, referencing style, and whether or not the publication uses color.
- The impact factor. This is calculated based on the number of times articles published in the journal have been cited in a year. It is one of several approaches used to assess the performance; a high impact factor raises the status of the journal.
- Open access (OA) publishing. This allows all readers free access to publications and enables researchers to share their results quickly. Authors pay fees to publish their papers. Not all journals use OA, but those that do will charge a fee. Check the amount and whether this is affordable. Also check whether the journal offers price reductions or waivers for researchers who lack funds. Further information about OA is available from NHS Networks (https://www.networks.nhs.uk)
- Publisher. The majority of publishing firms are open and honest in their dealings with authors. However, there are a small number that do not have good reputations. If you have concerns, for example very rapid or instantaneous acceptance, or fees you were not expecting, it is best not to consider publishing in their journals.

When you have chosen the most suitable journal for your research, read the guidance for authors carefully and follow them in planning your paper (Table 18.6). Send it to the journal with a copy of any copyright permissions required and the letter issued by the research ethics committee/independent review board that reviewed your study.

TABLE **18.6**

Tips for writing a research article.

Choose keywords that are compatible with the taxonomies used by Medline, NICE, and other major databases in order to encourage citation.

Tell the reader what the paper is about.

Stay within the word limit.

Less is more. Too many points and too much information will lead to superficiality.

Use plain language. Explain terminology likely to be unfamiliar to readers.

Design your own tables and figures to illustrate what you are saying, but explain them clearly.

If you want to incorporate tables, figures, or other items already published by someone else, obtain their written permission first.

Use the journal's referencing system.

Check spelling.

Proofread the final version.

18.5 An Agenda for Research

Research competence is an essential part of advanced practice. In acquiring research skills, advanced practitioners are able to develop a critical and systematic approach in all the other domains. Research informs and is in turn driven by clinical practice and patient need. Coaching and guiding similarly require a sound knowledge of the most robust evidence available. Research activities foster collaborative networks; leaders need research to ensure the success of their plans. Thus, research is not a separate field, but part of the integrated whole that is advanced practice.

Advanced practitioners have used their research skills to study both the emergence of their field and the needs of their patients. However, looking ahead, there is still much that requires their attention. The first is the need for continued research into the nature of advanced practice itself. This has expanded from nursing to include established and new allied health professions. Advanced practice roles have always worked across professional boundaries, but new, highly specialized roles are emerging that take practitioners well beyond their original professional practice. In some instances, for example in critical care and emergency retrieval, advanced roles now seem to have become hybrids, incorporating their original professional skills with others drawn from medicine or other fields. The introduction of consultant practitioners in professional career frameworks challenges the idea that advanced practitioners are the most senior professional role. Consequently, research is needed to determine and document:

- The nature of new and emergent advanced practice roles.
- The preparation and continuing professional education they require.
- How they contribute to patient care and treatment.
- How they relate to the current frameworks for nursing and allied health professions (NHS England 2016, 2017).

- The extent to which the competences regarded as the basis of advanced practice retain their currency or whether new competences are required.
- The poorly documented interface between advanced practitioners and their junior colleagues.
- The possibility that advance practice is becoming a new profession.

Second, health policies and new models of care such as those introduced by the Five Year Forward View and the NHS Plan (NHS England 2019) have the potential to radically alter how patients access and receive care. These changes challenge advanced practitioners to use their research skills to work collaboratively with patients, families and carers, health professionals, service providers, and commissioners to:

- Investigate the impact of new models of care on patients' access to and use of health services.
- Inform the development of inclusive strategies and resources that meet the needs of local people, including members of socially marginalized and culturally diverse groups, to help them:
  - Take charge of their own health
  - Prevent disease
  - Prevent the complications of disease
  - Manage long-term conditions.

18.6 Conclusion

As clinical and professional leaders, advanced practitioners can use their research skills in a variety of ways to benefit patients by challenging what is currently accepted, applying the best available evidence, and conducting original research. This chapter has proposed a number of pathways for research and development in advanced practice. The findings will facilitate the continued development of expert practitioners as clinical and professional leaders in their respective fields.

Key Questions

1. To what extent are you able to apply research skills in your daily practice? Give reasons.
2. What impact has your advanced practice role had on working relationships with your junior colleagues?
3. How can you promote critical appraisal skills among your colleagues?
4. What would you most like to change in your field of practice? How could research skills help you?

Glossary

Economic and Social Research Council (https:// esrc.ukri.org): the largest research funding body in the UK. The Council also provides a range of resources for research.

General Data Protection Regulations (GDPR): a European Union law which governs personal data

protection across all member states and the transfer of personal data to other countries. Further information about GDPR is available from the Information Commissioner's Office.

Health Research Authority (https://www.hra.nhs.uk): protects the interests and well-being of research participants, and oversees research ethics committees that provide independent opinions on ethical issues in research projects.

Information Commissioner's Office (https://ico.org.uk): an independent body that protects rights relating to the collection, use, storage, and other matters relating to information management. It covers a range of legislation, including the Data Protection Act 2018, the Freedom of Information Act 2000, and regulations governing privacy and electronic communications. It also investigates complaints about the misuse of information.

NHS Networks (https://www.networks.nhs.uk): helps NHS staff to develop networks, create forums for discussion, and share good practice.

South Asian Health Foundation (www.sahf.org.uk): a charitable organization that aims to improve the health of South Asian people in the UK. It provides a range of publications and conference events.

Vitae (www.vitae.ac.uk): provides professional development for researchers, especially for those embarking on doctoral study. It also works with universities and other organizations to improve research training and increase research capacity.

References

Ali, S., Gilani, A., Gill, J., Patel, V. (undated) Tips to prevent type 2 diabetes in South Asians. https://www.sahf.org.uk/resources (accessed January 14, 2019).

DePalma, J.A. (2009). Research. In: *Advanced Practice Nursing. An Integrative Approach*, 4e (ed. A. Hamric, J. Spross and C. Hanson), 217–248. St Louis: Elsevier Saunders.

Economic and Social Research Council (2018). What is impact? https://esrc.ukri.org/research/celebrating-impact-prize/what-is-impact (accessed January 14, 2019).

Foot, C., Gilburt, H., Dumm, P. et al. (2014). *People in Control of Their Own Health and Care. The State of Involvement*. London: King's Fund.

Gray, M. (2014). Evidence-based practice. In: *Advanced Practice Nursing. An Integrative Approach*, 5e (ed. A. Hamric, C. Hanson, M. Tracy and E. O'Grady), 237–265. St Louis: Elsevier Saunders.

Hains, M. and McGee, P. (2006). The working men's project. *Diversity in Health and Social Care* 3 (1): 43–45.

Hanif, W., Khunti, K., Bellary, S., Bharaj, H., Karamat, M., Patel K., Patel, V., (2014). Type 2 diabetes in the UK South Asian population. An update from the South Asian Health Foundation on behalf of the Diabetes Working Group of the South Asian Health Foundation. https://static1.squarespace.com/static/5944e54ab3db2b94bb077ceb/t/5a5b79a6419202b5496b82fd/1515944362018/Type-2-Diabetes-UK-South-Asian.pdf (accessed January 14, 2019).

Ingham-Broomfield, R. (2011). A nurses' guide to the hierarchy of research designs and evidence. *Australian Journal of Advanced Nursing* 33 (3): 38–43.

McGee, P. (2013). Measles, mumps and rubella. *Diversity and Equality in Health and Care* 10 (2): 123–125.

McGee, P. (2015). Cervical cancer. *Diversity and Equality In Health and Care* 12 (2): 77–80.

Murad, M.H., Asi, N., Alsawas, M., and Alahdab, F. (2016). New evidence pyramid. *BMJ Evidence-Based Medicine* 21 (4): 125–127.

NHS England (2014). The Five Year Forward View. https://www.england.nhs.uk/wp-content/uploads/2014/10/5yfv-web.pdf (accessed January 14, 2019).

NHS England (2016). Leading change. Adding value. A framework for nursing, midwifery and care staff. https://www.england.nhs.uk/wp-content/uploads/2016/05/nursing-framework.pdf (accessed January 14, 2019).

NHS England (2017). *Allied Health Professions into Action. Using Allied Health Professionals to Transform Health, Care and Wellbeing*. London: NHS England.

NHS England (2019). The NHS Long Term Plan. https://www.england.nhs.uk/long-term-plan (accessed January 20, 2019).

NHS Health Education England (2015). The handbook to the NHS constitution. Available www.gov.uk (accessed 8.1.18)

NHS Health Education England (2017). Multi-professional framework for advanced clinical practice in England. https://www.hee.nhs.uk/our-work/advanced-clinical-practice/multi-professional-framework (accessed January 14, 2019).

Poorman, E. (2016). Staying current in medicine: advice for new doctors. *NEJM Knowledge*. Nov.10. https://knowledgeplus.nejm.org/blog/staying-current-in-medicine-advice-for-new-doctors accessed January 14, 2019.

Rabiee, F., Robbins, A., and Khan, M. (2014). Gym for free: the short-term impact of an innovative public health policy on the health and wellbeing of residents in a deprived constituency in Birmingham, UK. *Health Education Journal* 4 (6): 691–704.

Royal College of Nursing (2018). *Advanced Level Nursing Practice: Introduction RCN Standards for Advanced Level Nursing Practice, Advanced Nurse Practitioners, RCN Accreditation and RCN Credentialing.* London: RCN.

Sackett, D., Rosenberg, W., Gray, J. et al. (1996). Evidence based medicine: what it is and what it isn't. *BMJ* 312: p71.

Vitae (2018). Demonstrating research impact. https://www.vitae.ac.uk/doing-research/leadership-development-for-principal-investigators-pis/intellectual-leadership/demonstrating-research-impact (accessed January 14, 2019).

CHAPTER 19

Conclusion: The Future for Advanced Practice

Paula McGee and Chris Inman

Birmingham City University, Birmingham, UK

Key Issues
- Sustainable Development Goals for health
- Full practice authority
- The relationship with medicine
- The preparation of advanced practitioners

19.1 Introduction

Earthrise is a photograph, taken on Christmas Eve, 1968, by William Anders, one of the astronauts aboard the Apollo 8 mission. It shows the Earth rising above the lunar landscape, a blue globe shining in the darkness of space. This was the first time that any human being had looked back at the Earth from space. It was not a scheduled photograph, more a spur-of-the-moment snapshot that was broadcast live (National Aeronautics and Space Administration 2017). *Earthrise* changed forever human ideas about the Earth. It revealed not just the planet's beauty, but the stark reality that it is unique; if it is damaged or destroyed, there is nowhere else to go. It challenged human beings to clean up their act, take better care of the environment in which they live and the natural resources that they use. This is by no means even partially achieved, but the intention remains and there is global commitment "to protect the planet from degradation … through sustainable consumption and production sustainably managing its natural resources" (United Nations 2015, p. 5).

Earthrise may seem a long way from advanced practice, but care of the planet is inextricably linked with human welfare. Together they formed the basis of the Millennium Development Goals (World Health Organization [WHO] 2000) and the subsequent Sustainable Development Goals (United Nations 2015). Human welfare, of which health is one major aspect, exists

---

Advanced Practice in Healthcare: Dynamic Developments in Nursing and Allied Health Professions,
Fourth Edition. Edited by Paula McGee and Chris Inman.

TABLE **19.1**

A summary of Sustainable Development Goal No. 3.

Decrease	• Preventable maternal and neonatal mortality • Epidemics • Early mortality arising from noncommunicable diseases • Deaths from road traffic accidents and environmental hazards such as pollution.
Increase	• Access to effective medicines and good-quality healthcare, including sexual and reproductive health services • Investment in the healthcare workforce • Capacity for early warning and response to national/global health threats
Promote	• Mental health and well-being.
Support	• Research and development of new medicinal products, including vaccines.

Source: Summarized from United Nations (2015, p. 20)

within the physical environment of the planet, but also the social and psychological environments in which poverty, gender inequality, violence, disease, lack of food and water security, and lack of education are among the many factors that prevent individuals from achieving "their potential in dignity and equality and in a healthy environment" (United Nations 2015, p. 5). All of these factors have the potential to negatively affect health, but accessible, available, and appropriate healthcare can do much to mitigate or prevent illness, suffering, and premature death. Health and healthcare are global priorities and rights (WHO 2014).

Sustainable Development Goal No. 3 sets out the targets to be met by 2030 (Table 19.1). These form an agenda for governments to address through their own health policies and the deployment of their resources in service provision. However, attainment of this goal is dependent on the capability of the healthcare workforce to meet demand; it must be *available, accessible, acceptable,* and be of an *appropriate quality* (WHO 2014, p. vi). For well over 20 years, advanced practitioners have shown that they are able to fulfill these requirements. This book has demonstrated their ability and versatility in developing new forms of practice in highly technical environments such as critical care, in primary care, and among the socially marginalized. In doing so, they have challenged established ways of working in order to provide better patient care and treatment. Nevertheless, they are still a fairly recent phenomenon and it is not yet certain what the future holds. This chapter presents our vision of what that future should include. We discuss this in relation to three topics: full practice authority, the relationship with medicine, and the preparation of advanced practitioners. The first two relate mainly to nursing as the profession which has global reach in advanced practice. However, we argue that the points raised may apply to advanced practice in other professions and recommend research to address this. The preparation of advanced practitioners is a more general topic, and we have therefore included both nursing and allied health professions.

19.2 Full Practice Authority

If advanced practitioners are to play their full part in providing care and treatment, they must be allowed to practice to the full extent of their abilities. Full practice authority refers to the right to assess, diagnose, and treat health problems, including the prescription of medicines, and to order and interpret diagnostic tests (Phillips 2018). This is in line with the scope of practice published by the International Council of Nurses (ICN 2008), which made clear that each country should develop appropriate legislation to enable advance practitioners to engage in these activities. Numerous reports testify to the obstacles that advanced practitioners encounter in their day-to-day workplaces, but it has to be acknowledged that it is a waste of money and effort to train them and then restrict what they may do (see, e.g., Jokiniemi and Haatainen 2012). Moreover, restrictions on advanced practitioners deny their patients access to other services and may cause delays in treatment. For example, if the advanced practitioner's signature is not accepted on referrals or formal documents, then the patient will have to consult another professional, which may mean additional expense in healthcare systems that are not free at the point of delivery. The implication here is that authority to perform certain tasks resides only with medical practitioners. In areas in which doctors are in short supply or simply absent, patients may have to travel long distances, and the challenges this presents may deter them from seeking further help.

There is some evidence that these issues are receiving attention. In the USA, there is a grave shortage of doctors willing to work in primary care, especially in the more remote areas. The Patient Protection and Affordable Care Act 2010 required everyone to have health insurance; enrolment into Medicaid rose dramatically. All of this increased the need for available primary care. As a result, 14 states have now passed legislation that allows full practice authority to advanced nurse practitioners and regulation by the state Board of Nursing; a further 11 place some restrictions on newly qualified practitioners. The remainder still restrict practice by requiring medical supervision in some form (Phillips 2018). Our vision is that, in future, all suitably prepared advanced nurse practitioners will be allowed full practice authority in every country. We also recommend further research into the potential for advanced allied health practitioners to have full practice authority and the form that this should take. Career progression and development are additional considerations. Several chapters in this book, particularly chapters 6 and 15, have addressed the consultant role in both nursing and in allied health professions in the UK. Consultant nursing posts have also been introduced in Australia. The introduction of these roles indicates another level of practice. In this context, advanced practice may be a stage in an upward career trajectory, or, as indicated in chapter 11, a stepping stone to completely new roles. We recommend further research into the impact of consultant practitioner roles compared with those of advanced practitioners and the preparation that advanced practitioners aspiring to consultant roles will require. We also recommend further research into the effects of these two roles on professional and assistant practitioner practice and the implications for patient care.

19.3 The Relationship with Medicine

Individual doctors can be very supportive of advanced nurse practitioners with whom they work and utilise their skills. Working relationships developed over what may be long periods of time lead doctors to trust the advanced practitioner, value that person's expertise, and treat them as an equal. However, this trust and respect may not extend any further into relationships with other medical practitioners even in the same organization, who may not be aware of or who may be dismissive of the advanced practitioner's expertise. Collectively, there is now some variation in the policies of doctors' organizations toward advanced nurse practitioners. The American Medical Association (AMA) remains implacably opposed them practicing without medical supervision, arguing that doctors should retain overall authority for patient care and treatment (AMA 2015). In contrast, the British Medical Association (BMA 2002) has cautiously recognized the possible advantages of advanced nurse practitioners acting as the first point of contact in primary care, and more recently added that they could reduce the number of doctors required (BMA 2016). The Royal College of General Practitioners (2015), in conjunction with the Royal College of Nursing, has published competences for advanced nurses working in that field.

Cautious responses to advanced nursing practice are understandable in the context of the long traditional history of medical responsibility for patients' welfare. It is perfectly reasonable that doctors feel this responsibility and that they should be reluctant to cede this to other professionals if they are uncertain about their level of preparation and/or ability. Nursing as a profession has not always helped itself. To give just one example, Loretta Ford and Henry Silver, a pediatrician, co-founded the first nurse practitioner program, but the American Nurses Association does not, initially, appear to have been supportive (Dunphy et al. 2004). Nevertheless, the course was a success and the education of nurse practitioners is now well established. Finally, medical practitioners' responses to advanced nursing practice can be understood in the context of change. Medicine and nursing occupy a particular space in healthcare services; each has a specific function, but there is overlap between them. The impact of social changes, health policies, new knowledge and technology, and new approaches to training and careers have all brought immense changes to practice in both professions. In this context, there is the potential to feel threatened by a perceived possibility of loss.

Despite these misgivings, "there are no data to suggest that nurse practitioners in states that impose greater restrictions on their practice provide safer and better care than those in less restrictive states or that the role of physicians in less restrictive states has changed or deteriorated" (Fairman et al. 2011, p. 194). There is, however, plenty of evidence that advanced nurse practitioners promote evidence-based practice (Gerrish et al. 2011), provide more timely care, and improve the management of deteriorating patients (McDonnell et al. 2014); they can also reduce length of stay and costs (Newhouse et al. (2011). Moreover, training advanced nurse practitioners "is the fastest and least expensive way to address the primary care shortage" (Fairman et al. 2011, p. 195).

Doctors and nurses need to reaffirm the complementary of their roles; both are indispensable to patients and to health services in general. Advanced nurse practitioners also have to unite and learn to act in unison. At present, there are far too many special interest groups and associations. Differences in or lack of professional regulation and title protection mean that, in countries such as the UK, no one knows how many advanced nurse practitioners there are. As a result, the advanced nurse practitioner voice is fragmented; it lacks a unified, well-articulated statement of what advanced practice is and sound evidence of what it achieves (Apold and Pohl 2014). As a profession, medicine has proved adept at avoiding these problems. Our vision is that advanced nurse practitioners will discover and use their collective professional power not to pursue conflict with doctors, but to achieve parity as equal but different providers of patient care and treatment. We also recommend further research both to examine the interface between advanced and medical roles and explore the impact of advanced allied health roles on working relationships with medical practitioners.

19.4 The Preparation of Advanced Practitioners

The delivery of good-quality patient treatment and care is contingent on the competence and capability of the workforce to employ clinical and technical expertise, and to do so in a manner that respects the dignity of all those seeking help. Interpersonal competence is crucial in forming and sustaining therapeutic relationships, and professionals and patients can work together to manage or resolve health problems. A competent and capable workforce requires comprehensive preparation to enable health professionals to achieve the aims set out in the Sustainable Development Goals and to meet the unpredictable and often complex needs among local populations in places where they live and work (Table 19.1). Thus primary care is now the main arena for the practice of healthcare, with hospitals reserved for specialized investigations and treatments and those with life-threatening conditions.

This has implications for the preparation of advanced nurse and allied health practitioners. They must be able to practice in primary care settings, particularly with patients who have multiple health problems and complex needs, and who, despite all these, are living longer lives. They need generalists who can help them to balance the demands of their conditions, prevent deterioration, and improve their quality of life. Care homes and hospices need professionals who can provide care and treatment for their clients. Workplaces also need practitioners who can educate staff and managers about hazards, the prevention of accidents, and the promotion of well-being. In short, what is required is holistic practice which addresses physical and mental health needs.

Problems in mental health are a global issue. There is an acute shortage of "health workers trained in mental health and a lack of investment in community-based mental health facilities" (WHO 2018). Stigma, ignorance, and fear often contribute to reluctance to seek help, and ill-prepared professionals may not recognize the implications of a patient's story or the symptoms they experience. Suicide accounts for at least 800 000 deaths each year, with adolescents and young adults being the most vulnerable (WHO 2018). Our vision is that all advanced practitioners, irrespective of their profession, will receive preparation in recognizing the signs of common mental health problems and work across the current boundaries between health and social care to provide appropriate and timely interventions and ensuring that early intervention becomes the norm. We also recommend research which:

- Evaluates the competence and capability of advanced practitioners to deliver safe, effective and efficient primary care services.
- Critically examines the preparation of advanced practitioners in order to clarify whether a full Masters' or Doctoral degree is essential.

286 Chapter 19 Conclusion: The Future for Advanced Practice

Finally, our vision is that advanced practitioners will remain at the forefront of their respective professions, providing direct care to patients, constantly challenging themselves and others to improve, and leading pioneering new developments that become standard care for every patient.

References

American Medical Association (2015). Physician-led Team-based Care. https://www.ama-assn.org/practice-management/payment-delivery-models/physician-led-team-based-care (accessed January 14, 2019).

Apold, S. and Pohl, J. (2014). No turning back. *Journal for Nurse Practitioners* 10 (2): 94–99.

British Medical Association (2002). *The Future Healthcare Workforce*. HPERU Discussion Paper no. 9. London: BMA.

British Medical Association (2016). *Safe Working in General Practice. One Approach to Controlling Workload and Dealing with the Resulting Overspill through a Locality Hub Model*. London: BMA.

Dunphy, L.M., Youngkin, E.Q., and Smith, N.K. (2004). Advanced practice nursing: doing what had to be done – radicals, renegades and rebels. In: *Advanced Practice Nursing. Essentials for Role Development* (ed. L.A. Joel), 3–30. Philadelphia: F.A. Davis.

Fairman, J., Rowe, J., Hassmiller, S., and Shalala, D. (2011). Broadening the scope of nursing practice. *New England Journal of Medicine* 354 (3): 193–196.

Gerrish, K., McDonnell, A., Guillaume, L. et al. (2011). The role of advanced practice nurses in knowledge brokering as a means of promoting evidence-based practice among clinical nurses. *Journal of Advanced Nursing* 67 (9): 2004–2014.

International Council of Nurses (2008). *The Scope of Practice, Standards and Competencies of the Advanced Practice Nurse*. Geneva: ICN.

Jokiniemi, K. and Haatainen, K. (2012). Advanced nursing roles: a systematic review. *Nursing and Health Sciences* 14: 421–431.

McDonnell, A., Goodwin, E., Kennedy, F. et al. (2014). An evaluation of the implementation of the advanced nurse practitioner roles in an acute hospital setting. *Journal of Advanced Nursing* 71 (4): 789–799.

National Aeronautics and Space Administration (2017). *Earthrise*. https://www.nasa.gov/multimedia/imagegallery/image_feature_1249.html (accessed January 14, 2019).

Newhouse, R.P., Stanik-Hutt, J., White, K.M. et al. (2011). Advanced practice nurse outcomes 1990–2008: a systematic review. *Nursing Economics* 29 (5): 1–22.

Phillips, S. (2018). 30th annual APRN legislative update. Improving access to healthcare one state at a time. *Nurse Practitioner* 43 (1): 27–54.

Royal College of General Practitioners (2015) *General practice advanced nurse practitioner competences*. London, RGCP.

United Nations (2015). Transforming our world. The 2030 agenda for sustainable development. https://www.un.org/development/desa/dspd/2015/08/transforming-our-world-the-2030-agenda-for-sustainable-development (accessed January 14, 2019).

World Health Organization (2000). Millennium Development Goals. https://www.who.int/topics/millennium_development_goals/en/ (accessed January 14, 2019).

World Health Organization (2014). A universal truth: no health without a workforce. https://www.who.int/workforcealliance/knowledge/resources/hrhreport2013/en (accessed January 14, 2019).

World Health Organization (2018) Mental Health ATLAS 2017. https://www.who.int/mental_health/evidence/atlas/mental_health_atlas_2017/en (accessed January 14, 2019).

INDEX

advanced clinical practice framework, 14
advanced nursing practice
  characteristics of, 20–22
  controversial issues in
    admitting and discharging patients from
        hospital, 32–33
    making a diagnosis, 32
    organisational constraints, 155
    prescriptive authority (*see* non-medical
        prescribing), 32
    regulation (*see* professional regulation)
  credentialing (*see* professional regulation)
  Development
    Australia
      clinical nurse consultants (*see* consultant
          practitioners)
      current issues in, 57–58
        remote and rural areas, 59–60
        standards framework, 54
    Europe
      The Netherlands, 29–30, 225–227
      Republic of Lithuania, 31
    Jamaica, 29
      Gulf region, 26
    North America
      Canada, 22, 26, 27, 29, 42
      United States, 4, 7, 20, 27, 30, 143, 224,
          242, 283
    Singapore, 30
    South America (PAHO), 26–7
    Africa, 27–28
    United Kingdom
      England, 13–14
      Northern Ireland, 13
      Scotland, 12
      Wales, 12–13
  definition of, 21, 53, 94
  drivers for, 23–24
  educational preparation (*see* professional
      preparation)
allied health professionals (AHPs)
  advanced practice

current issues in, 92–96
framework for, 89–90
paramedic practice, 92
physiotherapy, 90–91
applying for an advanced practice post, 183–184
assistant practitioners, 95
Association of Advanced Practice Educators,
    167, 237, 240

barriers to advanced practice, 34
  lack of role clarity, 34
  Relationships with other professionals, 34–5
  Public acceptance, 35

capability, 14–15
care/direct care
  assessment, diagnosis and management of
    acute respiratory distress syndrome, 163–164
    contraception for street workers, 226–227
    dysphagia in children, 117–120
    fractured humerus, 193, 196, 197
    heart failure, 47, 48
    health promotion, 52
    fractured thumb, 54–56
    sickle cell anaemia, 261–262
    urinary tract infection, 148–154
  physical examination, 48, 55, 148–154, 237,
      239, 240–241
Clinical Commissioning Groups (CCGs), 69
competence, 5–6
  challenging professional boundaries, 93
  cultural, 259
  in general practice, 8–10
  generic, 5–6, 44, 45
  maintaining competence, 33
  pioneering innovations, 10–12
    management involvement in, 10–12, 58,
        90, 123, 174, 215, 244, 255, 285
    patient involvement in, 10–11, 270–271
  professional maturity, 6–8
consultant practitioners
  Australia, 58–59, 227

Advanced Practice in Healthcare: Dynamic Developments in Nursing and Allied Health Professions,
Fourth Edition. Edited by Paula McGee and Chris Inman.
© 2019 John Wiley & Sons Ltd. Published 2019 by John Wiley & Sons Ltd.

consultant practitioners (*cont'd*)
  in nursing, 30
  paramedic practice, 72
  physiotherapy, 91–92
  radiography, 90–91
  speech and language therapy, 103, 110–111
  UK, 227–230

general practice
  General Practice Forward View, 70–175

health policy
  factors influencing, 67–71
  Five Year Forward View, 67–71, 68, 69–70, 89,
    256, 272, 278
  NHS Plan, 68–69, 71, 175, 272
  policy advocacy, 71
  policy competence, 71, 259–260
  policy literacy, 71

International Council of Nurses (ICN), 24–5, 283
interpersonal competence (see listening)
      listening, 6–7, 148, 154–155, 161,
        253–254

leadership
  clinical, 68, 72, 74, 122, 193, 208–209, 247,
    256–257, 261
  operational, 258
  organisational, 259–260
  professional, 29, 53, 72, 74, 103, 122–123,
    208–209, 227, 257–279
  strategic, 40, 260
  team leadership, 256–257, 260

Millennium development goals, 208, 281

National Health Service (NHS)
  apprenticeships, 15, 29, 92, 95, 246–247
  budget, 67, 69, 175, 215
  constitution, 67, 69, 175, 215
  influence of

health policies, 67–71
  nursing strategies, 71–73
  nursing organisations, 73–77

plan 68, 71, 72, 166, 175, 256, 278
professional preparation, 7–8
  apprenticeships, 15, 29, 92, 95, 246–247
  doctoral level programs/degrees, 7–8, 105,
    227, 228–9
  Master's curriculum/level/degrees 7–8, 12,
    13, 15, 40–41, 44, 46, 53, 60, 71–72,
    74, 91–94, 177, 224–225, 237–238,
    246–247.
  in the Netherlands, 42–44, 46, 225–227
  radiography, 104–105
  standards for initial nurse education, 14
professional regulation
  credentialing, 21, 30, 31, 33, 36, 75, 76,
    77–79
  in the Netherlands, 30, 42
professional standards authority (PSA), 75
  continuum of risk, 75
  dual registration, 77
  statutory registration, 75–77
  voluntary registration, 76–77
protected titles
  Australia, 53
  Netherlands, 42
Public Sector Equality Duty, 206, 212, 214

research skills
  critical appraisal tools, 266–268
  evidence based practice, 268–270
  impact, 271
Royal College of Nursing (RCN), 73–74, 95,
    177, 198, 206, 252, 284
  advanced nursing practitioner forum, 167
  credentialing, 13, 76, 77–79
  standards for education, 5, 66, 73–74

sustainable development goals, 4, 281, 282, 285